‘Giles Clark was a friend, colleague and inspiration. When I had a clinical problem that was giving me sleepless nights, Giles was my go-to person. I looked up to him more than anyone else of my generation. It is fantastic that his collected writings are now made available in this carefully curated book. Giles was an original thinker whose deep humanity shines through his clinical and philosophical writings. What he has to tell us about – for example – narcissism, transference-countertransference, the mind-body problem and Jung/Spinoza/Santayana is absolutely remarkable.’

Professor Andrew Samuels, *Author of Jung and the Post-Jungians*

‘The richness of this collection of writings honours our esteemed and much loved colleague Giles Clark. This volume shares the development of his thinking and experiences, bringing alive his heart and humanity in the face of suffering. We have been blessed with the presence, mind and deep clinical experience of Giles Clark. His innovative thinking has been part of the rich environment for the development of Jungian trainees and analysts who have been invited into deepening understandings on key concepts like the psychoid, recycling madness, narcissistic and borderline relations, symbolising and not symbolising in the clinical setting, with embodied countertransference a key interaction. This volume shares the abundance of his significant contribution to the psychoanalytic community.’

Joy Norton, *President, Australian and New Zealand Society of Jungian Analysts*

Collected Writings of Giles Clark

This timeless and thought-provoking volume makes available the collected writings of Giles Clark (1947–2019), whose original clinical theory constitutes a major contribution to the areas of analytical psychology, psychoanalysis and philosophy.

Clark's work influenced generations of analytical psychologists, psychoanalytic psychotherapists and trainees in England, Australia and elsewhere. His oeuvre covers important themes such as psychoanalysis as a deeply relational, mutually transformative and intersubjective endeavor; how, as wounded healers, analysts learn the art of recycling their own madness so as better to assist their patients; the clinical treatment of borderline and narcissistic disturbances and personality disorders; and psychosomatic issues as manifest and experienced in transference and countertransference relations in the analytic field. The book also explores the relevance of Spinoza, Santayana, Jung and German Romantic philosophers to analytical psychology and psychoanalysis, not merely in historical or theoretical terms but as a vital resource to guide clinical practice as demonstrated through a series of compelling case studies.

The *Collected Writings of Giles Clark* will be of great interest to Jungian analysts, analytical psychologists and psychotherapists in practice and in training, as well as anyone interested in understanding the interface between depth psychology, philosophy and neuropsychology, and in the mind-body problem more generally.

Judith Pickering is a psychoanalytic psychotherapist, Jungian analyst and couple and family therapist in Sydney, Australia. She is the author of *Being in Love: Therapeutic Pathways Through Psychological Obstacles to Love* (Routledge, 2008); *The Search for Meaning in Psychotherapy: Spiritual Practice, the Apophatic Way and Bion* (Routledge, 2019).

Geoffrey Samuel is a retired social, cultural and medical anthropologist. His books include *Mind, Body and Culture* (1990), *Civilized Shamans* (1993) and *The Origins of Yoga and Tantra* (2008). He is interested in mind-body interaction and healing in anthropological theory, in Buddhist practice and in dialogue between traditions of knowledge.

Collected Writings of Giles Clark

Recycling Madness with Jung, Spinoza and Santayana

Edited by Judith Pickering and Geoffrey Samuel

Routledge
Taylor & Francis Group
LONDON AND NEW YORK

Designed cover image: Two Faience Hippos, Gift of Edward S. Harkness, 1917, The Metropolitan Museum of Art

First published 2025
by Routledge
4 Park Square, Milton Park, Abingdon, Oxon OX14 4RN

and by Routledge
605 Third Avenue, New York, NY 10158

Routledge is an imprint of the Taylor & Francis Group, an informa business

British Library Cataloguing-in-Publication Data
A catalogue record for this book is available from the British Library

Library of Congress Cataloging-in-Publication Data
Names: Clark, Giles, 1947-2019, author. | Pickering, Judith, 1959– editor. | Samuel, Geoffrey, editor.
Title: Collected writings of Giles Clark : recycling madness with Jung, Spinoza and Santayana / edited by Judith Pickering and Geoffrey Samuel.
Description: Abingdon, Oxon ; New York, NY : Routledge, 2025. | Includes bibliographical references and index.
Identifiers: LCCN 2024015487 (print) | LCCN 2024015488 (ebook) | ISBN 9781032187044 (paperback) | ISBN 9781032187068 (hardback) | ISBN 9781003255826 (ebook)
Subjects: LCSH: Jungian psychology. | Psychoanalysis. | Mind and body.
Classification: LCC BF173 .C528 2025 (print) | LCC BF173 (ebook) | DDC 150.19/54—dc23/eng/20240528
LC record available at https://lccn.loc.gov/2024015487
LC ebook record available at https://lccn.loc.gov/2024015488

ISBN: 978-1-032-18706-8 (hbk)
ISBN: 978-1-032-18704-4 (pbk)
ISBN: 978-1-003-25582-6 (ebk)

DOI: 10.4324/9781003255826

Typeset in Times New Roman
by Apex CoVantage, LLC

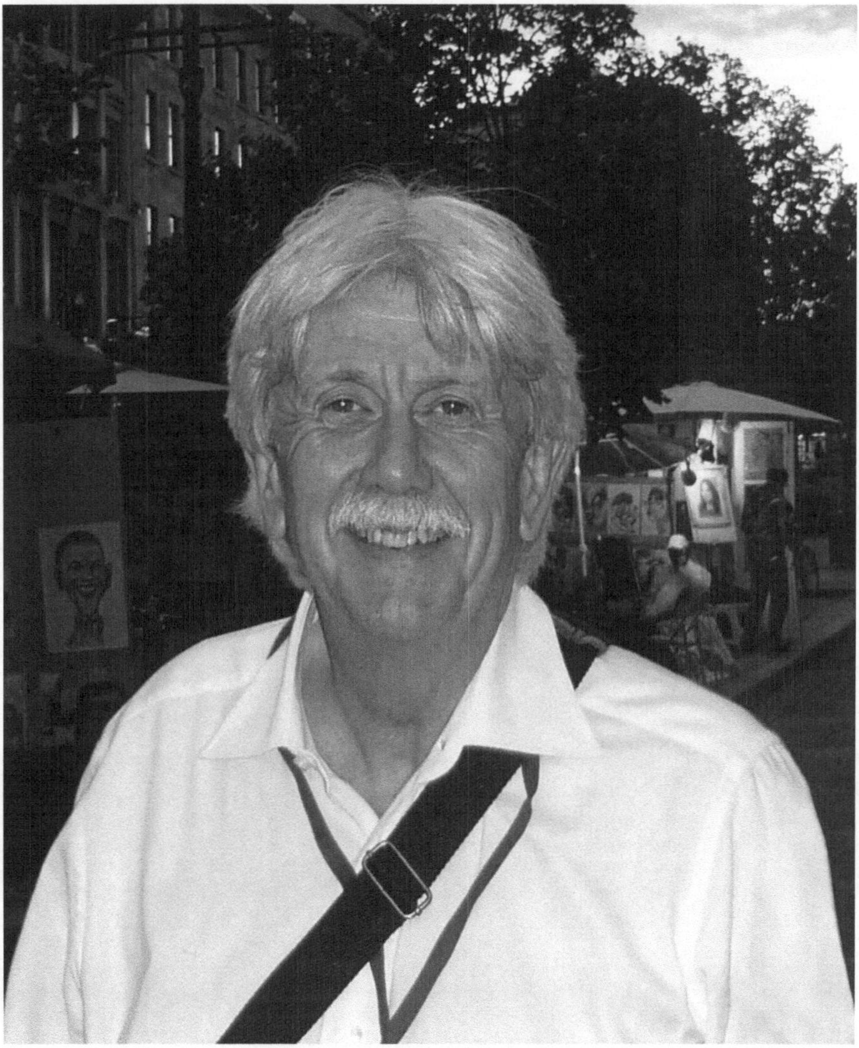

Amor aeternae necessitatis naturae
summa laetitia et acquiescentia est
Baruch Spinoza

Contents

Acknowledgements

Sed omnia praeclara tam difficilia, quam rara sunt.

– Baruch Spinoza

This book has been a labour of love but, like any great endeavour, at times difficult. We have needed support on many levels; emotional, intellectual and practical. Many colleagues, family and friends have generously given their time and expertise. Here we wish to thank the following: Ann Addison, the late Glenda Cloughley, Sally Gillespie, Andrew Gresham, Robert Hinshaw, Sally Kester, Jean Knox, Jonathan Marshall, Cheryl Moskowitz, Steven Nadler, Joy Norton, Naomi Parkinson, David Russell, Andrew Samuels, Craig San Roque, Leslie Stein, Maria Teresa Savio Hooke, Brendon Stewart and David Tacey. We extend heartfelt gratitude to the many friends and colleagues who have given generous help and support, including Sue Austin, Robert Bosnak, Patrick Burnett, Marguerite Castello, Jacinta Frawley, Anne Noonan, Joy Norton, Leon Petchkovsky, Ann Pickering, Brendon Stewart, Maree Thomas. We thank his colleagues in ANZSJA, the IAAP, UWS, APS, Jung Societies,Temenos and many more who remain anonymous.

We thank Angela Hobart, Maya Hobart and Betina Hermes and others at the Centro Incontri Umani, a cross-cultural research centre in Ascona, Switzerland, where Giles presented the first draft of Chapter Nineteen in July 2018.

Had he been alive, he would have warmly thanked his patients, trainees, supervisees and colleagues across disciplines and across the world. He would have shown profound appreciation to all his family and friends. We are acutely aware we have missed many who have given help in untold ways and extend our gratitude to all those who remain unnamed.

We thank our editors at Routledge: Kate Hawes, Alexis O'Brien, Manon Berset and Katie Randall, and Jayachandran Rajendiran at Apex CoVantage, for ongoing encouragement, care, patience and hard work behind the scenes. Anne Morris Bannerman has compiled the index with grace and a careful eye to detail.

We thank our families, particularly Naomi and Miriam Parkinson and Santi Rozario for ongoing support. Geoffrey appreciates Santi's patience in putting up with yet another lengthy academic project and the consequent disturbances to family life.

Lastly and very deeply, we thank Giles' family: Amelia Clark, Christian Clark, Brigid Clark, Lucy Clark, Annika Clark and Janet Clark, for their ongoing help, inspiration and encouragement for this project.

Publication permissions

We gratefully thank the following publishers for permission to reprint previously published papers by Giles Clark.

To Harvest Journal for permission to reprint the following three papers:

Clark, G. (1978). 'A Process of Transformation: Spiritual *Puer*, Instinctual Shadow and Instinctual Spirit'. *Harvest Journal*, 24: 24–39;
Clark, G. (1983). 'A Black Hole in Psyche'. *Harvest Journal*, 29: 67–80;
Clark, G. (1987–1988). 'Animation through the Analytical Relationship: The Embodiment of Self in the Transference and Counter-transference'. *Harvest Journal*, 33: 104–114.

To John Wiley and Sons, Ltd. and the Journal of Analytical Psychology[1] for permission to reprint:

Clark, G. (1995). 'How Much Jungian Theory is There In My Practice?'. *Journal of Analytical Psychology*, 40(3): 343–352, © Wiley Publishing;
Clark, G. (1996). 'The Animating Body: Psychoid Substance as a Mutual Experience of Psychosomatic Disorder'. *Journal of Analytical Psychology*, 41(3): 353–368, © Wiley Publishing;
Clark, G. (2006). 'A Spinozan Lens onto the Confusions of Borderline Relations'. *Journal of Analytical Psychology*, 51(1): 67–86, © Wiley Publishing.

To *Psychoanalysis Downunder: The Online Journal of the Australian Psychoanalytical Society* for permission to use:

Clark, G. (2007). 'Using a Jungian Inheritance of Lack and Loss: Psychosomatic Infection, Mourning and Irony in the Analysis of Borderline Relations'. Lecture for the 150th anniversary of Freud – November 2006. *Psychoanalysis Downunder*. 7A. www.psychoanalysisdownunder.com.au/issue-7a

To the Australia and New Zealand Society of Jungian Analysts (ANZSJA) for permission to use:

Clark, G. (2008). 'The Active Use of the Analyst's Bodymind as it is Informed by Psychic Disturbances'. In *The Uses of Subjective Experience*. A. Dowd, C. San

1 Copyright is retained by Wiley Publishing, 9600 Garsington Road, Oxford OX4 2DQ and 350 Main Street Malden, MA 02148, USA. DOI: 10,IIII/1468–5922.12886.

Roque and L. Petchkovsky, eds. E-book: ANZSJA. https://anzsja.org.au/wp/wp-content/uploads/2016/04/ANZSJA-UsesOfSubjectiveExperience.pdf

To Routledge for permission to use:

Clark, G. (2010). 'The Embodied Counter-Transference and Recycling the Mad Matter of Symbolic Equivalence: a Re-evaluation of Samuels' Idea of the "Embodied Counter-Transference"'. In *Sacral Revolutions: Reflecting on the Work of Andrew Samuels: Cutting Edges in Psychoanalysis and Jungian Analysis*, G. Heuer, ed. London: Routledge, pp. 88–96.

To Robert Hinshaw, Pramila Bennett Emilija Kiehl, Toshio Kawai, Misser Berg, Daimon Verlag and the International Association for Analytical Psychology (IAAP) for permission to include two papers originally published as conference proceedings:

Clark, G. (2012). 'Herder's force: pluralism, expressivism, mind-body relations and empathy'. In *Montreal 2010. Facing Multiplicity: Psyche, Nature, Culture: Proceedings of the XVIIIth Congress of the International Association for Analytical Psychology*. P. Bennett, ed. Einsiedeln: Daimon Verlag; and

Clark, G. (2015). 'Psychoid Relations in the Transferential/Counter-Transferential Field of Personality Disorders'. In *Copenhagen 2013: 100 Years On: Origins, Innovations and Controversies. Proceedings of the 19th Congress of the International Association for Analytical Psychology*. Kiehl, E. ed. Einsiedeln: Daimon Verlag, pp. 850–859.

To *The Atlantic Monthly* for permission to use a quote from de Saint-Exupery, A. (1942). 'Flight to Arras. III'. Lewis Galantière, trans. *The Atlantic Monthly*, March, 1942 Issue, pp. 313–333.

Judith Pickering and Geoffrey Samuel

Preface

JUDITH PICKERING AND GEOFFREY SAMUEL

Giles Andrew De Brassey Clark (1947–2019)[2] was a highly original and well-respected clinician and theoretician in the areas of psychoanalysis, analytical psychology and philosophy. His critically-tested theoretical contributions influenced generations of analytical psychologists, psychoanalysts and psychotherapists as well as trainees in England, Australia and Europe. His analytic practice spanned over 40 years, from 1976 to 1994 in London and from 1995 to March 2019 in Sydney.

He was also an anthropologist, philosopher and historian of ideas with vast erudition across a range of fields. He loved classical and contemporary music, art history, architecture, literature, poetry, film, politics, shirts, cricket, nature documentaries . . . and hippos, whose visceral muckiness, growls, wheezes and chuffs he managed to weave into clinical writing on primitive psychoid and borderline states and associated embodied countertransference experiences.

Born in Mayfair, London on December 17, 1947, Giles, an only child, grew up in rural Essex, in what once had been a mill house. His father had been a pilot in the RAF, then worked in insurance for Lloyds as well as serving as a church warden at the local Anglican church. Giles' mother was a talented amateur painter. He was sent to boarding school at Cothill House, then to Sherborne School. He then went to King's College, Cambridge, where he studied anthropology. His university studies were preceded by a year in India, where he first taught English at The Doon School in Dehradun and then commenced field work studying firstly the Jains and then Zoroastrians. A spinal neurofibroma led to emergency repatriation back to England and involved a major operation on his spine and over a year in hospital. Chronic pain dogged him throughout his life and drew him to Nietzsche, psychoanalysis, Jung, Spinoza and Santayana and a lifelong concern with mind-body problems.

2 The reader is referred to the excellent obituary: Colman, W., S. Austin, L. Petchkovsky. (2020). 'Obituary'. *Journal of Analytical Psychology*, 65(31): 609–614. We also acknowledge with deep gratitude our indebtedness for the information generously offered by his family: Christian, Amelia and Janet Clark.

In around 1971, Giles moved to Zürich to train as a Jungian analyst, personally encouraged by Ingaret Giffard and Laurens van der Post. In Zürich, where, he wrote his training thesis (Clark, 1977), his thesis advisor was Dr. C.T. (Toni) Frey-Wehrlin, who was a highly respected analyst and supervisor at the Zürich Institute in the 1970s, and founder of the Klinik am Zürichberg, a small psychiatric clinic established with the goal of employing a Jungian approach in the clinical setting. As related in Chapter Nineteen, Giles later came to realise that this thesis was 'a covert description and account of myself and of my own analytic experience', with the associated need to 'earth' and embody those aspects of himself that were somewhat ethereal and schizoid. This is a theme we find reiterated in the first three chapters of this book.

It was also in Zürich that he met his future wife, Janet Weir, an Australian woman. He and Janet married on September 20, 1975, in Chelmsford, Essex. During this time, he was back and forth between London and Zürich, completing his analytic training and undertaking final exams (coming first in both Basic Principles and Psychopathology). His last exams in psychiatry, individuation and pictures were taken in May and June 1977.

In London, he first joined the Association of Jungian Analysts (AJA), as well as a discussion group known as 'The Saplings', which included Bani Shorter, Neil Micklem, Sheila Powell, Mary Williams and his life-long friend Andrew Samuels. Later, he left the AJA to join the Independent Group of Analytical Psychologists (IGAP). He also became a vital member of the 'Umbrella Group', which sought to overcome splits and divisions between the four different analytical psychology groups in London.

As well as working full-time as an analyst, he gave seminars for all the major English Jungian training groups and was a highly respected supervising analyst. He was greatly interested in tracing the philosophical ancestry of Jung's psychology, from Kant through Absolute Idealism, Schelling and 19th-century German psychiatry. His earlier fascination with the philosophy of Nietzsche[3] later came to be replaced with that of Spinoza and Santayana, as well as many neo-Spinozan thinkers and scholars of Santayana.

In 1995, he, along with Janet and their two children Christian and Amelia, migrated to Sydney, Australia. Here, Giles took a vital role in analysing, supervising, lecturing, writing and training. His contribution to the development of the Australian and New Zealand Society of Jungian Analysts (ANZSJA) was pivotal, and he worked tirelessly both as a training analyst and as Convenor of Training from 1995 to 2004.

Inspired by the spirit of Herder's heteropathic[4] *Einfühlung*, Giles continued to leap across disciplines, cultures and analytic divides, seeking to bring together

3 In Chapter Nineteen, Giles mentions writing a 'disastrous' final thesis on Nietzsche at Cambridge University. He also discusses Nietzsche at some length in his Zürich diploma thesis.

4 Empathy based on appreciation of difference, as contrasted with idiopathic empathy, based on identification.

members of diverse psychoanalytic, philosophical and cultural lineages. He and the psychoanalyst Maria Teresa Savio Hooke were the original instigators in creating a professional body that included different psychoanalytic and analytical psychology groups and trainings, eventually leading to the formation of The Psychotherapy and Counselling Federation of Australia (PACFA). ANZSJA later became a foundation member of The Australasian Confederation of Psychoanalytic Psychotherapies.

Giles gave papers at conferences worldwide, including England, Australia, New Zealand, Switzerland, Italy, Austria, Russia, Canada and Denmark, for Psychoanalytic Psychotherapy groups and Jung Societies throughout Australia and New Zealand, at various Australian universities and for organisations such as Temenos in Canberra.

Between 2000 and 2008, while maintaining a full-time analytic practice, he was also a lecturer in Social Ecology and the Masters of Analytical Psychology at the University of Western Sydney, where he taught on 'The History of Ideas Pertaining to the Emergence of Depth Psychology' and 'The Mind-Body problem in Philosophy and Dynamic Psychology' among other topics concerning psychoanalysis, analytical psychology and philosophy. The Masters of Analytical Psychology degree at UWS was located in a Social Ecology programme, which, from its early years, had an ethos of adult education and social and cultural engagement. Important themes included sensibility to the Australian landscape, to the spirit of place and to the history of settlement and its impact on Australian indigenous peoples. Over time, Jungian and post-Jungian approaches came to be an important part of Social Ecology, taught collaboratively by a UWS staff and local Jungian analysts. The programme trained a sequence of Masters and research PhD students, and there were plans to introduce a professional doctorate, in which Giles was also involved. By the mid-2000s, however, the cultural and political climate had changed and Jungian studies were eventually phased out. For a while, however, the UWS programme offered Giles an ideal context for his innovative and trans-disciplinary approach to the Jungian heritage.

Giles was well known for his humility, kindliness, friendliness and generosity of spirit. A deep thinker, he listened with the 'third ear' of intuition, enabling what Spinoza called 'knowledge of a third kind' to emerge. Those who sat in his presence, those whose path he crossed – whether patients, supervisees, students, colleagues, friends, children of colleagues, osteopaths, shop-keepers, book-binders, strangers, homeless beggars, café owners – all felt a cord of connection, their unique essence valued.

He was an avid collector of rare books, as well as antiques, old clocks, works of art: well-wrought *objets d'art*. He began collecting as an idle pastime at school, rummaging around in old junk shops and finding many a great treasure. He said this yen for collecting and his love of rare books represented a nostalgic longing for home, having been sent to boarding school at such a young age. Such mementos transmitted a story: of the one who made it, the one who gave it, where it was found and what it symbolised. His love of architecture particularly focused on cathedrals; Wells Cathedral in the West of England being a special place of pilgrimage.

Although not 'religious', nor perhaps even 'spiritual' (he had a healthy suspicion of modern usages of 'spirituality' if implying philosophical mind-body dualism and etherealising), he was a true contemplative in the tradition of Spinoza and Santayana. He often quoted Santayana's 'My atheism, like that of Spinoza, is true piety towards the universe and denies only gods fashioned by man in their own image, to be servants of their human interests' (Santayana, 1922, p. 246). He also liked the expression that Spinoza was a 'God-intoxicated atheist'[5] and applied it to himself. He continued his interest in Zoroastrianism, which had begun during his time in India and which he had studied further in Zürich.

He was deeply concerned about political and social injustice, the plight of the oppressed, environmental devastation and climate change.

As well as a good friend, wise analyst and exceptional mentor, he was a devoted family man. His family, in-laws, out-laws, godchildren, grandchild and friends, as well as his colleagues, all speak of his kindly eye, his twinkling eye and his perceptive eye that knew when to intervene and when to sit back, watch and wait; his generous eye that knew just what gift would really make the recipient's heart sing. They remind us he was not just an influential analyst and 'armchair' philosopher but had a great sense of humour. He loved British sketch comedy, such as Peter Cook and Dudley Moore. His children recall with nostalgia the wonderful road trips taken to the tunes of Talking Heads and, aptly, Hot Chocolate's 'Heaven's in the Back Seat of My Cadillac'.

A major area of investigation throughout his professional life concerned psychosomatic and 'psychoid' issues as manifest in and experienced through transferential relations with those suffering from personality disorders. Another was the application of neo-Spinozan and other philosophical thinking to the development of analytic theory and practice in the realm of affective mind-body problems. He sought to demonstrate how neo-Spinozan philosophic systems deepen the theory and practical management of difficult psychotherapeutic work with severe emotional personality disorders, psychotic, borderline and narcissistic states. He showed how psychodynamic theory and practice may be enhanced through recourse to the rational, deductive metaphysics and ethics of Spinoza and also how interdisciplinary activity between psychoanalysis and philosophy creates a mutually informative relationship between the two disciplines. Yet he always warned that one must not rely on a top-down approach but immerse oneself in the lived, emotionally confusing and psychosomatically infectious domain of the analytic relationship, which requires embracing radical otherness, not knowing, the unknown and unknowable.

His oeuvre, as represented in this book, covers the following important themes: the application of Spinoza's concept of the *conatus* and dual-aspect theory of mind-body relations to psychoanalysis, psychosomatic contagion and psychoid states in the analytic field; psychoanalysis as a mutually transformative and intersubjective endeavour;

5 This expression was perhaps first used by Peter Cave (2006, p. 21), referring back to Novalis' earlier description of Spinoza as a 'God-intoxicated man' (*ein Gotttrunkene Mensch*).

the theory and clinical treatment of borderline and narcissistic disturbances and other personality disorders; the vital role of analytic reverie, uncertainty and negative capability tempered by insight, reason and interpretation and a capacity to think in the midst of the most destructive borderline attacks; the pre-symbolic, symbolic and developmental failures in symbolising function; the analyst as wounded healer and the recycling of madness (sanity as madness put to good use, following Santayana); love, primary love and the influence of lacks and loss in the early relations between infant and parent on the capacity to love; a new theory of *jouissance*. In the papers in this book, Giles also explores the relevance of Spinoza, Santayana and German Romantic philosophers to psychoanalysis and analytical psychology, not merely in historical or theoretical terms but as vital resources to guide clinical practice.

Psychoanalytic influences include Freud, Jung, Winnicott, Bion, Klein, British Object Relations and recent post-Freudian, post-Jungian, post-Kleinian and Lacanian theory. Here, we could name Erik Rhode, Thomas Ogden, Michael Fordham, Christopher Bollas, Andrew Samuels, Ann Addison, Jean Knox, Jan Wiener, Michael Eigen, Roderick Peters, Nathan Field, Susie Orbach and Warren Colman, among many others. Philosophical influences include first and foremost Baruch Spinoza and George Santayana, but also Johann Gottfried von Herder, the Absolute Idealists, the neo-Spinozan work of Stuart Hampshire, Jonathan Bennett, Don Garrett, Aaron Garrett, Alan Donagan, Genevieve Lloyd, Gilles Deleuze, Warren Montag and Yirmiyahu Yovel, Charles Jarrett, Stephen Nadler, Michael Brodrick, John Lachs, Michael LeBuffe, T.L.S. Sprigge, Diane Steinberg and others.

Certain seminal papers were published in journals such as *Harvest Journal* and *The Journal of Analytical Psychology*. However, many papers included in this book were previously unpublished despite being regarded as vital contributions to analytic training and the development of post-Jungian and post-Freudian clinical thinking.

Giles' tireless generosity in helping students, trainees, supervisees and colleagues publish their work was often at the expense of his own work being published. However, a long-term goal was to publish his writings as a body of work. From 2017, he was part of a small writing group dedicated to such a purpose. Tragically, an undiagnosed late-stage cancer intervened in February 2019, but in the three short weeks between diagnosis and tragic death on March 23, 2019, he was greatly comforted by the undertaking from members of the writing group to endeavour to continue his *conatus* towards the self-preservation of his life's work in the form of this book. It was a vital last wish that his life work be published.

Our editorial approach

Citing Archilochus' metaphoric comparison of the fox who knows many things while the hedgehog knows one big thing, Giles saw himself more as a hedgehog than a fox. He reworked his central concerns repeatedly over the course of his professional life. This means that many of his papers contain material in common with other papers. It was not always easy to decide whether to make individual papers available in their original form or whether to take out repeated material on the same topic, particularly where there are verbatim repetitions.

For Giles, writing was a form of intellectual container/contained relationship in Bion's (1962) sense, in which he took in, mused upon and recycled his ideas, using writing as a form of cogitation. It was through his reading, writing, listening and conversing that he worked out what he thought, then went on reconsidering his ideas. Just as he spoke of recycling madness, so, too, he recycled his own writings. He also recycled certain key case studies, each character exemplifying a particular pathology. Often, when Giles was giving a paper in his later years, he would have a folder at hand with the relevant clinical cases and a handout of his *jouissance* grid and explanations. Here, we have included the cases and grid the first time they appear and generally referred the reader back on later occurrences. In situations where the clinical case and other repeated themes were integral to the later chapter, we have included some of the material again.

Our general approach has been to remove direct repetition as far as possible while keeping each chapter in a form which makes sense as an independent item. With published papers, we have kept them for the most part as is, apart from some light copy editing and corrections. However, with a few papers, particularly those published as part of the proceedings of IAAP conferences, there were also longer versions in Giles' files, and in some cases, he had added to a given paper repeatedly over the years. Where we felt important material had been omitted due to restrictions of word length, we have included some of this additional material.

With unpublished papers, we have, in some cases, amalgamated unpublished papers on the same topic, where there is a substantial overlap between their contents. Such amalgamations are indicated in the footnotes at the start of the relevant chapters.

Giles' writing style is conversational, relational, embodied and vivid, with a sense of compassion as well as irony, of courage as well as heteropathic empathy and negative capability. We have been at pains to retain his voice and only apply the kind of light editorial touch with which we felt he would have been happy had he been able to compile his life work himself with a trusted editor.

We have also chosen to arrange the chapters chronologically so as to show the development of his ideas over his lifetime, rather than group the papers by theme.

References

Bion, W. (1962). *Learning from Experience*. London: William Heinemann.

Cave, P. (2006). 'Spinoza: Cursed Be He By Day, and Cursed Be He By Night'. *Philosophy Now*, 56(July/August): 20–23.

Clark, G. (1977). *The Transformation of 'Spiritual Image' and 'Instinctual Shadow' into 'Instinctual Spirit': Pan, Wild Man, Green Man, and Animals as Symbols of the Instinctual Shadow of the Introverted, Spiritually-Fascinated 'Puer' and of Its Transformation.* Diploma Thesis, C. G. Jung Institute, Zürich.

Santayana, G. (1922). 'On My Friendly Critics'. In *Soliloquies in England, and Later Soliloquies*. London and Sydney: Constable & Co.

Introduction to Collected Writings of Giles Clark

GEOFFREY SAMUEL AND JUDITH PICKERING

Giles Clark was 23 when he journeyed to Zürich in 1971 to undertake analytic training, and 28 when he returned to London in 1976 and began work as a practising analyst. The published and unpublished items in this book cover his entire career, and while they do not include everything that he wrote, we have done our best to ensure that all the major themes of his writing are fully represented. The first item, Chapter One, was based on his training thesis at Zürich, while the final chapter, Chapter Nineteen, was originally written for a workshop in Ascona, Switzerland, in 2018 and contains his reflections on his career as a whole. The book ends with some notes jotted down in his diary while in hospital in the final weeks of his life.

As Warren Colman, Sue Austin and Leon Petchkovsky note in their obituary (Colman et al., 2020, p. 609), Giles arrived back in London at a time of crisis and dissension in UK Jungian affairs. Jung died in 1961, and the already fractious relationships among Jung's circle in Zürich were amplified by disagreements among the growing body of Jungians and post-Jungians throughout the world. The first Jungian body in the UK was the Analytical Psychology Club, formed in 1922 and modelled on the club which had developed around Jung in Zürich in 1916. A society of medically-oriented analysts was created within the club in 1936 and, with Jung's approval, formulated standards for training. This led in 1945, after the end of the war, to the formation of the Society of Analytical Psychology (SAP), under the direction of Michael Fordham, and the inauguration of a clinically-oriented training program (Kirsch, 2000, pp. 32, 38–43).

The clinical emphasis at the SAP went along with collegial links with many UK psychoanalysts and analytically-oriented psychiatrists and with the adoption of clinical and theoretical approaches from the object relations school within British psychoanalysis (Bowlby, Fairbairn, Guntrip, Winnicott, Klein, Bion, etc.; see Solomon, 2008, pp. 128–136). In Zürich, the approach was different. In Thomas Kirsch's words, 'the influence of Jung's own interest in archetypal symbolism and mythological amplification of dreams held sway longer over clinical traditions than in other training centres' (Kirsch, 2000, pp. 20–21). There were other significant contrasts: Fordham and his colleagues placed more emphasis on

DOI: 10.4324/9781003255826-1

psychological development in early childhood (hence the label 'developmental' for their approach).[1] They also emphasised the transference/countertransference relationship between analyst and analysand. For Fordham and the 'London school' more generally, transference and countertransference were key components of the healing process in analysis.

In London in 1976, tensions between proponents of Fordham's 'developmental' approach and those who were more committed to the 'classical' perspective of Zürich were at their height (Samuels, 1985; Kirsch, 2000). In 1977, not long after Giles' return to London, these tensions led to a split in the SAP and the creation of the Association of Jungian Analysts (AJA), a breakaway group of 'classical' Jungians under Gerhard Adler. The two societies were eventually accepted as separate members of the International Association for Analytical Psychology (IAAP), which had been formed in 1955 to provide an international professional association and accrediting body for Jungian analysts, but in 1976, this resolution of the tension between them was still some years in the future.

As a Zürich graduate from a non-medical background, Giles became a member of the AJA. However, he maintained good relations with both sides and undertook a prolonged supervision with the late Camilla Bosanquet, a leading member of the SAP (she had been its chair from 1972 to 1975). Giles also became involved in various mediating efforts between the groups, including 'The Umbrella Group' modelled on a similar venture that had taken place in relation to the Freudian tradition some years earlier (Kirsch, 2000, pp. 51–53; Colman et al., 2020, p. 610).

Thus, Giles' early writing took form within a field of forces and possibilities defined by the opposition between the SAP and AJA, between the 'developmental' and 'classical' approaches, as well as by the growing archetypal approach represented by James Hillman's work. With the exception of Chapters One and Two, published in 1978 and 1983, Giles' work is closer in orientation to the SAP and the 'developmental' school than to the 'classical' school or to Hillman.[2] As his work came to focus increasingly closely on clinical issues, and in particular on the seriously disturbed borderline and narcissistic patients with whom he was working in London, it was the developmental school that gave him the resources he needed to make sense of his clinical encounters. The object relations theorists, particularly Klein, Segal, Winnicott and Bion, are also key references in his work. Transference and countertransference are also issues of major significance for Giles. The ways in which they work out at the bodily and emotional level, as much as in terms of rational thought, are an important theme in many of these chapters.

1 The labels 'developmental' and 'classical' were introduced by Andrew Samuels (1985), along with a third term, 'archetypal,' for the school later associated with James Hillman.

2 Hillman had left the C. G. Jung Institute under a cloud in 1969, but he remained in Zürich and was working and publishing on *puer-senex* issues and the *puer aeternus* during the period of Giles' studies in Zürich. Giles uses Hillman's 'Essay on Pan' (Hillman, 1972) at length in Chapter One and in the diploma thesis on which Chapter One was based. He mentions Hillman somewhat more critically in Chapter Two.

If clinical work was at the centre of Giles' writing, as of his professional life, Giles also had a strong theoretical and philosophical orientation. His sustained interest in Santayana, the German philosophical tradition and, above all, Spinoza can be seen as his way of building up an alternative philosophical basis for analytical psychology. Giles was interested in spiritual and mystical questions, but he evidently wanted a more personally adequate philosophy than was offered by the classical Jungians. He saw Jung as having important insights into processes within the mind-body totality and was particularly interested in Jung's writing on the psychoid (see what follows), but he needed, perhaps, something cooler, more rational, more compatible with contemporary scientific knowledge than the classical Jungian perspective. This desire for a *rapprochement* with science emerges particularly in the final chapters, in his discussion of Antonio Damasio's neuroscientific rewrite of Spinoza.

Thus, Giles gradually constructed a personal orientation to the field, one that took important insights from Jung and from the Jungian and Freudian traditions more generally, and set them within a wider philosophical framework.

The Harvest papers: Chapters One to Three (1977 to 1987)

We see the early stages of this process in Chapters One to Three. These three chapters, dating from 1978, 1983 and 1987, were all published in *Harvest*, the journal of the London Analytical Psychology Club, which had continued to exist as a shared resource for the various Jungian groupings. The first two chapters began as talks to the Club, and the first was derived from his 1977 Diploma Thesis for the C. G. Jung Institute, Zürich. All three chapters demonstrate Giles' early concerns with analytical work with the pathology of the *puer aeternus* or 'eternal youth'. As we move through the three chapters, however, we also see Giles' increasing focus on clinical work with borderline pathology and his growing involvement with the 'developmental' approach and the object relations theorists.

The references to the three chapters alone tell much of the story. Chapter One's references are either from 'classical' and 'archetypal' Jungians (including Jung himself) or from figures outside the analytic field. There are no 'developmental' Jungians and no Freudians. Chapter Two's references include several items by Jung and one by Marie-Louise von Franz, but the remaining items include Freudian writers (Atwood, Stolorow, Kernberg), along with Jungians associated with the developmental school. Chapter Three references Jung, Wilfred Bion, Melanie Klein and Andrew Samuels. It is no surprise that when Samuels, a good friend of Giles, arranged the Jungians of his time in a continuum between 'developmental' and 'archetypal' extremes in his 1985 book, *Jung and the Post-Jungians* (Samuels, 1985, p. 20), he placed Giles (and himself) firmly towards the 'developmental' end of the continuum.

Chapter One, however, originally given as a talk a year after Giles returned to London, is still largely within the classical Jungian orbit. It is closely based on his Diploma Thesis at the C.G. Jung Institute in Zürich, which he had completed the year before.[3] The thesis is about the psychopathology of a sub-type of the *puer aeternus*, described by Giles as an 'over-idealistic and spiritually-fascinated young man who has split off and repressed his feeling and sensation functions, his awareness of his own body and its needs, and above all his sexuality'. Through analysis, the *puer* is able to integrate his ethereal, disembodied form of spirituality with the shadow and the more sexual, instinctive self. The symbolic images of Pan, Wild Man, Green Man and Animals refer to different 'levels' of the 'instinctual shadow' as well as different stages in the process of integration. Green Man, as Lord of the Animals, is seen as 'a transcendent symbol incorporating both image and instinct', which may aid the making of a more healthy relationship with the 'animal passions', that is, one's instinctual, sexual side. Such a development helps transforms the *puer's* split-off spirituality and 'its instinctual shadow' into a more integrated 'instinctual spirit'. Thus, the *puer* may be able to sense the 'spirit' in his instinctual nature as well as accept the animals that represent the autonomy of his instinctive side.

The thesis is some 183 pages in length with references. The *Harvest* article, Chapter One of the present book, is much shorter, but the contents are taken more or less word for word from the thesis, and present its central argument. In the full thesis, the sections on Pan, the Wild Man and the Green Man contain much amplificatory material on related figures in classical mythology and folklore, including extended sections on Gilgamesh, Cernunnos, *Gawain and the Green Knight* and the Green Man carvings in mediaeval English churches. The thesis also includes four short case studies, followed by a section on Nietzsche as a type-example of a disastrous split between body and intellect. Nietzsche, along with Max Beckmann, had been the subject of Giles' final-year thesis at Cambridge (see Chapter Nineteen) and remained one of his favourite authors, though he never, as far as we know, wrote about him at length in later years.

The animal material in the thesis is also considerably longer than the corresponding passage in Chapter One. This section is particularly interesting in light of the later development of Giles' ideas. In both the thesis and the *Harvest* article, he quotes Aniela Jaffé at length on the need to integrate the animal soul or instinctual psyche: 'the animal soul is the condition for wholeness and a fully lived life'. He also ended the thesis with a quote from Goethe about integrating the divine and animal aspects of humanity. In Giles' later work, he moves away from the language of instinct and archetype to view the 'animal' aspects in terms of psychoid processes, but the animals and their animating function remain important in his mature writing.

The following two chapters also concern *puer aeternus* cases, but the style is already significantly different, doubtless reflecting Giles' early experience as a practising analyst in the UK.

3 The full thesis was entitled *The Transformation of 'Spiritual Image' and 'Instinctual Shadow' into 'Instinctual Spirit: Pan, Wild Man, Green Man, and Animals as Symbols of the Instinctual Shadow of the Introverted, Spiritually-Fascinated 'Puer' and of its Transformation* (Clark, 1977). In Chapter Nineteen, Giles refers to it as *The Wild Man and the Green Man.*

Chapter Two enters the terrifying realm of psychological black holes within the psyche experienced by patients such as 'Robert', the case described in the chapter. This 'empty centre' appears as 'an unassimilable evil or intolerable object of anxiety and dread that negates life [and] causes chronic psychic atrophy, dissolution and a disappearing of psychic life'. The analyst's dilemma is that healing, integration of splits, individuation and movement towards wholeness may seem or actually be impossible in such cases. Giles explicitly poses his material as a challenge to the 'constructivism and optimism' of orthodox Jungian psychology and discusses the case in terms of *puer* pathology. 'Although the *puer* is indeed cut off from worldly reality and *senex* demands (as Hillman and others have stated) . . . it is more important to see that he is cut off from his own psychic reality'.

Giles goes on to evaluate a variety of Freudian and Jungian approaches to narcissistic disorders for their usefulness in understanding cases such as that of Robert. He ends by suggesting that

> the original or primal . . . unity, which in healthy enough circumstances, is enabled to develop and grow towards a living wholeness of many ambivalent parts, can sometimes instead get chronically stuck, can never move out to meet reality, and so turns to devouring and disappearing into itself as if into a black hole, becoming nothing.
>
> (Chapter Two, p. 50)

It is worth noting that this paper, given first at the Analytical Psychology Club, London, in 1982, then published in *Harvest* in 1983, predates later psychoanalytic use of the metaphor of psychic black holes.

Chapter Three, Giles' third paper for *Harvest*, some five years later, moves into a more optimistic territory and also re-introduces the animal/animation theme, here in the form of one of Giles' favourite animals, the hippopotamus.[4] 'Andrew', the case study in this chapter, shares some features with Robert, including the black hole in the psyche, but he is less cut off than Robert and more able to build a workable relationship with the analyst. Andrew's transference and Giles' countertransference connect when each, in turn, dreams of a large, hermaphroditic hippopotamus. The hippopotamus, both a great mother and erotic animal spirit, offers healing for Andrew's black hole; the animal symbols bring what was previously unalive and unlivable to life and to the possibility of relationship. In contrast with Robert's analysis, Andrew's is relatively successful, and he is able to achieve a considerable degree of healing and individuation.

The analytic relationship here is intersubjective, mutually infectious, with both analyst and analysand unconsciously communicating imagery as well as partaking of a third area both between them and between internal life and external reality.

4 The only reference to animals in Chapter Two is to the significant absence of animal imagery in Robert's fascinations and dreams.

Archaic animal symbols pertaining to the sympathetic nervous system are shareable, affecting analytic relations at a primitive level. The hippopotamus-goddess

> is the animating *anima*-animal in him and between us. Such archetypal pre-person images are intra-physical as well as intra-psychic. Their power to heal and bring to life can only be realised in relationship, in mutually experienced, emotionally loaded images and sensations. Thus, I think the transcendent function in the transference/counter-transference recreates the symbolising process and brings life where previously it could not be.
>
> (Chapter Three, p. 62)

This sense of the transference/countertransference as deeply physically embodied and accessible through emotional states and dreams more than rational thought and also as central to the healing process runs through all of Giles' later writing. His case studies are mostly drawn from a small group of analysands with borderline and narcissistic personality disorders with whom he worked in his private practice in Victoria in London.[5] They include Pat with her crazed zonal and gender non-identity (Chapter Five); self-harming Jewish Rose with her intergenerational inheritance of unmet displacement (Chapter Seven); borderline Jim, the sadomasochistic skinhead and cathedral-body fucker (Chapters Six, Seven, Nine, Ten and Thirteen); narcissistically brittle, ever-defended and ever-righteous Christine (Chapters Nine, Thirteen and Sixteen); and the uptight and unimaginative Adie, determinedly stuck in a state of non-symbolising, non-play and non-imagination to avoid mourning intolerable loss (Chapter Ten).

It may be useful to provide here a list of diagnostic conditions for borderline personality disorder written by Giles for his students in Australia:

1. Faulty development of symbolising function and reality principle and thus a very low distinction between fantasy and reality. Therefore also actions and reactions as concretisations/literalisations of fantasy;
2. Impulsivity;
3. Unreasonable expectations of compliance;
4. Interpersonally exploitative;
5. Lack of empathy;
6. Inappropriate and intense rage (lack of control of anger/frustration);
7. Envy, spoiling and destructiveness;
8. Affective instability and marked reactivity of mood;
9. Transient, stress-related paranoid ideation and severe dissociative symptoms;
10. Identity disturbance, including fragile sense of self and unstable self-image;

5 In the original papers, Giles does not always use the same fictitious name for each person, but we have aimed to keep the same name throughout in this volume, so have occasionally changed the names given in the original.

11. Extremes of idealisation and devaluation in interpersonal relationships;
12. Frantic efforts to avoid real or imagined abandonment: clinging, adhesiveness, identification;
13. Extreme jealousy, and, therefore, sexual invasions;
14. Occasional self-mutilation/self-harm.

These were the patients around which much of Giles' career and most of his writing are oriented.

Chapters Four to Nine: Giles' mature synthesis (1996–2005)

Five of the six papers in this group were published in one form or another, three of them (Four, Five and Seven) in the *Journal of Analytical Psychology* (*JAP*). This was the house journal of the SAP and the 'developmental' school. It was initially founded in 1955 as a clinically-oriented journal for English-speaking Jungians under Fordham's editorship, though by Giles' time, it had become more open to other approaches (Kirsch, 2000, p. 43). Giles' first two articles in the *JAP*, around the time of his move to Australia, mark a new level of maturity in his work. The second, which won the Michael Fordham Prize, is among his best-known writings. These two chapters continue to refine the arguments about 'animation' and transference in Chapter Three. They also introduce new and significant themes, including Giles' personal take on Jung's concept of the psychoid and on dual-aspect identity theory, which he derived from the philosopher Baruch Spinoza. In Chapter Seven, Giles' third and last *JAP* paper, some years later, he discusses his use of Spinoza in more detail.

The contents of Chapters Four and Six are complementary rather than sequential, and together, they give us a picture of where Giles had arrived in his intellectual understanding of the analytic process by the time he moved to Australia. The title of **Chapter Four** suggests an evaluation of Jungian theory in relation to Giles' evolving practice. The chapter gives us this, but it also presents Giles' personal understanding of the nature and purpose of analysis:

> I see analysis as a particular and peculiar relationship through which we both endeavour to understand consciously, in new ways, the most possible meanings for our unconscious history (which is also environmental) and our nature . . . The object of this unconscious experience is always fearful, touching on primitive anxieties. It feels unbearably sad, out of control and above all dangerous. It is neurotic and potentially psychotic.
>
> (Chapter Four, p. 65)

Understanding can generate a sense of freedom and power to change. Giles suggests that this is more a 'healthy illusion' than reality. Psychotherapy nevertheless offers a way to manage 'two fundamental primitive fears . . . the fear of loneliness and lack of meaning . . . [and] the concomitant, opposite fear of dangerous desire and power'. He outlines four motivating aims for seeking therapy. The first three are the desire for change (beneath which is a desire *not* to change), the desire for understanding from another person (under which is a desire to remain hidden) and the desire for self-preservation (which conceals a desire to break down and lose control). For each of these, analysis can help one to accept the limits of change, of understanding and of one's drive for self-preservation. The fourth desire is the unrealistic desire for an 'absolute and eternal loving relationship'. In reality, there may be obstacles, 'fearful defeats and lifeless places', that obstruct the full achievement of a mature and realistic relationship. Nevertheless, Giles suggests that the process of analysis offers enough to be worthwhile.

Giles' position here, as he hints, owes more than a little to his explorations of Spinoza's work.[6] He contrasts his approach with a classical Jungian view in which there is a built-in teleology to the analytic process, a specific meaning to be unveiled. This, and the accompanying tendency towards reification and hypostatising, he no longer finds helpful. The unconscious is not an entity with its own will and intent; it is an energetic and dynamic process. Jung, he suggests, understood this, but some of his followers have made his theories into a 'school of wisdom'; not a bad thing in its own right, but not always helpful for the analytic process. The analyst needs some theory, but it should be open and generative rather than closed and dogmatic, particularly in relation to healing the psyche-soma split. Here, Giles offers his own concept of the 'consubstantial animating body' as a way of making sense of the healing process that he described for Andrew in Chapter Three, for Pat in Chapter Five and other case studies later in the book. We hear more about the 'consubstantial animating body' in the following chapter.

Giles, as a self-confessed 'cheerful pessimist', was acutely aware of the limits to change and the limits of free will, but he had an animal faith in the necessary illusion of free choice, in what Spinoza referred to as 'free necessity' (e.g. Kerr-Lawson, 2000, pp. 246–248). In his work with very difficult cases, he also observed that there are times when psychosomatic damage may be irreparable, and there may be limits to the degree of full healing. In addition, we all have a need to mourn our lacks and losses and find a degree of acquiescence:

> Thence, what have always been intolerable lacks, losses, limitations and frustrations can be painfully grieved and perhaps mourned, and meaningful causal links can be made, and so there may emerge a more realistic symbolic functionality.
>
> (Chapter Twelve, p. 178)

Chapter Five is built around the, at times, quite terrifying, but ultimately constructive, clinical encounter with the first of Giles' borderline patients to

6 Note the reference to a 'seventeenth-century model of human nature,' to the *conatus* and to that very Spinozan term 'acceptance' (*acquiescentia*), also the reference to Deleuze and neo-Spinozan philosophers at the end of the paper.

appear in the book, 'Pat'. In this chapter, Giles spells out the argument about the consubstantial animating body and Jung's concept of the psychoid in some detail. We also hear a little more about Spinoza, though for a full account of Giles' growing engagement with Spinoza's philosophy, we will have to wait for Chapters Six and Seven. Chapter Five begins with Jung's hypothesis of a '"psychoid" level or quality of the unconscious psyche' (Jung, 1970a, *CW* 8, paras. 368–9, 380) and his related idea that psyche and matter may be 'two different aspects of one and the same thing' (*CW* 8, para. 418). This concept of the psychoid was to become a major theme in Giles' later work.

Jung introduced his concept of 'psychoid processes' in a 1946 presentation at the Eranos meeting in Ascona, the forum in which he first presented many of his more innovative ideas from the 1930s onwards. That year's Eranos meeting was unusual in that it was devoted to the relationship between science and nature. It was the first time that natural scientists had been invited to take part in the discussions at Eranos (Vajdová, 2021, p. 244). Jung responded with a remarkable essay which was devoted to the problems of understanding psychological knowledge, particularly knowledge of the unconscious, within a scientific framework. The original German title was 'Der Geist der Psychologie' (Jung, 1947); it was first published in English as 'The Spirit of Psychology' (Jung, 1954). It was later revised and augmented and is now known in English as 'On the Nature of the Psyche' (Jung, 1970a).

In this essay, Jung returned to the term 'psychoid', which he had suggested to Freud as a term for the unconscious many years before, in 1907 (Addison, 2019, p. 16). Versions of the term psychoid had been used in somewhat different ways by Hans Driesch and by Jung's own mentor at the Burghölzli, Eugen Bleuler. Jung differentiates his usage from both Driesch's and Bleuler's. Jung's 'psychoid' is adjectival, referring to a class of processes of a 'quasi-psychic' nature, distinct from and intermediate between the merely vitalistic or organic and the specifically psychic (1970a, *CW* 8, para. 368). In his essay, he uses the image of a spectrum, analogous to the spectrum of colours, between the biological and the psychic:

> Just as the 'psychic infra-red,' the biological instinctual psyche, gradually passes over into the physiology of the organism and thus merges with its chemical and physical conditions, so the 'psychic ultra-violet,' the archetype, describes a field which exhibits none of the peculiarities of the physiological and yet, in the last analysis, can no longer be regarded as psychic, although it manifests itself psychically.
>
> (*CW* 8, para. 420)

In 'On the Nature of the Psyche', the term 'psychoid' is used, among other things, to clarify the concept of the archetype. The ideas and images associated with the archetype are part of the psyche. However, the archetype itself is not strictly psychic at all but belongs to this underlying layer of psychoid processes. Psychoid processes are described as forming a spectrum between the biological and the psychic, and Jung further distinguishes between individual and shared aspects of the psychoid unconscious.

Jung also referred to psychoid processes in a number of letters, in his late essay *Synchronicity: An Acausal Connecting Principle* (Jung, 1952, 1970b) and in the book *Mysterium Coniunctionis* (Jung and von Franz, 1955–6, Jung, 1970c). In *Mysterium Coniunctionis,* we get a rather different image from that of the spectrum. Here, Jung writes of a series of levels going down or back through the various evolutionary stages to the 'transcendental mystery and paradox' of the nervous system:

> For just as a man has a body which is no different in principle from that of an animal, so also his psychology has a whole series of lower storeys in which the spectres from humanity's past epochs still dwell, then the animal souls from the age of Pithecanthropus and the hominids, then the "psyche" of the cold-blooded saurians, and, deepest down of all, the transcendental mystery and paradox of the sympathetic and parasympathetic psychoid processes.
>
> (Jung, 1970c, *CW* 14, para. 279)

Here, the psychoid level lies beneath the animal (and animating) spirits that had preoccupied Giles in much of his earlier work. In either case, psychoid processes serve to describe a range of processes that are neither mind nor body, between psyche and soma, but also serve to connect the two together. This had already led Jung in 'On the Nature of the Psyche' to a suggestion which was to be of particular significance for Giles:

> Since psyche and matter are contained in one and the same world, are moreover are in continuous contact with one another and ultimately rest on irrepresentable, transcendental factors, it is not only possible but fairly probable, even, that psyche and matter are two different aspects of one and the same thing.
>
> (Jung, 1970a, *CW* 8, para. 418)

For Giles, this opened the way for him to read Jung's work as implying a dual-aspect substance monism[7] similar to that of Spinoza. Mind and body, psyche and soma, were two aspects of the same underlying process.[8]

7 Giles generally used terms such as 'double identity' or 'double-aspect identity theory' both in relation to Spinoza's and Santayana's work and to his own. As Ann Addison has pointed out, Spinoza's position is not strictly speaking an identity theory, but a form of what is usually called dual-aspect monism (personal communication, 2023). We have changed these references accordingly to avoid confusion.

8 Jung was himself exploring dual-aspect monism approaches in the mid to late 1940s in his correspondence and discussions with the physicist Wolfgang Pauli, discussions which probably underlie his comment in 'On the Nature of the Psyche'. Jung cites a letter from Pauli in the Supplement to his

Giles' sense of the psychoid builds on Jung's but has its own specific identity. For Giles, the concept of the psychoid can be understood as referring to a dynamic, embodied, psychosomatic, interpersonal experience that encompasses both psychic and somatic elements. This is the basis of the consubstantial animating body, shared between the analyst and analysand, which we met in Chapters Four and Five.

This shared level of emotion and affect is particularly evident when working with deeply regressed patients who confuse inner and outer, subject and object, reality and fantasy. In such cases, the analyst can be infected by the analysand's animating fantasies and their need to use the analyst as a psychotic object. The analyst may experience this as chaos, disorder, raw emotion and feelings of illness and struggle to find a way out of this shared world of psychoid animation. However, success may assist the patient to find their own way to a more satisfactory psyche-soma relationship. The case study of the borderline patient 'Pat' in Chapter Five exemplifies many of these themes, including the concluding realisation that 'this terrible animating body, which is so fierce, disharmonious, sickening and dissociated is in fact what brings life and unites us'.

Giles' interpretation of the psychoid as an animating mind-body process, potentially shared between analyst and analysand, became an ongoing theme throughout much of his subsequent work. Spinoza's dual-aspect theory ('mind as idea of the body') provided him with a basis for interpreting the concept of psychoid as itself, implying a dual-aspect theory, and so understanding his clinical experience in terms of an underlying mind-body unity. For Giles, the psychoid always refers simultaneously both to 'sensuous body matters, processes and relations' and to 'mental image, idea and emotion'. In clinical contexts

> the psychoid realm is one of psychosomatic mutuality, a pre-verbal relational field that is a conduit for urgent communication, often sickening or seductive, but demanding internal recycling into a more integrated co-ordination and a separation out of identification into differentiation.
>
> (Chapter Twelve, p. 178)

Mind and meaning emerge from bodily relations yet remain identified at both the physical and mental level of their common psychoid substrate. They are emergent, vital organic forces. Transferentially/countertransferentially, the dual aspect of the psychoid bodymind realm makes for 'consubstantial' psyche-soma experience at the level of the autonomic nervous system, which emerges out of, between, around us both in analysis, whence it calls out to be moved from somatic sensation or somatisation to a functional symbolic ordering, and so to a more relational state.

If, as Giles himself thought, there was 'one big thing' underlying his work, it can probably be seen most clearly in this central connection between Spinoza's mind-body dual-aspect approach, Jung's psychoid process and Giles' own sense of the

1947 article (see 1970a: *CW* 8, para. 439, also Atmanspacher, 2012, pp. 109–111; Atmanspacher and Fuchs, 2014).

possibility of analytic progress and the 'recycling of madness' (see what follows) for positive ends by entering and working with the consubstantial, animating body formed by analyst and analysand together. We return in a little while to some of the further implications of this perspective.

Chapter Six is an unpublished paper from 1999, 'Mind-body intimacies and pains'. This takes up the position articulated in Chapters Four and Five, that psychopathology can communicate and reveal mind-body relations and asks what kind of ethic this might generate. Giles suggests 'an emergent ethic which is not just a socio-cultural code but is post-synoptic, in that it is ratio-centric yet not fixed, open to differences, to perpetual reforming and to unconscious (emotional) complexity' (Chapter Six, p. 88). Put otherwise, the objective of Giles' work with his borderline patients is to achieve 'a good-enough life which incorporates the cunning of unconscious reason and unreason (even destructive chaos)'. To attain this, as we have already learned, analysts need to be open to the contagion of the borderline states at a physical level and to allow themselves to be affected by it.

In this chapter, Giles argues that Spinoza's dual-aspect theory, as elaborated and interpreted by neo-Spinozan philosophers such as Gilles Deleuze, provides him with a vital tool. If, as Spinoza puts it, 'the mind is the idea of the body', then the ideas of the mind correspond to the affections of the body. He discusses the Spinozan feminist scholar Genevieve Lloyd's argument that since bodies and their powers are shaped by socially imposed limitations, female minds are shaped by the limitations imposed on female bodies. He argues that the family and 'the deep pathologies of unconscious destructiveness and disorder' also shape the mind as an 'idea' of the body and that this idea is 'subjectively complex, fantastically distorted, only semi-conscious, largely unconscious, but energetic/libidinal'. Merleau-Ponty, Winnicott, Orbach and Deleuze and Guattari's *Anti-Oedipus* are all brought in to reinforce this general position, as are Bion's beta-elements. All this, as in Chapter Four, helps to counter unhelpful aspects of Jungian metapsychology (in particular, hierarchy and splitting). In Giles' work, he is dealing with a disrupting, destructive, unpredictable realm of emotion that he must somehow encounter and incorporate. 'This is work in the paleo-mammalian and reptilian psychoid realms, not of so called "normal" neuroticism'. Working with a pre-given set of categories and distinctions simply gets in the way of accepting the fluid and disordered nature of the situation. Two clinical vignettes, 'Annie' and 'Jim', illustrate mind-body relations as communicated through embodied transference-countertransference relations.

Chapter Seven, which was originally presented at the *Journal of Analytical Psychology*'s 50th Anniversary Conference in Oxford in 2005 and published in the journal the following year, takes a similar overall position but provides a more fully-worked out presentation of how Giles was using Spinoza. Again, the key point is the clinical utility of the dual-aspect mind-body position when working with difficult borderline patients. Two of Giles' most compelling and dramatic case studies, 'Rose' and 'Jim', appear here and illustrate Giles' theory of an analytically co-created, co-transformative psychoid animator. (Jim repeatedly recurs in Giles' later writings.) Giles' reflections on counter-transferential interactions are woven into a neo-Spinozan conceptual system, including Spinozan theories of substance, mind-body univocalism, passion and action, and the *conatus* as representing the endeavour to preserve one's being. Giles expands Spinoza's 'mind is the idea of the body' which is moved by desires, pleasures and pains (*cupiditas*, *laetitia* and *tristitia*) into a wider complex of internal and interpersonal emotional relations (including ideas of bodies and body relations) that make for a *jouissance* of affects and the tensions between them. Here, *jouissance* is understood to be part of the *conatus,* and the *conatus*-as-*jouissance* is a dynamic incorporation of all the emotions of the 'bodymind'. He introduces a diagram, the *jouissance* grid, which is intended to depict dynamic psychic and somatic (psychoid) affects, emotions or 'passions' and their relations. In later years, he often gave out this grid and its associated dot points in lectures and training seminars, the points being slanted towards the given topic.[9]

Towards the end of this chapter, we find the first mention in the book of another of Giles' recurrent themes, the one that we have adopted for the subtitle of this book, 'recycling madness'. Giles suggests that it is because the analyst has been wounded and is weak in particular areas and has learned to 'recycle' that weakness productively that he or she is able to receive the countertransferential information and to work with it. Santayana famously wrote of 'normal madness' and 'sanity' being 'a madness put to good uses' (1910, cited in Coleman, 2009, p. 269). Such 'madness put to good uses' morphs into Giles' seminal concept of recycling madness. Through their own training analysis, analysts have hopefully been enabled to recycle their various forms of madness, understand their complexes, recurrent issues, normal neurosis and even psychotic pockets. In turn, this enables analysts to understand better and help others suffering similar as well as different forms of mental illness. Related to this, Giles repeatedly argued that analysts as wounded healers heal through their own wounds, 'through their survival, management and recycling of their own wounds and madness. This contains and processes the maddening wounds of the other' (Chapter Twelve, p. 185). It is the analyst's areas of both emotional and physical vulnerability that are open to being disturbed by the patient, and such wounds are the openings through which countertransferential information is received.

Chapter Eight consists of the first part of a paper presented in late 2006 and published in *Psychoanalysis Downunder* 7A, the online journal of the Australian Psychoanalytical Society, in February 2007. This is another coming to terms with Giles' relationship to Jung, but here, more in terms of the ongoing consequences of Jung's own psychic life. In the material included in the book, Giles situates his post-Jungian inheritance within the history of psychodynamic theory. Jung's theories emerged out of his childhood lacks and losses: Jung's mother's reactions to the tragic loss of several stillborn siblings and infant mortality, Jung's subsequent existential loneliness and the magical retreats he created to cope. The Freud-Jung

9 As noted previously, to avoid unnecessary repetition, when the grid recurs in later chapters, we have referred the reader back to the original diagram and earlier explanations.

split, after their intense, short-lived friendship, was never resolved and continues as an ancestral split in the psychoanalytic world. Giles' criticisms of Jung's perspective here are similar to those in previous chapters and again aligned with the general position of the 'developmental' school: early development does not receive enough attention, and an adequate clinical approach needs to draw on object relations and post-Freudian theory, particularly that of Klein, Winnicott and Bion in order to flesh out clinical practice on a developmental basis. The first part of Giles' paper ends with an evaluation of the positive side of the Jungian inheritance: Jung's emphasis on psychic reality is a corrective to materialism, and his openness to psychotic experience is significant. Giles has found Jung's philosophical ancestry and the pluralistic foundation of an Idealist-Romantic intellectual and cultural ancestry personally productive. Jung's own life, particularly his capacity to live through and recycle his own familial madness and put it to good clinical use, continues to offer inspiration. The second part of this paper has been omitted because it repeats earlier material in which Giles applied his considerations concerning his Jungian inheritance by 'earthing' them in his clinical experience of working with borderlines, reusing the case of Jim.

The last chapter in this group, **Chapter Nine**, derives from a paper presented at an ANZSJA conference in 2007 and subsequently published in e-book form. The general position here is similar to that in the other chapters of this group. The chapter focuses on the active use of the analyst's bodymind, embodied countertransference, imagination, analytic reverie, interpretive thinking and linking as vital clinical elements, particularly in relation to borderline and narcissistic relations. 'Jim', the explosive sadomasochistic skinhead, receives further analysis and we meet 'Christine', an artist and art teacher with 'brittle narcissistic defences, self-delusions and illusions'. The venomous envy and resentment underlying such cases inevitably infect the analyst, who needs to think their way out of such infection and bring about a degree of transformation and healing for the analysand.

Jim's case is supplemented by a fictionalised clinical exchange between a borderline and an analyst to show how analytic work with borderlines features a fused psychoid unity, which demonstrates 'the mind is the idea of the body'. A phenomenological summary of narcissistic relations and the case of Christine show how the analytic task is to address primitive anxiety, interpersonal terrors and shames lurking behind narcissistic defences.

The set of ideas articulated in this group of papers, derived primarily from Jung and Spinoza, were at the core both of Giles' analytic practice with his highly disturbed borderline and narcissistic analysands, and of his understanding of the analytic process. They allowed Giles to see his countertransferential reactions to the transference as providing both vital evidence of his patient's inner world and as leading to intuitive responses, which were able to move the analysis forward. These responses came from the shared psychoid processes (or psychoid field) in which he and the analysand were engaged. Whereas a 'normal neurotic' has achieved enough symbolic control or insight into his or her situation to enable the analyst and analysand to work directly in words with the analysand's symbolic material to access and reference the underlying psychoid (bodymind) processes, with the borderline, narcissistic and psychotic patients with whom Giles was mostly working, this was not possible.

Giles' model of the psychogenetic process within these very disturbed patients essentially derives from the object relations tradition (Klein, Winnicott, Bion and Segal, in particular). While it is a *sine qua non* for Giles that there may be 'endogenous' causes within any particular case, his focus is on psychogenetic processes in early life in which distorted or inadequate family interaction has made it impossible for the subject to have achieved proper symbolising, and so to gain a measure of insight into and control of his or her situation. Instead, they are caught up in tensions between uninterpreted forces (beta-elements, in Bion's vocabulary), which they are unable to resolve or integrate. Giles speaks of this situation as a *beta confusa*, deliberately conflating Bion's beta-elements with the *massa confusa* of Jung's alchemically-inspired description of the transference in 'The Psychology of the Transference' (Jung, 1993).

For these patients, since things are not yet clearly articulated at the level of the conscious psyche, it is necessary to find some access to the underlying levels of the psychoid unconscious with its unintegrated beta elements. In Giles' psyche-soma dual-aspect model, the transference-countertransference processes are manifestations of these unconscious, unsymbolised or partially symbolised psychoid processes, and they offer a way of accessing them and working with them. The analyst's job here is to remain in the situation, to model a 'healthy' ability to deal with psychic and psychoid forces for the analysand and to remain open to the intuitive moments through which a leap of insight into the *beta confusa* may emerge. Giles sees these insights as related to Spinoza's 'third type of knowledge' or to Bion's use of Poincaré's 'selected facts' (Bion, 1962, p. 72).

Giles' '*jouissance* grid', which occurs in several of these papers, provides a diagrammatic representation of the unbalanced forces while also pointing to the potentiality of balance and integration between them. Giles' highly disturbed analysands are unable to symbolise this material, at most achieving a limited degree of 'symbolic equations' (here, Giles borrows from Hanna Segal), and so also unable to articulate it clearly in language. However, the psychoid processes of transference and countertransference enable a sensitive analyst to pick up what is going on through awareness of his or her own emotional responses, dreams and intuitive insight. This approach to analysis may, if all goes well, bring about a forward movement towards integration. Giles is particularly sensitive to moments which indicate symbolic insights by his patients, often as a result of his own 'intuitive' responses to the tensions of the analytic situation.

The animal (and 'animating') levels with which we are concerned here correspond to the realm of the *anima/animus* and other archetypes in the Jungian model. Giles, however, finds the prescriptive and hierarchical approach of the classical Jungian tradition less helpful, preferring to remain open to the actual experience of the psychoid levels through transference and countertransference in the specific analytic situation. Since the unintegrated and unbalanced material is at a level corresponding to animal rather than human levels of functioning, it often emerges in animal imagery (as with the hippo in Chapter Three, the bull in Chapter Five and the elephant in Chapter Fourteen). Such imagery hopefully has the potential to animate and bring to life stuck and frozen situations and to bring about movement towards integration and wholeness.

The later chapters in the book, representing Giles' later work, present different aspects of this overall picture. They generally rearticulate Giles' overall perspective (or *Anschauungsweise*, to use one of his favourite German terms) while presenting new material which explains and elaborates in detail particular aspects of his *Anschauungsweise*. This leads to a certain amount of repetition, which we have generally removed or summarised. Some, intended as teaching material, are relatively didactic in form, presenting Jungian or object relations theories from which his ideas developed or with which they may be contrasted. Others, including many of the conference papers, go into more detail about the model itself, including its relation to Spinoza, German idealist and romantic thinkers and other theorists, particularly in the neo-Spinozan tradition.

The American philosopher George Santayana's work is referenced and discussed in several places. He is significant for Giles primarily as articulating and describing a picture of 'ordinary madness', being madness put to good use, in which a healthy individual has developed a viable way of living through and with his or her internal psychic and psychoid processes. This generally involves adequate symbolising (what Bion, 1962, referred to as alpha function)[10] through which the intrinsically 'mad' psychic and psychoid material has become integrated. It is facilitated or enabled by 'good enough' parenting and other positive features of the early childhood environment (Winnicott, Segal, Bion). Giles' task as an analyst dealing with highly disturbed patients where this process has not taken place is to help them move towards it to whatever degree possible.

This is the 'recycling madness' to which the title of the book alludes. It involves developing a common symbolic language through the analytic process by which the analysands can start to grasp and work with their highly disordered and chaotic internal life.

Chapters Ten to Eighteen: published and unpublished papers, 2008 to 2017

A key part of Giles' professional life related to Jungian analytic training, and he wrote and rewrote a substantial body of material for training seminars for Jungian analysts. Several of the later chapters included here originated as presentations for

10 Alpha function is a term left deliberately undefined by Bion, but it describes how primitive, inchoate and unprocessed fears, named beta elements, when taken in and contained by mother/analyst in a state of reverie, undergo a metamorphosis whereby they are metabolised and transformed into that which can be thought, which he calls alpha elements (Bion, 1962).

ANZSJA training seminars and related occasions (Chapters Ten, Thirteen, Fourteen and Eighteen). Often, these training seminars began with material taken from earlier items but moved on to explore implications not in the earlier version or onto new ground altogether. Other chapters here began as seminars or conference papers for the Jungian or wider psychoanalytic community in Australia (Chapter Eleven and Seventeen) or as papers for conferences of the International Association for Analytical Psychology (Chapter Fifteen for the 2010 Montreal Conference and Chapter Sixteen for the 2013 Copenhagen conference). The remaining chapter (Chapter Twelve) appeared in a celebratory volume in 2010 for Giles' friend Andrew Samuels.

There is much new material in these chapters; Giles presents several more case studies, further exemplifying his understanding of borderline and narcissistic conditions and how they can be treated analytically. Among other things, there are detailed presentations of the symbolising process and how it can go wrong (Chapter Ten), of the problems of romantic relationships (Chapter Eleven), of unconscious structures and defences (Chapter Thirteen), psychosis (Chapter Fourteen) and countertransference (Chapters Twelve and Sixteen). We also learn much more about Giles' views on the relevance to analytic work of the philosophy of Spinoza (Chapters Twelve, Sixteen and Seventeen), of the work of Johann Gottfried Herder, Friedrich Schelling and other 18th- and 19th-century German philosophers (Chapters Eleven and Fifteen) and of the writings of another of Giles' favourite writers, George Santayana (Chapter Eighteen).

Only three of these chapters (Twelve, Fifteen and Sixteen) were published in Giles' lifetime. Giles frequently revised and added to his papers, including the three published items, so much of his writing exists in multiple versions with substantial overlaps but also significant new insights. In places, we have rearranged and abridged his material to avoid extensive repetition of earlier matter. In some cases (Chapters Ten, Eleven and Seventeen), we have also combined material on related themes from different presentations.

Chapter Ten, on symbolising and on the inability to symbolise, is based on two papers from 2008 and 2014. Psychodynamic psychology views the capacity to symbolise as vital to psychological and interpersonal well-being. A clinical issue is how to help patients who suffer a lack of symbolising function, as well as psychological mindedness, self-awareness, empathy, imaginal capacity, play and relationality that goes along with its absence. Giles discusses the contrasting understandings of the symbolising function in the work of Freud and Jung and outlines Hanna Segal's concept of the 'symbolic equation' as well as other Freudian writers on symbolising function, such as Charles Rycroft and Ronald Britton. Jung's theory of symbolisation was that symbols express through images, ideas, language, rituals, dreams and fantasies, are internal dynamic forces and are images that move from the unconscious to conscious awareness.

Giles examines the origins of Jung's ideas, like those of Freud, in 19th-century German thought while emphasising the distinctiveness of Jung's own concepts of symbols and symbolisation. For Jung, the true symbol is 'an intuitive idea that cannot yet be formulated in any other or better way'. Such symbols connect back to earlier, repressed or split-off emotional experiences and. unconscious memories They are also coloured by and formed from an archetypal and impersonal level of the creative unconscious. Language is both a key vehicle for symbolic expression and a central context for the failure of 'healthy symbolising, memory and imagination'. Problems and confusions in this area can go back to the early family environment, and to a lesser or greater extent, we all have some problems in this area. Post-Jungian writers such as Michael Fordham and Warren Colman offer further insights into problems with symbolising.

In the later sections of the paper, Giles presents a new clinical vignette of Adie and also returns to Christine and Jim, whom we have met in previous chapters. How does the symbolising function begin to emerge from such unpromising ground? And how can the containing frame of analysis assist in this emergence? How can the analyst assist people with a range of pathologies in which the symbolising function (and so the capacity for self-awareness, imagination, empathy) has failed to develop or been damaged or atrophied? Giles concludes with a summary of his own perspective on symbolising in the form of 21 brief points.

Chapter Eleven ('Romantic catastrophes and other vital realities') is an amalgamation of three unpublished papers concerning love, all dating from 2009. The chapter considers the analytic relevance of the radical subjectivity of German Romanticism, Idealism and the early philosophy of Schelling, the psychoanalytic application of Spinoza's writings on love before analysing the ways in which borderline and narcissistic disorders stem from the early lack and loss of primary love.

Although the need for and struggle for love is intrinsic and perennial, can we love properly, healthily and generously, Giles asks, if we have not experienced primary love? Does such lack lead to narcissistic and borderline defences, to magical thinking involving the construction of an all-loving godhead or other ideologies or to suicidal impulses aimed at preserving the good? The vicissitudes of later love relations start with primary love and its lacks, losses and failures, but this is also the source of imagination, creativity and the development of symbolising function.

Chapter Twelve, originally published in 2010 by Routledge in a *Festschrift* for Andrew Samuels, elaborates on Samuels' seminal concept of the 'embodied counter-transference', a key idea in Giles' own work. The version we have included here includes some material that is not in the original publication. This was added by Giles in unpublished revisions before and after the paper was published. Building on the discussions in earlier chapters, Giles suggests that embodied countertransference can be seen as extending Jung's concept of the psychoid into psychosomatic states involving psychotic transference and psychosomatic contagion. This makes for a mutual field that is pre-symbolic, or a realm of 'symbolic equivalence' (Segal, 1957), where beta-disordered fragments may yet eventually become ordered into a functional alpha state. The analyst is psychically informed by this process, and thence helps the patient grieve and mourn his or her lacks, losses, limitations and angry frustrations, allowing for the possible emergence of a truer and more satisfying liveliness.

Chapter Thirteen on unconscious structures and defences began as an ANZSJA Professional Development Seminar given in Christchurch, New Zealand, in 2010. This is another presentation of Giles' understanding of transference and countertransference, with illuminating discussions of several of Giles' favourite themes, including the relationship between free will and necessity, the consubstantiating animating psychoid body and the 'affective psychic immersion' through which analytic progress can be made. Giles points out that Jung, unlike Freud, developed his ideas through working with psychotic and near-psychotic patients; this is why his psychology is particularly helpful when working with such cases. The later parts of the chapter revisit the cases of Christine and Jim, presenting new material about the later phases of Giles' work with them.

Chapter Fourteen is another of Giles' teaching papers, here on the topic of psychosis. The opening sections are on the difference between 'normal human madness' in Santayana's sense – the natural human desire to change what cannot be changed and to hold on to what cannot be held on to – and the more extreme psychotic and borderline conditions. These may have a neurological basis, but they may also be psychogenic, resulting from the 'normal, necessary defences of the self' being unable to cope or becoming self-destructive. Giles discusses some of the relational disorders in early life which can generate such conditions. But in such psychogenic cases, there is at least hope of a symbolic interpretation leading to positive change.

Psychotic and related conditions (borderline, narcissistic) are often experienced in terms of a monstrous, alien force, holding the individual in a state in which the world feels maddening and unmanageable. The psychotic and near-psychotic are caught up in overwhelming emotional chaos, and communication is also disordered. This is unlike more typical analytic situations, where the analyst can reflect back and clarify the analysand's own state of mind. With these psychotic and related conditions, as Giles has discussed elsewhere, the analyst is likely to be caught up in the psychological violence and disorder experienced by his patient, but in this chapter, Giles provides an interesting and valuable discussion of how the analyst can hope to cope with the projections and acting-out and can model a healthier way of being to the analysand. An extended case study ('Kim') exemplifies how trusting his intuitive knowledge of the patient's 'living nightmare' enabled Giles to 'be part of the process of re-cycling it'.

Chapter Fifteen is the first of Giles' two IAAP conference papers and derives from the 2010 conference in Montreal, though the version given here includes some material from longer, unpublished versions of the paper. In this chapter, Giles discusses the seminal work of Johann Gottfried Herder (1744–1803), particularly in relation to his reworking of Spinoza's ideas. Herder's version of Spinoza's *conatus* acts at the level of the group as well as that of the individual, leading to the potential incorporation of culture and aesthetics into Spinoza's rationalistic perspective. Other aspects of Herder's work anticipated Jung's psychoid in its integration of psychology and physiology, while his emphasis on *Einfühlung* ('empathy') raises critical issues for both cultural studies and analytic practice.

This chapter gives particular attention to Herder's vitalist rereading of Spinoza's God/Nature as an active force and his reworking of the *conatus*, a key Spinozan concept (see Giles' discussion in Chapters Seven and Twelve). These provide the basis for Herder's view of cultural pluralism and individual difference. Herder, like Spinoza, works with a sense of 'free necessity'. Giles also discusses Herder's approach to *Einfühlung* and closes with another discussion of his '*jouissance* grid', suggesting that his model of *conatus*-as-*jouissance* can be seen as a 'Herderian' reading of Spinoza, in which the *conatus* as an active force unites and energises the affects and passions of the bodymind with their mutual tensions. The diagram also helps to illustrate how the process can go wrong and shift into psychosis if the tensions become mutually destructive rather than vitalising.

Chapter Sixteen is the second of Giles' two IAAP conference papers and was presented at the 2013 Copenhagen conference. Again, we have added some material from longer unpublished versions. This expanded version is perhaps the fullest presentation of Giles' thoughts on psychoid processes. Giles presents his hypothesis that

> all intra-psychic and interpersonal psychic relations are psychoid relations . . . body and mind are a basic psyche-soma unit, an identity experienced and expressed through a dual aspect, different modes of 'bodymind' which is also a single psychoid substance.
>
> (Chapter Sixteen, p. 219)

He calls on George Santayana to provide reinforcement, referring in particular to Michael Brodrick's interpretation of Santayana's position as implying an 'amphibious psyche'. Further on, Giles brings in the neuroscientist Antonio Damasio to provide a neurobiological model of the psychoid processes (we hear more of Damasio in Chapter Eighteen). We then move to a long and detailed account of Christine's analysis, introducing much new material. Through it, Giles shows how the analyst's bodymind is open to the patient's bodymind, and so is able to reflectively think through, link up and interpret the patient's damaged relational lacks, which drive the patient's infectious projections and identifications. Twelve closing observations about narcissistic and borderline defences show their close interrelationships, as well as their aetiology, their resistance to change, their failures of symbolising function and psychoid *conatus,* as well as transference-countertransference dynamics in analysis.

Chapter Seventeen was put together from two unpublished and overlapping papers and represents a 'working through' of Giles' long-standing engagement with the application of Spinoza to psychoanalysis. We have taken out material repeated from earlier chapters and done some minor editing whilst retaining Giles' own words, including some inevitable repetition as he uses the process of writing as a vehicle to think through and clarify his ideas.

This chapter presents a psychoanalytic application of Spinoza's concepts of the *conatus*, mind-body relations, passion and action and knowledge of the third kind (intuitive knowledge). It adapts such concepts into psychodynamic language, including their representation in the psychopathology of difficult psychosomatic relations and how they might help to psychosomatically re-order these confused and destructive internal and external relations. It suggests that destructive disorders of the self might well demonstrate a so-called 'psychotic metaphysics' that can be understood from a Spinozan perspective (Rhode, 1994). Giles finds five inter-related Spinozan concepts to be particularly helpful in the analytic setting: the '*conatus*', 'the mind as the idea of the body', neo-Spinozan theories of 'emotions, passions and actions', the issue of 'free necessity' and 'intuitive knowledge'. Giles explains how Spinoza's *Ethics* seeks to demonstrate a monistic, single-substance metaphysics in which God is identified with nature and the human mind and human body are two aspects of one substance. As before, Giles relates this to Jung's psychoid. The *conatus* is identified as being an endeavour for self-preservation and for the power of mental and physical activity and agency; this striving can be unconscious, conflicted, counter-intuitive and multiple; it is also interpersonal, relational and social; it incorporates the endeavour to make or find 'meaning' and thus also to symbolising, as well as pertinent to the human realm. The *conatus* is also 'panpsychic' or substantially absolute and is, therefore, an aspect of our being 'part of nature'.

The tone of this chapter is personal and subjective: these are central passions for Giles, informing how he understood psychoanalytic reverie, insight and agency in the particular intersubjective environment of analysis and conditioned by his own significant intimate relationships.

Chapter Eighteen was given as an ANZSJA training seminar in Auckland in 2017. Giles also worked on this paper in preparation for a conference in Ascona in July 2018. The last editorial changes were made on May 18, 2018. It is his last theoretical paper. He suggested that the paper needs to be read alongside three of his published papers (Chapters Five, Seven and Twelve). Although psychoanalysis focuses on mind-to-mind communications (whether conscious or unconscious), Jung viewed psyche as fundamentally psychoid. Giles draws on Spinoza's *conatus* and dual-identity substance monism in postulating a psychoid *conatus*. The psychoid is seen here as simultaneously 'bodily matter and sense' and 'mental image and idea'. Implying dual-aspect substance monism, at the psychoid level, body, image and idea are a unit, experienced or expressed through a 'dual identity', the different 'attributes' of a single substance. Giles discusses Santayana's materialistic 'organic psyche' (Santayana, 1930), incorporating the emergence, development and ongoing flux of self-regulating and self-preserving processes, which he also sees as psychoid. Giles also draws on Brodrick's idea of psyche being amphibious and on John Lachs and Jessica Wahman, who showed how, for Santayana, the material psyche and spirit are distinct before putting forward his own psychoanalytic application of Spinozan monism, Santayana's organic psyche and the psychoid *conatus*. Damasio's neurobiological contribution to these matters is also considered. There are further elaborations of how and why the psychoid is so evident in borderline and regressed relations and their therapeutic treatment.

Giles' final paper and some last jottings

Chapter Nineteen is the most personal and autobiographical of all Giles' writings. The paper emerged out of encouragement from a small group of colleagues and friends who had formed a writing group with the purpose of encouraging one another to persevere with vital writing projects. The group attended a writers' retreat on the topic of life writing at the Centro Incontri Umani, a cross-cultural research centre in Ascona, Switzerland, in July 2018, and it was here that Giles presented this paper. He continued working on it throughout the last year of his life, right up to his untimely and unexpected death in March 2019.

The chapter contains an autobiographical narrative of how the author's bodily issues led him as a teenager to travel to India, where he first studied the body-denying Jains and then, as an antidote, the more embodied Parsee Zoroastrians. He urgently returned to England suffering from a terrible spinal neurofibroma which hospitalised him for a year. This led him to Nietzsche, Jung, psychoanalysis and a life-long interest in mind-body relations and the philosophy of Spinoza and Santayana. We see here how Giles' oeuvre was inspired not only by a professional lifetime working with severe borderline, narcissistic and psychotic disorders with their mass of infectious, primitive psychoid identifications but also by his personal experience with problematic physical matters. These physical difficulties were his 'faithful but savage pet dog'. Giles discusses some of his earlier papers and reflects on the central ideas of his work, but he closes with a gently self-deprecating quote from one of his favourite authors, George Santayana.

We have included a few jottings he wrote in his diary in his last weeks after the end of this chapter to bring the book to a close with his last thoughts on life, love and death, and added a bibliography of his writings.

References

Addison, A. (2019). *Jung's Psychoid Concept Contextualised*. London: Routledge.

Atmanspacher, H. (2012). 'Dual-Aspect Monism à la Pauli & Jung'. *Journal of Consciousness Studies*, 19(9–10): 96–120.

Atmanspacher, H. & Fuchs, C. (2014). *The Pauli-Jung Conjecture and its Impact Today*. Exeter: Imprint Academic.

Bion, W. (1962). *Learning from Experience*. London: William Heinemann.

Bion, W. (1967). *Second Thoughts*. London: Heinemann.

Clark, G. (1977). *The Transformation of 'Spiritual Image' and 'Instinctual Shadow' into 'Instinctual Spirit': Pan, Wild Man, Green Man, and Animals as Symbols of the Instinctual Shadow of the Introverted, Spiritually-Fascinated 'Puer' and of Its Transformation*. Diploma Thesis, C. G. Jung Institute, Zürich.

Colman, W., Austin, S. & Petchkovsky, L. (2020). 'Obituary'. *Journal of Analytical Psychology*, 65(31): 609–614.

Deleuze, G. & Guattari, F. (1985). *Anti-Oedipus*. London: Athlone Press.

Hillman, J. (1972). 'An Essay on Pan'. In *Pan and the Nightmare*. W. H. Roscher & J. Hillman, eds. New York: Spring Publications.

Jung, C. (1947). 'Der Geist der Psychologie'. In *Geist und Natur. Vorträge gehalten auf der Tagung in Ascona 26*. August bis 3. September 1946. O. Fröbe-Kapteyn, ed. Zürich: Rhein-Verlag (Eranos-Jahrbuch XIV/1946).

Jung, C. (1952). 'Synchronizität als ein Prinzip akausaler Zusammenhänge'. In *Naturerklärung und Psyche*. C. Jung & W. Pauli, eds. Zürich: Rascher-Verlag.
Jung, C. (1954). 'The Spirit of Psychology'. In *Spirit and Nature: Papers from the Eranos Yearbooks*. J. Campbell, ed.; R. Hull & R. Manheim, trans. Princeton, NJ: Princeton University Press (Papers from the Eranos Yearbooks. Vol. 1).
Jung, C. (1970a). 'On the Nature of the Psyche'. In *The Structure and Dynamics of the Psyche*. Vol. 8 of *The Collected Works of C.G. Jung*. R. Hull, trans. 2nd edn. London: Routledge & Kegan Paul.
Jung, C. (1970b). 'Synchronicity: An Acausal Connecting Principle'. In *The Structure and Dynamics of the Psyche*. Vol. 8 of *The Collected Works of C.G. Jung*. R. Hull, trans. 2nd edn. London: Routledge & Kegan Paul.
Jung, C. (1970c). *Mysterium Coniunctionis: An Inquiry Into the Separation and Synthesis of Psychic Opposites in Alchemy*. Vol. 14 of *The Collected Works of C.G. Jung*. R. Hull, trans. 2nd edn. London: Routledge & Kegan Paul.
Jung, C. (1993). 'The Psychology of the Transference'. In *The Practice of Psychotherapy*. Vol. 16 of *The Collected Works of C.G. Jung*. R. Hull, trans. London: Routledge & Kegan Paul.
Jung, C. & von Franz, M.-L. (1955/56). *Mysterium Coniunctionis: Untersuchungen über die Trennung und Zusammensetzung der seelischen Gegensätze in der Alchemie*. Zürich: Rascher-Verlag.
Kerr-Lawson, A. (2000). 'Freedom and Free Will in Spinoza and Santayana'. *Journal of Speculative Philosophy (N.S.)*, 14(4): 243–267.
Kirsch, T. (2000). *The Jungians: A Comparative and Historical Perspective*. London and Philadelphia: Routledge.
Rhode, E. (1994). *Psychotic Metaphysics*. London: Karnac Books.
Ryška Vajdová, I. (2021). 'On the Brink of the Expressible: Adolf Portmann Meets Carl Gustav Jung on Eranos Ground'. In *Adolf Portmann: A Thinker of Self-Expressive Life*. Filip Jaroš & Jiří Klouda, eds. Cham: Springer Verlag.
Samuels, A. (1985). *Jung and the Post-Jungians*. London: Routledge.
Santayana, G. (1930). 'The Psyche'. In *The Realm of Matter: Book Second of Realms of Being*. New York: Scribner.
Segal, H. (1957). 'Notes on Symbol Formation'. *International Journal of Psycho-Analysis*, 259(38): 391–397.
Solomon, H. (2008). 'The Developmental School'. In *The Cambridge Companion to Jung*. P. Young-Eisendrath & T. Dawson, eds. 2nd edn. Cambridge and New York: Cambridge University Press.

Chapter 1

A process of transformation

Spiritual *puer*, instinctual shadow and instinctual spirit

Harvest, 1978[1]

The aim of this chapter is to explore the process and symbols of the psychic transformation of a *puer aeternus*, or 'eternal youth', through the realisation and integration of certain specific qualities of his shadow. The type of *puer* in question is one frequently met with in analysis, namely an over-idealistic and spiritually-fascinated young man who has split off and repressed his feeling and sensation functions, awareness of his body and its needs, and above all his sexuality. I suggest that his heady spirituality is a repressive sublimation of his shadowy sexual instincts.

I divide the chapter into two parts. In the first part I define in detail this kind of *puer*. This entails describing the aetiology of his particular pathology – a typical anamnesis; then a classification of the split between his one-sided, ethereal spirituality and its shadow, namely his repressed, inferior and undifferentiated sensuous instincts. I shall show how this split epitomises the spirit-instinct polarity of opposites, and how out of this dialectic can emerge a synthetic 'instinctual spirit' in the form of a symbol of a transcendent Green Man figure.

In the second part, I differentiate the symbolic images I refer to as Pan, Wild Man, Green Man and Animals, and show how they can be seen as being different 'levels' of the instinctual shadow and different stages in its process of integration.

The *puer*'s intellectual fascination with ideas, images, symbols etc. is compulsive, driven by his repressed and frustrated instinctual needs. These fascinating images and ideas found in his dreams and fantasies are likely to be images of instinctual needs, although the *puer* in his ethereal spirituality does not see, understand or experience them as such. He represses the 'infra-red' meaning of his fascinations. Eventually, the neurotic imbalance cannot be maintained and the repressed instinct forces itself into experience, usually in an episode of 'acting out', which is, in effect, an actualisation of the instinctual meaning of the image. This stage can be called the regressive actualisation and realisation of the Wild Man. Such regression may, however, lead to the emergence of a constructive and progressive figure, deriving from a more impersonal, more archetypal level of the natural instinctual

1 Lecture originally given to the Analytical Psychology Club, London on September 15, 1977, published in *Harvest*, 1978. Minor editing has been applied (Eds.).

DOI: 10.4324/9781003255826-2

aspect of the Self: the Green Man. The Green Man is the Lord of the Animals and, so long as ego does not identify itself with the Green Man (which would be a form of inflation), he can become a transcendent symbol incorporating both image and instinct, and thus help ego-consciousness into a more useful and healthy relationship with the 'animal passions' – i.e. with the instincts, particularly sexual instincts. Such a development transforms the spiritual *puer's* original spirituality and its instinctual shadow into a more positive, transcendent 'instinctual spirit'.

What are the typical aetiological conditions in the anamnesis of our type of spiritual *puer*? They often involve an apparently over-loving, smothering mother who protects her son from his masculine sexuality and a weak father who is unable to relate erotically to his wife's feelings and to his own *anima*. Such a mother tends, in fact, to be so afraid of her son's masculine sexuality that, in effect, she rejects him in his sexuality. Her smothering love really hides a fear of expression of love or, in other words, her devouringness compensates for a fear of masculine sexuality. She could be seen as a schizogenic mother. The father, in his inability to relate to his wife's feelings and to his own *anima*, tends to retire into a private world, his weakness often appearing as 'strong and silent'. He may retreat into an alcoholic escape, which counteracts its own intentions, exacerbates his bad feelings or fear of his *anima*/wife and leads to aggressive behaviour against the wife.

In such schizogenic familial circumstances, one unconscious objective of the mother's denial of her son's masculine sexuality is to keep him 'virginal', by emasculating him, if not psychological castration. This would be a means to keep him from being a 'man for other women', and so keep him for herself. In other words, it is psychologically incestuous. Furthermore, the mother's incestuous love is made safer (vis-à-vis the taboo) by the son being made sexless, neuter or feminine. The anti-sexual tendencies of both parents lead the son to repress or suppress his own apparent frighteningly dangerous, dirty and taboo sexual instincts. The libido of these split-off instincts, as well as of the inferior attitude (extraversion) and functions (feeling and sensation) bound up with this, morphs into inflated narcissistic and overly 'spiritual' (ethereal) fantasies and ideas. When, however, he is faced with situations which make demands on him to express his extraverted sexual feelings and instincts (i.e. when sexually attracted to or by a woman), he will experience marked anxiety, or have feelings of alienation, which are a displacement of such anxiety.

Such anxiety or alienation is not only a fear of the taboo 'dirtiness' of his own sexuality; it often is projected onto the object of the demand, i.e. onto the sexuality of women. This fear of women's sexuality is also a projection of the devouring, smothering and castrating mother-image: the *vagina dentata*. But the anxiety is even more than this, and it can be further differentiated: an anxiety or fear of expressing extraverted sexuality also derives from a feeling of the vulnerability of the inferiority of that sexuality. Since his extraverted masculine sexuality has been repressed and not expressed, it is inferior and immature, if not infantile. Thus, it seems weak and vulnerable. Any expression of that sexuality would therefore be anticipated fearfully as firstly being a revealing of an insecure, infantile bit; and secondly as something likely to be rejected or even attacked as it would have been by mother (which would further compound and 'prove' the vulnerability). Under such conditions, a young man neurotically displaces or sublimates his split-off instinctual libido into narcissistic, spiritual fantasies and ideas.

I have noticed that when such young men first come into analysis they more often than not claim an 'interest in the archetypes', which all too often actually means an intellectual interest in second-hand ideas about archetypes, with no room for conscious awareness or personal experience of the subjective and unique nature of actual archetypal encounter. The compulsive fascination of this interest betrays a personal pathology, an out-of-control, frustrated and misdirected instinctual drive in conflict with the repressive conscious ideals and will.

Much of what Jung says about the introverted intuitive type seems to describe the character of the young men I am considering. In *Psychological Types* (Jung, 1921, 1971) Jung says that with the introverted intuitive,

> the intensification of intuition often results in an extraordinary aloofness of the individual from tangible reality . . . The moral problem arises when the intuitive tries to relate himself to his vision, when he is no longer satisfied with mere perception and its aesthetic configuration and evaluation, when he confronts the question: What does this mean for me? . . . What emerges from this vision in the way of a duty or a task for me? . . . The pure intuitive who represses his judgment, or whose judgment is held in thrall by his perceptive faculties, never faces this question squarely, since his problem is the 'know-how' of perception . . . . . What the introverted intuitive represses most of all is the sensation of the object, and this colours his whole unconscious.
>
> (Jung, 1971, *CW* 6, paras. 661–663)

In such passages, Jung touches on many characteristics that I shall be exemplifying, particularly the negative shadow qualities of the spiritually-fascinated *puer*, who is often attracted to Jungian analysis – or to their idealistic fantasy of it.

In their research study, 'Incidence of Psychological Types among Jungian Analysts Classified by Self and by Test', Katherine Bradway and Wayne Detloff found that:

> Jungian analysts as a group are markedly differentiated from the general (non-analytic) population in the higher incidence of introvert-intuitive types and the low incidence of sensation types.
>
> (Bradway and Detloff, 1976, p. 143)[2]

The low incidence of sensation types is also important since it would suggest sensation to be the most common inferior function of Jungian analysts. This is relevant

2 A finding replicated by Bradway and Detloff (1996).

in regard to the inferior sensation function as part of the shadow of the introverted intuitive, spiritually-fascinated *puer*.

The abstract, spiritual ideas that fascinate the *puer* tend to be intellectualised, disembodied spiritual images lifted both from their instinctual origins and projected right out of the body. They are not so much projected onto nature, but out into the ether. Split off from and devoid of their physical instinctuality and relatedness to any material nature they lack a sense of what Otto (1950) called the *mysterium tremendum*,[3] and cannot be sensually experienced or suffered at all. They are abstract ideas, affect-less images, symbols and structures. They inevitably derive their fascinating power from instinct or from the needs of the repressed instincts behind them; but of this, our *puer* is unconscious, for his physical instinctuality and sexuality make up his shadow. In his 1935 Tavistock lectures (Jung, 1977), Jung said:

> We do not like to look at the shadow-side of ourselves; therefore there are many people in our civilisation who have lost sight of their shadow altogether, they have got rid of it. They are only two-dimensional; they have lost the third dimension, and with it they have usually lost the body. The body is a most doubtful friend because it produces things we do not like; there are too many things about the body which cannot be mentioned. The body is very often the personification of this shadow of the ego.
>
> (*CW* 18, para. 40)

I suggest that 'body' here can be seen to mean the opposite of 'spiritual' and that the shadow of 'spiritual image' is instinct, nature and body. Is the opposition between image and instinct an essential condition of the human psyche? In 'On the Nature of the Psyche' (Jung, 1970a) Jung describes the 'psychic spectrum', drawing an analogy between the idea of archetypes and instincts and the colour spectrum. The psyche has an organic-material-instinctual pole and an archetypal and thence image-pole. The former is like the infrared end of the spectrum, the latter like the ultraviolet end. The latter is the image or (spiritual) meaning of the former. Jung says, 'Just as, in its lower reaches, the psyche loses itself in the organic-material substrate, so in its upper reaches it resolves itself into a "*spiritual*" form' (*CW* 8, para. 380). By 'spiritual form', Jung means the psychic archetypal image of the instinct. Purely instinctual functioning is compulsive: it is, as William Halse Rivers said, an 'all-or-none reaction' (Rivers, 1920). It is an innate and, therefore, inevitable, impulsive 'drive'. If this is so, the question is then: how can any instinct be repressed or suppressed as I am going to suggest it can? How, in fact, can the image lose its instinctual base? Can the image become so spiritual that it, so to speak, loses sight of itself as also being an instinctual image – an image of an instinct?

3 A reference to Rudolf Otto's (1950) description of the holy as having two aspects, the *mysterium tremendum* and the *mysterium fascinans* (Eds.).

On this point, Jung notes, 'the *partie supérieure*, which is best described as psychic . . . can be subjected to the will and even applied in a manner contrary to the original instinct' (*CW* 8, para. 376). This is what I mean by spiritual repression or suppression of the instinct. Consciousness or conscious ideals split the instinct off from the image; the image becomes spiritually inflated and loses all touch with its relatedness to its physical, instinctual roots. It even loses touch with sensation and becomes 'pure idea': an intellectual, spiritual fascination.

One way that a *puer* realises and becomes conscious of his sensuous-instinctual shadow is when his libido goes into his unconscious and its primitive instinctuality and intemperance are activated, compulsively 'driving' him to express and experience their affects through a compulsive acting out. But even then, the image-vs-instinct split may be so acute that he still will not see any connection between the two. He will feel that such *tremendum* of experienced compulsive instinctual sensuality could have nothing to do with the *fascinans* of the spiritual image. What he has not seen is that the increasing intensity of his fascinating spiritual images is proportionately related to the intensity and specificity of his instinctual acting out. In other words, his fascinating images are, in fact, images of specific sensational, physical, instinctual needs and drives. These very instincts are crying out to be realised, and in order to compensate for his one-sidedness, they force themselves to be realised. Only once he can connect the image to the compulsively acted out (and therefore experienced or realised) instinct can he begin to assimilate and integrate the shadow and transform it. In so doing, the compulsive quality of the shadowy sensuous-instinct and the spiritual image will both concurrently begin to transform.

The image is related downwards to the instinctual shadow, thus sacrificing its fascinating, over-spiritual quality, and instinct is related upwards to its image, thus losing its compulsive shadow quality. The synthetic gain is an instinctually-related image that has to do with a quite different sort of spirit, namely an 'instinctual spirit'. This instinctually related image is a transcendent symbol, the Green Man. In his definition of 'Symbol' in *Psychological Types*, Jung says:

> Since life cannot tolerate a standstill, a damming up of vital energy results, and this would lead to an unsupportable condition did not the tension of opposites produce a new, united function that transcends them. This function arises quite naturally from the regression of libido caused by the blockage.
>
> (Jung, 1971, *CW* 6, para. 824)

Then he goes on to say:

> If, for instance, we conceive the opposition to be sensuality versus spirituality then the mediatory content born out of the unconscious provides a welcome means of expression for the spiritual thesis because of its rich spiritual associations, and also for the sensual antithesis, because of its sensuous imagery. The

> ego, however, torn between thesis and antithesis, finds in the middle ground its own counterpart, its sole and unique means of expression and it eagerly seizes on this in order to be delivered from its division. The energy created by the tension of opposites therefore flows into mediatory product and protects it from the conflict which immediately breaks out again, for both the opposites are striving to get the new products on their side. Spirituality wants to make something spiritual out of it, and sensuality something sensual; the one wants to turn it into science or art, the other into sensual experience.
>
> (*CW* 6, para. 825)

Only when ego relates to the symbol and lets that symbol carry the tension of the opposites within itself is it functionally a transcendent symbol. This matter has to do with ego's relationship to the Green Man.

If our *puer* eventually transforms his instinctual shadow and assimilates the instinctual meaning of those fascinating images, they do not thereby lose 'spirit'. Instead, he discovers another meaning of spirit. Rather than incorporeal and ethereal, he finds that there is also a 'spirit' in his instinctuality, in the figures of the process of transformation of instinct – Pan, Wild Man, Green Man and Animals. There is a spirit in here, too, a spirit I shall call 'instinctual spirit'. This instinctual spirit is of necessity bound up with the *puer's* feeling, sensations, sexuality and extraversion.

In the *Shorter Oxford Dictionary,* there is another meaning of spirit other than something non-instinctual, incorporeal and ethereal, which is closer to my idea of 'instinctual spirit'. For spirit can also mean 'animating or vital principle in man and animals', or 'emotional part of a man', 'vivacity'; 'vital power of energy'; 'vigour'; 'a tendency, inclination or *impulse* of a specific kind'; 'the *sentient* part of a man'; etc. These two meanings of spirit (in-corporeal/ethereal and vital/instinctual) are similar to those distinguished by Hugo Rahner as 'Earth Spirit' and 'Divine Spirit' (Rahner, 1954).

While the instincts themselves cannot be assimilated into consciousness, the instinctual meaning of certain images or the instinctual images (Wild Man, Green Man and Animals) can indeed be integrated.

Symbolic images of the transformation of the puerile instinctual shadow Pan

In his 'Essay on Pan' James Hillman says:

> As God of all nature, Pan personifies to our consciousness that which is all or only natural, behaviour at its most nature-bound. Behaviour that is nature-bound is, in a sense, divine; it is behaviour transcendent to the human yoke of purposes, wholly impersonal, objective, ruthless. The cause of such behaviour is obscure; it springs suddenly, spontaneously. As Pan's genealogy is obscure so is the origin of instinct. To speak of instinct as an inborn release mechanism,

> or to speak of it as a chthonic spirit, a prompting of nature, puts into obscure psychological concepts the obscure experiences that might once have been attributed to Pan.
>
> (Hillman, 1972, p. xix)

What is this natural, ruthless, spontaneous and, to us, obscure behaviour? It is instinct: 'He (Pan) lives in the repressed which returns, in the psychopathologies of instinct which assert themselves' (p. xxiii). But Hillman goes on to say that Pan need not remain psychopathological, compulsive instinctuality but can offer a way to its transformation or modification:

> The figure of Pan both represents instinctual compulsion and offers the medium by which the compulsion can be modified through imagination. By working on imagination, we are taking part in nature 'in here'.
>
> (p. xxv)

What is this imagination that modifies Pan-as-compulsion or compulsive instinct? Hillman equates it with 'Pan's loves' – his nymphs, whom he chases but never catches. They are reflections, and they also turn into 'reflections', and thus reflections of or on himself, awareness of and modification of his nature (pp. xliv-xlix).

We can psychologically interpret the theme of Pan as an incubus-son who panics his mother into deserting him as meaning the sexuality of the son panics the mother, who thus rejects his sexuality, and this causes him to repress it. As he did with his mother, so too, Pan causes the nymphs he loves to flee from him in panic. But on fleeing and being chased, the nymphs then depersonalise themselves and turn into elements that Hillman considers to be reflections of Pan. The three main nymphs whom Pan desired were: Syrinx, who turns into a reed, sighing in the wind (Pan's pipes); Pitys, who turns into a pine tree; and Echo, who turns into reflected sound.

I interpret Pan's rapacious desire for and chasing of these nymphs who depersonalise themselves as the activated sexual instinct, but which has to act itself out (extravert) against an *anima* projection. This projected *anima* is so subjective and idealised that it cannot relate to a real woman. The rapacious desire is, in fact, masturbatory and narcissistic. The nymph Syrinx, who becomes a reed and/or pipe (which Pan can then play), is a symbol of phallic-masturbation, while the nymph Pitys, who becomes a pine tree, is another male, phallic symbol – and the pine cone is indeed an attribute of Dionysus. Echo, who becomes an echo of Pan's own voice, was, in fact, she who loved Narcissus himself in vain. Although the *puer*, in realising his sexual instincts (when they compulsively force him to act them out), will no doubt *use* a woman as a hook for those Pan-derived *anima* images, which are, in fact, narcissistic mirrors for seeing his own sexuality. This is a sort of chauvinistic, sexist stage in which a man can get stuck and fixed.

Wild Man and Green Man

There are severe didactic problems in discussing Wild Man and Green Man, the main problem being distinguishing them. The Wild Man and the Green Man (or 'Jack o' the Green') were medieval European names for two different but often juxtaposed characters, popular in allegoric literature. Their original sources were very different: the Wild Man belonged to a Teutonic folk tradition of the outlaw, whereas the Green Man was a Celtic mythological figure – a god or demon. An indication of this is the frequency of public drinking houses in German-speaking countries called *Der Wilde Mann* and the many British 'public houses' called 'The Green Man'.

What are the differentiating characteristics of the Wild Man and the Green Man in medieval literature and folk tradition? There are three essential differences:

1 The Wild Man is (or was) a *human* who has regressed to an animal state and to the wild. The Green Man is super-human, a divinity or demon.
2 The Wild Man, though originally human, is, as a Wild Man, primarily *animal*, or at least his animal qualities are emphasised and definitive: he is hairy and behaves like a wild animal. He is 'bestial man'. The Green Man, though a divinity or demon, is not an animal himself but may be 'Lord of the Animals'. In fact, in some ways, he looks more human than the bestial Wild Man.
3 Wild Man's animal hair is usually red. The Green Man is 'foliate'. That is, he either wears a green leafy mask, crown or body covering, or sprouts green leaves, often from his head or mouth.

To psychologically interpret these distinctions, the Wild Man's original humanity means that he has to do with the personal unconscious, whereas the Green Man's essential divinity makes him more of an impersonal archetype, closer to the 'Self'. The Wild Man is a symbol of a man's regression into undifferentiated wild 'animal' instinctuality. The Green Man is a quality and process of the unconscious *per se*. But as 'Lord of the Animals', and as a divinity or demon, the Green Man is also the controller and transformer of the bestial Wild Man. Perhaps this is why the Green Man often appears with or soon after the Wild Man both in medieval literature and in dreams: it is as though he (the Green Man) is that part of the 'Self' that attracts, relates to and can transform the regressive Wild Man.

Further amplificatory material on the Wild Man can be found: in the stories of Esau and Jacob; Nebuchadnezzar becoming like the beasts of the field; Merlin retiring, mad, to the forest; in the Grimms' Fairy Tales 'Iron Hans' and 'Bearskin'; in such monsters of folk-lore as vampires, werewolves, Frankensteinian monsters; etc.

Jung became aware of the two types of spirit, ethereal and vital, through his dreams, alchemical studies, and also his two spirits, Philemon and Ka, as recorded in 1961 by Aniela Jaffé in *Memories, Dreams, Reflections*. Jung speaks of how Philemon developed out of a fantasy of Elijah, Salome and a black snake. Philemon was pagan but was attributed with the colour blue – blue sky, blue water, blue kingfisher's wings; he was an image of the archetypal 'divine spirit' (Jung, 1967, pp. 207–209). Later, Jung tells us how Philemon became relativised by the emergence of another figure, Ka. Ka came from 'below', from 'out of the earth'. In Jung's painting of Ka, he appeared 'demonic' and 'Mephistophelian'; he represented 'a kind of earth demon or metal demon'. 'Philemon was the *spiritual* aspect or 'meaning'. Ka, on the other hand, was a *spirit of nature* like the Anthroparion of Greek alchemy – with which at the time I was unfamiliar' (Jung, 1967, pp. 208–209). In a footnote to this passage, Aniela Jaffé points out that the Anthroparion is a homunculus, and indeed she equates such a figure with the Daktyls (Daktyloi) (in Jung, 1967, p. 209, n. 5).

So Jung's Ka is an earth-bound, nature-figure with phallic implications. He is the complementary opposite of the 'spiritual' Philemon. Ka is Philemon's natural, 'instinctual shadow', i.e. spirit as natural, earthy and vital spirit in contrast to Philemon's more ethereal, 'blue' or divine spirituality.

Further on in *Memories, Dreams, Reflections,* Jung recounts his alchemical dream about the 'greenish gold' figure of Christ on the cross. He goes on to point out that the green-gold (*viriditas*) of the alchemists is an expression of the 'life-spirit', which is the *Anima Mundi* spirit that pours itself into everything, including matter. It is the *vitalising or animating spirit*; the natural, earthy spirit in the divinely spiritual Christ; incarnate spirit (Jung, 1967, p. 237).

Perhaps we can see here a psychic development that is strictly relevant to my thesis. Firstly, in Jung's fantasies of Elijah, Salome and the black snake, we notice Elijah's hairy-animal attributes. Salome is the *erotic anima* – the Eros principle; and the black snake is (amongst other things) a dark, shadowy, phallic sexual symbol closely related to Jung's childhood underground ithyphallic dream and his black Kabir mannikin figure.[4] Perhaps even Jung did not see the instinctual sexuality in these dreams.

In the figure of the green-gold Christ, we have a synthesis of the opposites spirit and matter, or spirit and instinct, something closer to the 'instinctual spirit' as opposed to pure 'spiritual image' and its 'instinctual shadow'. Jung associated the colour green with the sensation function, which he himself claimed was, for a long time, his inferior function and thus, an aspect of his shadow. It is perhaps also significant that he associated red (the redness of the hairy animal Wild Man) with feeling and with emotion. Feeling and, above all, sensation are likely to be the inferior functions of our *puer* and so belong to his instinctual shadow.

There is not space to amplify the themes of Wild Man or Green Man from exemplary source material. The structure and dynamics of the epic of Gilgamesh – with Gilgamesh's instinctual shadow in the person of Enkidu – offer a rewarding area for research into the psychology of the Wild Man syndrome. The medieval poem

4 For further associations, see Noel (1974).

'Sir Gawain and the Green Knight' is also perhaps one of the best sources for a deductive psychological study of the Green Man.

As literary source material mentioned previously shows, the Wild Man can be seen as a personal instinctual shadow figure, the Green Man as a more impersonal image of the transforming potentialities of the masculine instinctual spirit, perhaps a psychopomp of the Self. The Wild Man is a part that the ego has to learn to relate to; the Green Man can relate to ego; and can, as a transcendent symbol, incorporate the tension between the 'opposites' spirit and instinct.

Animals

We have seen how the Wild Man represents regression to a wild animal-like state of affairs, often manifest as a concrete sexual acting out and how the Green Man is a divine/demonic transcendent symbol of the shadow-side of the 'Self' who transforms the instinctual shadow contacted in the Wild Man state. In 'Symbolism in the Visual Arts', Aniela Jaffé says:

> The animal motif is usually symbolic of man's primitive and instinctual nature. Even civilised men must realise the violence of their instinctual drives and their powerlessness in face of the autonomous emotions erupting from the unconscious.
>
> (Jaffé, 1964, p. 237)

After giving many examples of animal symbols in mythology and world religion, she goes on to say:

> The boundless profusion of animal symbolism in the religion and art of all times does not merely emphasise the importance of the symbol; it shows how vital it is for men to integrate into their lives the symbol's psychic content – instinct. In itself, an animal is neither good nor evil; it is a piece of nature. It cannot desire anything that is not in its nature. To put this another way, it obeys its instincts. These instincts often seem mysterious to us, but they have their parallel in human life: the foundation of human nature is instinct.
>
> But in man, the 'animal being' (which lives in him as his instinctual psyche) may become dangerous if it is not recognised and integrated in life. Man is the only creature with the power to control instinct by his own will, but he is also able to suppress, distort and wound it – and an animal, to speak metaphorically, is never so wild and dangerous as when it is wounded. Suppressed instincts can gain control of a man; they can even destroy him.
>
> The familiar dream in which the dreamer is pursued by an animal nearly always indicates that an instinct has been split off from consciousness and ought to be (or is trying to be) readmitted and integrated into life. The more dangerous the behaviour of the animal in the dream, the more unconscious is the primitive and instinctual soul of the dreamer, and the more imperative is its integration into his life if some irreparable evil is to be forestalled.

> Suppressed and wounded instincts are the dangers threatening civilised man; the 'animal' is alienated from its true nature; the acceptance of the animal soul is the condition for wholeness and a fully lived life. Civilised man must heal the animal in himself and make it his friend.
>
> (Jaffé, 1964, pp. 238–239)

Jaffé's argument here implicitly harks back to one of Jung's major influences, Goethe, who likewise sought to understand the relationship between the 'divine' and 'animal' aspects of human life.[5] The previous passage from Jaffé supports the basic idea of this paper that animals symbolise instincts and ego's relationship to instincts. The issue in question is: If Wild Man represents regression to the animal, and if Green Man is the 'Lord of the Animals', then what happens to 'animal-instinctuality' in this entire process? It seems to me that the Green Man differentiates the animal from the Wild Man so that the *humanity* of the Wild Man returns to consciousness, now related to, but not contaminated by, compelled by or devoured by 'the animal'. In other words, the ego itself becomes more of a master of the sensuous-sexual instincts rather than cut off from them. How does ego do this? The answer is through the transcendent symbol of the Green Man.

The Wild Man is an *image* of regression to the animal level of instinct where ego has been swamped or devoured by repressed, shadowy, compulsive instinctual drives. The Green Man is an *image* of the 'Self's' progressive tendency to differentiate, to grow from and to 'use' animal instincts: a symbol of what Jung, in a paper first written in 1916, calls the 'transcendent function' (Jung, 1970b). And animals are *images* of those animal-instincts which are recognised as useful sources of energy, instinctual libido, basic sensations and sexuality, etc. These animal instincts can be ridden and, to a certain extent, directed, as a person can ride and direct a horse. But a rider must always remember that the animal ridden has its own autonomous existence and strength, which one must respect in order to utilise it to one's advantage. Psychologically, this is done by recognising the meaning of animal-images and remembering that one's ability to control these instincts is derived from the transcendent symbol, the Green Man, and is not the prerogative of ego.

It is essential that ego does not identify itself with the Green Man-as-transcendent symbol, for doing so would lead back to either the original inflation or the regressive, concrete acting out. Ego must recognise that this transcendent symbol is other and greater than ego itself, that it is related to the 'Self'. This recognition, in turn, should help relativise ego's feeling of control over the animal instincts, for it is the Green Man who is the real master or Lord of the Animals, not ego. In fact, ego needs

5 E.g. 'Perhaps in this way we shall attain the high philosophical goal of perceiving how the divine force in man is joined in all innocence with animal life' (cited in Kerényi, 1976). This quotation serves as the Epigraph for Kerényi 1976 and was presumably taken by the author from this source. We have not been able to identify Goethe's original. The author makes one change; the Kerényi volume has 'divine life' not 'divine' (Eds).

the Green Man in order to relate to the animal instincts. Respect for the Green Man's 'otherness' implies respect for the animal instincts' ultimate autonomy.

Orpheus

Having said all this, I must add a moral qualification based upon an ambivalence that is exemplified in the story of Orpheus. Orpheus was a musician whose music expressed his state of harmony with nature, a harmony so perfect that he charmed even trees and animals. He was indeed in touch with and related to nature and perhaps instinct, but all the same, he remained one-sided. He was too idealistic, his music was too magical, and above all, he could not relate to women, particularly after his second loss of Eurydice, where after he refused to have anything more to do with any women. This looks like a puerile suppression of *anima*-relatedness. It seems to me to have been an apt punishment that, as a result of this cutting-off of his relationship with the feminine, he was torn to pieces by the women of Thrace in a Dionysian orgy. Furthermore, it seems even more appropriate, and a sign of his basic unrelatedness to his own body, that after his death, his disembodied head went on singing (of Eurydice), and his lyre went on playing – on Lesbos.

Orpheus is a golden *puer aeternus* who has idealised and sublimated the Dionysian wildness of natural sexual instincts, and so it is psychically inevitable that he is ultimately devoured by the repressed shadow of this 'perfect' idealism in the form of Wild Women who tear his body to pieces. The story of Orpheus, therefore, emphasises my point that animals and animal-like instincts cannot be totally mastered by ego. That is inflated idealism – like Orpheus's magic. It is both inflation and negative sublimation of instinct by an all-too-spiritual ego. It is just such a suppression of instinct and re-inflation of an idealistic ego that is our *puer's* constant danger. The transformational process that I have described is often beset with recurrent regression, re-suppressions, inflations, defeats and failures. So long as there is no total defeat, it is worth suffering the *repetitio* – even as a ritual. Out of such acceptance, further progress might grow. Our *puer* may then move from being a mother's boy split off from his shadowy masculinity and phallic instincts to being a man related to his own potent and vital masculine spirit, which is an instinctual spirit that in turn relates him to earth, matter, reality and to women. He can even begin to experience genuine embodied Eros. The fantastic child, replanted in his nature, can now begin to grow up as a man in the world.

References

Bradway, K. & Detloff, W. (1976). 'Incidence of Psychological Types among Jungian Analysts Classified by Self and by Test'. *Journal of Analytical Psychology*, 33(2): 134–146.

Bradway, K. & Detloff, W. (1996). 'Psychological Type: A 32-year Follow-Up'. *Journal of Analytical Psychology*, 41(4): 553–574.

Hillman, J. (1972). 'An Essay on Pan'. In *Pan and the Nightmare*. W. H. Roscher & J. Hillman, eds. New York: Spring Publications.

Jaffé, A. (1964). 'Symbolism in the Visual Arts'. In *Man and His Symbols*. C. G. Jung & M. L. von Franz, eds. London: Aldus Books.
Jung, C. (1921). *Psychologische Typen*. Zürich: Rascher & Cie.
Jung, C. (1947). 'Der Geist der Psychologie'. In *Geist und Natur. Vorträge gehalten auf der Tagung in Ascona 26. August bis 3. September 1946*. O. Fröbe-Kapteyn, ed. Zürich: Rhein-Verlag (Eranos-Jahrbuch XIV/1946).
Jung, C. (1967). *Memories, Dreams, Reflections*. Recorded and edited by A. Jaffé. Translated from the German by R. & C. Winston. London: Collins (Fontana Library).
Jung, C. (1970a). 'On the Nature of the Psyche'. In *The Structure and Dynamics of the Psyche*. Vol. 8 of *The Collected Works of C.G. Jung*. R. Hull, trans. 2nd edn. London: Routledge & Kegan Paul.
Jung, C. (1970b). 'The Transcendent Function'. In *The Structure and Dynamics of the Psyche*. Vol. 8 of *The Collected Works of C.G. Jung*. R. Hull, trans. 2nd edn. London: Routledge & Kegan Paul.
Jung, C. (1971). *Psychological Types*. Vol. 6 of *The Collected Works of C.G. Jung*. H. Baynes, trans. London: Routledge & Kegan Paul.
Jung, C. (1977). 'The Tavistock Lectures: On the Theory and Practice of Analytical Psychology'. In *The Symbolic Life*. Vol. 18 of *The Collected Works of C.G. Jung*. R. Hull, trans. London: Routledge & Kegan Paul.
Kerényi, C. (1976). *Dionysos: Archetypal Image of Indestructible Life*. R. Manheim, trans. Princeton, NJ: Princeton University Press (Bollingen Series, LXV, 2).
Noel, D. (1974). 'Veiled Kabir: C. Jung's Phallic Self-Image'. *Spring*, 1974: 224–242.
Otto, R. (1950). *The Idea of the Holy*. J. Harvey, trans. London: Geoffrey Cumberlege/Oxford University Press.
Rahner, H. (1954). 'Earth Spirit and Divine Spirit in Patristic Theology'. In *Spirit and Nature: Papers from the Eranos Yearbooks*, R. Manheim, trans. Princeton, NJ: Princeton University Press.
Rivers, W. (1920). *Instinct and the Unconscious: A Contribution to the Biological Theory of the Psycho-Neuroses*. Cambridge: Cambridge University Press.

Chapter 2

A black hole in psyche

Harvest, 1983[1]

In psychological terms, this paper is about the possible failure of psychic life or about the impossibility of any movement towards wholeness. It is a *senex* perspective onto and into a psychic dualism where a phenomenologically un-alive or empty centre is seen to be an unassimilable evil or intolerable object of anxiety and dread that negates life, sometimes literally (it is fatal) but above all within the realm of the self where it causes chronic psychic atrophy, dissolution and a disappearing of psychic life. In more analytical terms, what follows is an attempt to describe various levels of defences against apparent psychic annihilation or self-dissolution, to consider the nature of an annihilating object or archetype and thereby to offer some speculative ideas on the psychodynamics of necessary splitting.

The questions I am asking are: To what extent can fear of annihilation and actual self-dissolution be dealt with reductively? What is the symbolism of this fearful inner object? Has it to do with negative parental images or with the child's own unassimilable annihilating impulses; is it, in fact, just a sophisticated introject – and if not, what is it? To what extent is a psychic disappearing and becoming nothing (the image here is one of disappearing into a black hole) real and irreversible? In other words, is this a form of psychic death instinct and does this say something about the archetype of evil?

I argue that we are dealing with a threatening nothingness that cannot be integrated, a quality that is anathema to the life instinct, a death instinct which must be distinguished from an ordinary fear of dying, or even more extreme forms of death anxiety or phobia. Paradoxically, this apparently bad object is actually no-object; it is conspicuous by its absence and may have to do with parental absences and abandonments. This 'actively not-there bit' has to do with the unconceived and unconceivable, therefore, the unborn and unbearable, the unalive and unlivable. As one patient called it: 'a nothingness that vaporises the meaning of life'.

Analytically, I can neither parent this unalive bit, nor midwife it, nor love it, nor angrily shock it into life. At best, I can maintain the patient's splits and defences

1 Lecture originally given to the Analytical Psychology Club, London, on September 16, 1982, and published in *Harvest*, 1983. Minor editing has been applied (Eds.).

DOI: 10.4324/9781003255826-3

within, but sometimes I can only sit and watch helplessly as the defences become self-defeating. I am talking about cases where internalised parents can never join, where certain opposites can never be integrated and where healing can never take place. I am talking about holding, not healing. I may also be talking about failure of therapy, the hopeless case, or even the hopeless life.

I am going to present a clinical example and then consider the case from the perspectives of various metapsychological models and clinical theories. In particular, I shall utilise ideas about pathologies of the *puer aeternus* and *puella* and schizoid splitting and defences against a massive depressive anxiety. I shall try to discern the nature and object of this depressive anxiety by looking at narcissistic character disorders, in which I consider the possibility of catastrophic damage to the self and its unity. In discussing the symbolism of the self and images and fantasies of apparently anti-self processes such as annihilation, dissolution, disappearing into a black hole and of 'not being here', I shall consider the relationship – or lack of it – between metapsychology and clinical theory, and show how the Jungian idea of psychic reality offers a radical synthetic solution to the dichotomy. At the same time, I shall declare the subjectivity of the metapsychological structures that I am using with this sort of case and its phenomenology.

Much of this is addressed to those of us who are drawn to the constructivism and optimism of orthodox Jungian psychology, a psychology which sees meaning and purpose in neurosis and an ideal of integrating and transforming the weak or underdeveloped, bad or shadowy parts into a new whole. This model can impose a one-sided model of progress or growth on the psyche and thereby lead to over-simple value judgments of psychic states and movements. It can also be used defensively to sentimentalise, idealise and so consciously deny the psychic realities of the unchangeable, above all, the unchangeably 'bad'. This defensive idealising of psyche and denial of psychic realities is especially the tendency of the *puer* and *puella* types. But the case I shall be taking here exemplifies the *puer* in extremis, whose ethereal escapism and pneumatic flights are pathological, irreversible and fatal yet inevitable and necessary. With these types, body and/or body image is split off together with an earthy sexual identity, and so I see in the pathology of the *puer/puella* a sort of spiritual Manichaeism which can be symptomatically catered for by an excessive, intellectual and impersonal fascination with such Jungian paradigms as the archetypal worlds of Gnosticism etc. Therefore it is not insignificant that the man who dreamt the dream I am about to relate, and who I shall call Robert, was a scholar of the Albigensian heresy with a special interest in the Manichaean influence that lay within it.

'Robert'

Robert was 29 years old when he first came to see me, offering no overt presenting problem other than what he called 'the big numinous dream *par excellence*', which he found 'interesting' and knew that I would too 'because you are a Jungian analyst'. In certain respects, the whole of this paper is an interpretation and amplification of this dream, whose meaning Robert himself could not assimilate since it had to assimilate him.

Robert's dream

> I am in a jungle. I see an enormous snake on the jungle floor. It turns round on itself and starts eating its tail, forming an uroboros. I am disgusted to notice that it is actually chewing its tail, gnawing and crunching at itself. Then, this noisy eating stops and its tail just starts silently disappearing into thin air so that there is an increasing gap between its mouth and the end of its body. I then notice that the ring of ground under the loop of the snake's body is disappearing as the body disappears. When the whole snake has vanished altogether, there is, therefore, what looks like a circular band cut into the earth where the snake has been. But in fact, this is a circular abyss, which is bottomless. As I realise this, the core is swallowed up and I know that the bottomless pit is actually a black hole as in space. Then I think or say or hear, 'black holes can't eat; they have no stomachs'. Slowly or quickly, the jungle around gets sucked into the black hole, and I notice that as it moves towards it, the atmosphere becomes cold and the scene loses any jungle-like qualities. Then, the whole world disappears into the black hole. The entire cosmos would go next, but at this point, I woke up.

I impulsively asked Robert, 'And what about you? in the dream'. 'Oh, I'm all right – I'm the dreamer. It wasn't a nightmare. In fact, I don't have nightmares'. He said he thought it was a dream about the empty centre of a serpentine mandala, which is a symbol of the self. Then he added: 'Don't worry – you don't have to interpret it, but I knew you'd find it interesting. It tells you what an interesting unconscious I've got, doesn't it?' I felt this statement was both a defensive request against further interpretation, especially of the dream's instinctual or infantile body zone meanings, and symptomatic of his need to give this dream to me as an inflated present which I had to receive and keep as such, in no way return or reduce by interpreting it. Although fascinated, Robert otherwise seemed to be emotionally unaffected by the dream, and fearless of it.

In her interpretation of Apuleius's *Golden Ass*, Marie-Louise von Franz says that when the mother complex has taken on the form of a destructive dragon and no fight takes place with it,

> this conveys that the 'devouring mother' has now taken on her deepest, coldest and most destructive form, and has disappeared into the bowels of the earth . . . Nothing happens anymore on the level of consciousness . . . If an archetype takes on the form of a snake or a dragon, it means it is in such deep layers that it manifests only in the sympathetic nervous system, and the conflict . . . cannot be assimilated into consciousness: there will not even be any more important dreams. It is the stillness before the storm.
>
> (von Franz, 1970, Chap 8, p. 10)

The word 'stillness' was very pertinent to Robert's case because, for him, there was no subsequent psychic 'storm', but rather a series of dreams about a lethally deepening stillness and a physical decline. The dreams were, in order, about: a still-born baby, a mutant or monster birth, a miscarriage and then several about abortions. Finally, there was a dream in which:

> A voice in a dark room whispers to me, 'I am being aborted backwards, I am being aborted backwards'.

He told me by way of association with this dream that people sometimes used to tell him that 'he didn't seem to be there'. Then he said, 'and perhaps they're right; sometimes I wonder if I'm really here at all'. On saying this, he shivered, the only outward manifestation of any feeling or emotion Robert ever showed me: cold fear or fear of the cold and empty centre of himself and anxious dread at his devouring internal void.

At the end of his time with me, Robert developed symptoms which I mistakenly thought to be hysterical but which were certainly psychogenic. He developed migraines, his eyesight suffered, his sense of taste and smell atrophied and his legs tingled and ached. He went to hospital and a social worker later told me that the diagnosis was general debility based on poor diet and vitamin deficiency. When he left the hospital three years ago, this social worker described him as being 'a shadow of his former self' and said she felt he was 'drifting away like a male anorexic'. For the next two years, he led a totally solitary life, occasionally communicating with me by letter, but then he fell ill again, a cancer was diagnosed and after four months in hospital, he died.

Men like Robert and their female counterparts are extreme pathological types, but I think I can see the psychotic reality of his fate partially in everybody. Most of us win where he lost. So why do the Roberts of this world lose, and why are their splitting and defences ultimately in vain and self-defeating? I can start to answer this question by considering *puer* pathology in more detail.

The pathology of the *puer aeternus*

The psychic reality of the *puer aeternus* is voyeuristic, masturbatory and second-hand, which can mean fearful, hysterical and provisional. The bad and depressing matters that he is evasive of and defensive against include real related sexuality, violent feelings, aggression and assertiveness, non-sentimental affection, love and its emotional demands, sadness and loneliness and above all, anxiety or panic at a depressingly empty self-image. These underlie the overt neurotic gains: substitute sexuality, idealistic spirituality, sentimental affectations, social clowning or charm and an inflated idea of being magically omnipotent. Although the *puer* is indeed cut off from worldly reality and *senex* (older man) demands, it is more important to see that the intra-psychic root of this is that he is cut off from his own psychic reality.

He is fascinated by an idea of psychic and instinctual reality. He is actually frightened of psyche as an experiential reality, and rightly so, because distorted, maltreated or frustrated instincts must turn destructive and devour the person in the end. Everything is etherealised into beautiful or awesome images or fascinating ideas, and in so far as ego identifies with these objects, there is a massive but hollow ego inflation. Thus he provisionally and defensively lives floating in the Gnostic's 'pneumatic sphere', which in true Manichaean dualistic fashion splits an idealised realm of spirit off and away from the dark matter of earth and body, thereby equating spirit with the salvation of the good and matter with evil bondage. Furthermore, the *anima* or *anima* of such a *puer* or *puella* is split, unstable, immature and incapable of relating because it becomes a vehicle carried away by its own load: the spirit. As Nathan Schwartz-Salant says of these personalities,

> while their anima or anima functioning can have a spiritual character, it will be undeveloped and archaic in human relatedness and in dealing with negative emotions. It will especially be unstable under the impact of exhibitionistic energies, which are usually keenly warded off for fear of inflation.
>
> (Schwartz-Salant, 1982, p. 172, n. 61)

Robert had, on the one hand, an idealised *anima*, a virginal, porcelain, almost bodiless/ethereal *anima* whom he called 'star sister', and a sado-masochistic woman of his masturbatory fantasies, who would laugh at him if he did not forcibly teach her to love his fantasy prowess. The idealised sister *anima* saved him from needing to act out the sado-masochistic side, and in the end, even the idealised *anima* got re-sublimated into his intellectual fascinations. In this way, his *anima* totally failed to relate him to the world, to his own sexual drives and/or his emotional needs and reactions. Only some of his dreams revealed his more penetrating-aggressive or exhibitionistic instincts and impulses, but these he managed to interpret only theoretically, never to assimilate emotionally; he was terrified of them.

To summarise, animated connection to psychic reality and body-sense is atrophied or lacking. There is no 'connecting *anima*' to relate head to body and idea to self-image, and so no assimilation of instinctuality. But the atrophied *anima* is so spiritualised that instinct, body and even life itself becomes its forbidden shadow and by ignoring or stopping psychic images of body and life, the *anima* is so-to-speak sucked into the killing and death of its own shadow (i.e. life). Then, by killing its own shadow, it inevitably kills itself. This, I think, is what is happening when the fascinations and dreams themselves cease to reveal a chthonic, animal, body zonal or sexual imagery. Instead, they become increasingly images of outer space, of flight and of disappearing objects, but are sometimes at least initially accompanied by a generalised anxiety in the face of an immense void: although again, of course, the *puer*/*puella* may well utilise intellectual defences, for example finding satisfactory meanings for the void such as Nirvana or 'empty centres of mandalas'. But then we must ask: what is happening, as in the case of Robert, when even the anxiety seems to disappear? I often imaginally and non-literally saw Robert's inner infant or child as being autistic and auto-destructive. In some ways, he had a 'not there' child. Donald Meltzer et al. (1975) have argued that autism is psycho-pathologically closer to obsessional states than to the psychoses and has to do with a withdrawal from and a dismantling of objects in order to manage massive depressive anxiety; the result is that mental life disappears. This here equates with Robert's managing of his own depressive anxiety of dread of not being here, of disappearing and his impotent rage at being abandoned. I am here using an idea of autism within the symbolic child in the adult, autism as an analogue. Such patients as Robert have unrelatable, archetypal or object images that seem to disappear into the nothingness that they really are, carrying the personality and perhaps the person with them. Where can we discern such unfilled/unfillable holes in their development? Where are the gaps in their family environment – both outer and inner?

The half-alive ones

Eva Seligman describes patients who feel themselves to be but half alive, appearing 'to dwell, as it were, in a state of permanent twilight, of non-differentiation, inexorably trapped' (Seligman, 1982, p. 1). Such half-alive ones may have a phobic fear of being 'almost irresistibly pulled back into the powerful, but suffocating, dark embrace of . . . mother' but also 'a longing to come alive and develop [their] own atrophied identity' (Seligman, 1982, p. 1). She observes that the absence of a parent, usually a father, is a causal thread running through these patients, together with an omnipresent mother who is an ego-damaging figure. The father might have been physically present but was experienced as being unavailable, allowing himself to be obliterated by wife and child, who themselves are in unconscious collusion to prolong their mutual unconscious omnipotence and inter-dependency in a conflict-free dyad, avoiding the family triad.

In some ways, the aetiology of certain cases that I am considering is similar to this, but in other ways, more extreme. At a primal level, extremely schizoid *puer* and *puella* types are unalive and disappearing; they are unwanted, unparented and abandoned; they are the unconceived and unborn, and thereafter, inconceivable and unbearable. The father is usually actually absent, and there is no father substitute. The mother is anti-child and so anti-mothering. She may be physically absent much of the time as well as emotionally absent all of the time. She is anti-erotic, herself an arch-*puella*, and is perceived (and may be described) by the patient as enigmatic or 'nor really there'. 'Father' is just an idea, sometimes idealised, sometimes rendered an utterly terrifying *imago* by the mother's *anima* descriptions of him. In other words, as an inner object, he can be either good or bad, but he is really a totally fantastic introject with no outer object. Any unconscious, incestuous desire for an erotic mother or a penetrating, inspiring and guiding father finds neither an outer nor an inner response, vainly tries to turn into hysteria/hysterical symptoms, and ends up forming somatic symptoms which damage the body and may kill it.

Negative feelings and aggressive-greedy impulses arising out of frustrated needs, out of sibling and oedipal rivalries and jealousies can never be realised or expressed. The mother, if and when she is around, forms anti-father collusions with the younger sibling/s, thus both keeping the patient out of this collusion and pushing him or her into the no-man's land of the non-father. This means that the latent jealousy can never turn into clinging to mother later on because mother is too untrustworthy, too wounding or destructive, because, like father, she is experienced as absent and 'not there'.

The asexual marriage of both parents is, of course, exactly what the mother's *animus* and the father's *anima* both want. Mother is ambivalent about wanting to be penetrated and fertilised by the outer and inner male; thus, she chooses the strongest and most silent type of man she can find, namely an idealised man who is not going to be around enough to be real, and who, when he is around is hated for a) having been absent and b) spoiling the ideal by being all-too-real when he is around. These men themselves carry idealised families from a distance, and their hatred of real woman/wife is often displaced when actually with the family.

The child who feels utterly abandoned in this situation can neither create good inner parents or objects with whom to identify nor bad objects to fight. The child has had little mirroring and, at times, feels like a 'living abortion', unwanted originally and forever unwanted. With this drastic precondition, there is, at one level, nothing born into life that can die or even have the privilege of wanting to die: where there is no *eros,* there can be no *thanatos*. Instead, there might be an unconscious wish never to have been so mis-born or mis-conceived, mixed with an unconscious fear of disappearing back to pre-conception. Could this be the meaning of Robert's dream of being 'aborted backwards'? Certainly, the rest of such a person's existence seems to be spent aborting itself out of psychic reality and out of life itself, which is, of course, self-defeating. As another similar though less chronic female analysand once said to me: 'I feel like a mistake who should be returned; perhaps God forgot to fill me up with enough life'. Anxiety about this depressingly unconceived and unconceivable area is naturally repressed and split off; its libido sublimated into intellectual or spiritual fascinations that are empty of real inner or outer relatedness.

An empty world and an empty centre are interesting and liveable with as an intellectual idea, but as a psychic reality, it is truly dreadful and precludes psychic life and development. It feels so appallingly awful and lonely that the child/patient must retreat into an inflated alienation and dares not consciously experience or acknowledge either the loneliness or the panic that such uncontainedness and abandonment must induce. The anxiety about this chronic aloneness derives from a sense of being so fundamentally and intrinsically unwanted that one loses all trust in others and in one's own existence, which is felt to be unneeded and unnecessary. Furthermore, extraverted rage at being abandoned has, therefore, to be repressed utterly; you cannot attack if there's no enemy, and/or you had better not attack if the enemy (parents) is bound to obliterate you. On top of this, the more any good object or good self-image becomes unreal, the less and less there is to fight for.

Michael Fordham (1974) says that patients in a psychotic transference (who are fighting for the good) empty themselves into the analyst; patients in a narcissistic transference seem to put their emptiness into the analysis (for there is no analyst) and so empty it, making the analysis a non-analysis, reflecting (like a vampire's mirror) their own non-being. Robert Hobson talks of no-being as 'frozen isolation, empty silence, a being neither dead nor alive'. He continues

> No-being is partly expressed in the paradox 'I am no-one' – a terrible saying when spoken with deep seriousness and not with a mild, deprecatory and resentful tone of voice. There are no images that I can call 'me', 'mine' or 'my own' . . . The odd sentence 'I have no being' carries with it the implication 'No-one is there'. I have no sense of contact with another person who can confirm that 'I am me', capable of having an identity separate from the world of people and things 'out there'. Even my body is alien. There is a threat of non-being – a loss of the capacity to speak the word 'I'. Non-being (like death as distinct from dying) cannot be experienced directly but in no-being there is some strange mysterious uncanny sense of the unknown, of an annihilation in which 'I' cease to be. In my view this disintegrating anxiety is the basic problem in all psychotherapy.
>
> (Hobson, 1974, p. 76)

As I said earlier, I experience this condition of no-being in the emptied-out analysis of the so-called narcissistic transference (which looks and feels like a non-transference). Narcissistic character disorders pertain to a primal wounding of self-image or self-structure and dynamics, and analytical psychologists such as Rosemary Gordon (1980), Rushi Ledermann (1979, 1981, 1982) and Nathan Schwartz-Salant (1982) have all contributed vitally to a Jungian clinical perspective on narcissistic disorders, while Mario Jacoby (1981) has recently written about the similarities and differences between Jung's and Kohut's ideas of self. Schwartz-Salant rightly states that, in narcissistic character disorders,

> we are dealing with a disturbance in the development of the ego-Self relationship, rather than with symptoms stemming from instinctual processes breaking through ego defences, as in the psychoneuroses.
>
> (Schwartz-Salant, 1982, p. 9)

But this is not to say that the disturbance is any the less primary or thorough. As Béla Grunberger suggests, 'narcissism is a psychic agency present at or even before birth, as absolute and forceful in its demands as an instinct' (1979, p. 105). Gordon points out that 'Kohut suggests that the pathology of the self may precede, indeed may cause, the pathology of drives and of structures' (1980, p. 251).

One reason why Kohut (1971, 1977) appeals to some Jungians is that his view of the self (and its disorders) is essentially positive and purposive. Otto Kernberg has a more pessimistic prognosis for narcissistic disorders, which I feel better explains

Robert's case. Kernberg especially stresses the role of repressed envy, rage and hatred:

> These patients experience a remarkably intense envy of other people who seem to have things they do not have or who simply seem to enjoy their lives . . . They are especially deficient in genuine feelings of sadness and mournful longing; their incapacity for experiencing depressive reactions is a basic feature of their personality.
>
> (Kernberg, 1975, pp. 228–229)

> [The narcissistic patient's] attitude towards others is either deprecatory – he has extracted all he needs and tosses them aside – or fearful – others may attack, exploit and force him to submit to them. At the very bottom of this dichotomy lies a still deeper image of the relation with external objects . . . It is the image of a hungry, enraged, empty self, full of impotent anger at being frustrated and fearful of a world which seems as hateful and revengeful as the patient himself.
>
> (1975, p. 233)

Kernberg goes further and says that not only does this impotent anger rob external object relations of vitality, but the internal world becomes impotent too. 'Internalised object representations acquire the characteristics of real, but rather lifeless shadowy people' (1975, p. 233):

> [Narcissistic patients] need to devaluate whatever they receive in order to prevent themselves from experiencing envy. This is the tragedy of these patients: that they need so much from others while being unable to acknowledge what they are receiving because it would stir up envy.
>
> (1975, p. 237)

Kernberg emphasises that conscious experience of this envy and expression of its rage is impossible (no object can be attacked). This is because the parents were not-there in themselves and would not/could not let the infant/child be there in his otherness and own-ness. As Schwartz-Salant explains:

> When parents lack a sense of their own identity they become sensitive to how their child likes *them*, or how it adds or detracts from *their* esteem. Not only will they be unable to mirror the child's emerging personality, but they will want to be mirrored by the child, who feels this keenly.
>
> (1982, p. 48)

In other words, the parents make the most unfulfillable unconscious demand on the child/infant, namely: 'Don't be yourself: be my unknown and unfulfilled needs. You are here to become my existence, my identity; you must not and do not exist for yourself'. They are, in effect, wanting the real child to go away, and as he/she grows up, so the more they will resent him/her, reject and abandon the emerging person.

The end result of this wrong-way mirroring is that the child feels hated, not receivable, abandonable and thus its potential worth annihilated. The subsequent sense of identity will be very poor at best; at worst, they will not dare form any positive life-oriented self-image. All subsequent feelings of being envied or hated merely prove to them their lack of right to exist, and so the special narcissistic defences are erected against further injury. Kohut calls this defensive unconscious structure (which functions in inflated and unworldly fantasy) the 'grandiose self'. In more Jungian terms, Schwartz-Salant calls this resultant fused ego-self structure 'defensive *uroboric*', which I see as a false ego identified with a pre-image or pre-object self archetype which is itself stuck and sucks ego development or potential ego development backwards into it. This means that the stuck primal self takes on the unreality of the false ego which it devours, and so becomes a source of non-identity or false identity, a 'false self'. Because of the lack of inner reality, the narcissistic character is terrified of meeting this lack and is afraid of any emotional interaction with the unconscious (Schwartz-Salant, 1982, p. 66).

In such cases, one has a crippling fear, and it may be well founded, that entering the unconscious, losing one's ego structures and attitudes, leads to absolutely nothing; there is no regeneration, no rebirth, just an amorphous non-existence. Kernberg says that the resultant incapacity to deal with other people as real or to properly assess personal capacities becomes a tragic dominant of these patients' lives and gets worse with age.

With narcissistic character disorders specifically, the 'false self' archetype is vast and empty and hungry and transferred onto self-carriers called 'self-objects' by Kohut. For an analyst to be regarded as vast and empty and hungry is both inflating and deflating, but it is also alienating and depersonalising. This is bound to induce a considerable degree of resentment in the analyst, and so he can soon find that he is carrying the patient's split-off rage which may also incorporate the negative parental images. The narcissistic patient will, of course, defend himself against any recognition of these projections and/or their external reality, perhaps either by running away or, like Robert, by fading away.

With Robert, I sometimes shared his metaphysical interests and let him see and use me as a fellow-traveller, or in Kohut's terms, as an idealised self-object, and sometimes I showed him that I felt exasperated by him. But I also found him boring and once found myself telling him that there was a 'yawning void between us'. This yawning void (which indeed often nearly put me to sleep) can be seen as a product of Robert's fear of and fending off of his need for a mirroring self-object, as Mario Jacoby has described. Or it can be seen as a product of the black hole within him and between us in the emptiness of the narcissistic non-transference.

In his Nietzsche seminars, Jung says that the self is both body and psyche. He says that if one does not live in the body, if one does not represent the self in life in its uniqueness, then the self rebels. 'The self wants to live its *experiment* in life', and if it is not willingly embodied, it manifests negatively in somatic symptoms and phobias (Jung, 1989, p. 413). Obviously, in narcissistic characters, there is always an aspect of the self that is not living the experiment of life and has accordingly turned negative. The analyst may hope to give some sense of self or self-image to these patients via his own body-consciousness, but sometimes all these good mirroring, body-conscious, self-carrying, cohesion-forming or raging positions of the analyst seem to fail to embody the patient's self. His self will not go into life, and the black hole endlessly aborts the personality backwards. The pre-object self can meet no object and form no self-image, and so it fails to work constructively and actually self-destructs.

In the end, I do not know whether this black hole is part of self, a damaged and split self or is beyond or even anti-self. But I take it as psychically real, an archetypal symbol. This is where, as a Jungian, I would diverge from both Kohut and Kernberg. Ultimately, these archetypal factors actively behave as inner objects far more powerful than personally acquired sophisticated introjects. So, what is the black hole symbol? Can the self be self-destructive, can it go backwards? What if the self sends up not only *scintillae*[2] but also black holes which seem to extinguish the *scintillae*? Can the self have a black hole within itself, or disappear into one? Is this a Jungian perspective onto an idea of a death instinct, which is different from *thanatos* in that I am talking about something that precludes life rather than backs out of life, although this preclusion of life also threatens the alive bits?

These questions pertain to metapsychology, so beg certain other questions. Can there be archetypes of metapsychological possibilities? Are there archetypes of the dynamics of the psyche and the self, archetypes of development and non-development? Like Wolfgang Giegerich, James Hillman and others, I think there are.

In psychodynamic theory, the term metapsychology is generally used to refer to those propositions which attempt to 'explain' clinical analytic observations in terms of hypothetical energies, forces and structures which are presumed actually and objectively to exist. Metapsychology deals with the material substrate of subjective experience; it is couched in the natural science framework of impersonal structures, forces and energies; while clinical theory, on the other hand, deals with intentionality and the personal meaning of subjective experiences seen from the perspective of the individual's unique life history.

Therefore, it has been stated that metapsychology is completely inappropriate for the elucidation of the data of the psychoanalytic situation but that clinical theory is uniquely applicable. Furthermore, metapsychology can be used as a system of reification and, at worst, a distorting subjectivism. Atwood and Stolorow (1993), Storr (1973) and others have accused Jung of treating psychic complexes as though

2 See Jung's discussion of *scintillae* (sparks) in 'The Nature of the Psyche'. He understood this alchemical term to refer to fragments of illumination from the self into unconscious levels (Jung, 1970, *CW* 8, paras 387–393) (Eds.).

they were living personalities or partial personalities, and then worse: seeing as universal what are his own inner objects.

These criticisms miss the point of Jung's idea of psychic reality, in which the symbol can transcend ego-self dichotomies and in which an archetype is both personal and typical. Furthermore, psychic bits do behave as if they were personalities and effect the ego personality in all sorts of ways. It is analytically constructive and integrative to treat psychic reality *as if* it existed in the same mode of being as external realities and determines in a real way our conscious perception of external reality. The symbolic image is not the psychic reality, but it is the only possible, appearance of it.

I am not suggesting that intra-psychic or even anti-psychic black holes exist as in space, any more than the *scintillae* exist as actual sparks. They are different but homologous. But Robert's symbol was of an archetypal black-hole-like process, and together with dreams, fantasies and ideas of 'aborting backwards', 'not being here' and 'disappearing altogether', etc. and his Manichaeism, these surely say something about his psychic reality – or unreality.

As his analyst, I saw him disappearing, and I saw how he was not there – as did others. This split that cannot be integrated is inevitable and perhaps vital because the annihilating black hole was psychically real, and no one clasps or incorporates a black hole, although it may suck you into it; so, in fact, you had indeed better steer clear of it. The black hole process concerns elements of the self that were never allowed to be and so seem unconceived and unconceivable. In the language of ontology, it is an essence real in its own mode of non-being and actively threatens being with unbecoming.

I see Robert's Manichaean/Albigensian interest as his subjective metapsychological model of his split psychic reality. But it is a paradoxical if not tragic split because, like all Manichean *puer*s, he consciously regarded life, world and body as fearful and bad, incorporating evil. Yet the real destructive 'evil' was the opposite: his unconscious depressive anxiety and dread of non-existence (which can be sublimated into 'spirit' by a Manichaean *puer*).

My own subjective metapsychology (based, I acknowledge, on my own pathological defences) accepts that we all split off unacceptable psychic evil, but thinks that pathology depends upon what is perceived and experienced as evil, and why. There is another archetypal religious model which is both sympathetic to splitting and sympathetic to me, and in my on-going countertransference, I oppose this to Robert's Manichaeism. This is a Zoroastrian belief that good and evil are opposed and mutually exclusive entities in themselves, not dependent upon their symptoms, manifestations or carriers. In other words, good and evil are the ultimate and absolute dualistic essences or substances, not equated with spirit and matter or any Cartesian division. In fact, matter and life are to be perceived and valued as good, whereas evil (which includes 'death' though not dying) is that which is antagonistic to matter, body, life and psyche. Furthermore, to the Zoroastrian the idea that God incorporates any destructive or dark quality – in other words, for God to be regarded as ambivalent – is the greatest heresy. God is thus not omnipotent because of the counter force of evil which is innately driven to annihilate God's creation. It is easy to interpret this religion as pre-ambivalent and so schizoid and pre-depressive or relatively undeveloped and unsophisticated. But this would be to impose the personal on the collective and the phylogenic on the ontogenic, let alone the microcosm on the macrocosm. Although this Zoroastrian dualism appears totally antithetical to our ideas of psychological health, which usually means an integration of shadow, a process of un-splitting towards ambivalence and wholeness, I suggest that it posits an archetypal model of one possible psychic reality: either the split nature of the self or perhaps the existence of anti-self. In itself, this is not an unhealthy psychic reality or archetype. But if and when the death instinct of anti-self is fundamentally stronger than the other dynamics of the self, then psychic life shall not be able to go forward, but the reverse. The losing life instinct is then bound to repress and sublimate the dreadful object of its anxiety, turning the anti-life and anti-matter reality into a 'Manichaean' ideal.

Robert's splitting included but was also more than *puer* flights from psychic reality, paranoid schizoid defences against bad objects and integration of a depressive ambivalence. Rather, they were a necessary splitting, vital to his provisional survival because they were a temporary evasion of his real feelings of pointlessness. Robert's potential wholeness was emptiness. As Jung said,

> there are without doubt individuals who are not at bottom altogether viable and who rapidly perish if, for any reason, they come face to face with their wholeness. Even if this does not happen, they merely lead a miserable existence for the rest of their days as fragments or partial personalities, shored by social or psychic parasitism. Such people are, very much to the misfortune of others, more often than not inveterate humbugs who cover up their deadly emptiness under a fine outward show. It would be a hopeless undertaking to try to treat them with the method here discussed . . . The only thing that 'helps' here is to keep up the show, for the truth would be unendurable or useless.
>
> (Jung, 1992, *CW* 7, para. 188)

As a structure, the self can be seen as the totality of the personality, conscious and unconscious, psychic and physical, which, through dynamic processes (arising out of libido from its tension of opposites), creates an increasing consciousness of its own many-sidedness and wholeness. Therefore, any symbol of this titanic tension of opposites is immensely potent and creative. In symbols of the self, we see the solution to these clashing and ego-tearing instincts and contrary impulses, among which we endlessly get re-positioned in the struggles of ego-development and increasing consciousness.

But if symbols of the self have to do with processes of wholeness and a synthesis or transcendence of opposites, then what is the symbol of disintegration, disappearance, dissolution and annihilation? Surely, this literally dreadful symbol reveals insoluble splits and opposites that cannot be transcended; it negates the healing dynamic of the self.

I do not see how this can be called the dark side of the self, for the latter must be an integrable part of the whole. The black hole symbol and its syndrome must, therefore, be either symptomatic of a primarily wounded self, with a greater part of the self stuck in a pre-image state of non-being, or it must be the archetype of something essentially other than and contrary to self, an anti-self which I feel it is not psychological heresy to call evil, or at least intra-psychic evil. It is like a state of death before and in life which can never be integrated into a psychic wholeness, because instead, it assimilates life and so precludes dying. Jean Laplanche and Jean-Bertrand Pontalis define the death instinct as being

> opposed to the life instincts, striv[ing] towards the reduction of tensions to zero-point. In other words, their goal is to bring the living back to the inorganic state. The death instincts are to begin with directed inwards and tend towards self destruction but they are subsequently turned towards the outside world in the form of the aggressive or destructive instinct.
>
> (Laplanche and Pontalis, 1973, p. 97)

But tragically, characters like Robert cannot even get to turn these instincts outwards and so they remain self-dissolving. Jung said in a letter of 1956 to Rudolf Jung:

> I have in fact seen cases where the carcinoma broke out . . . when a person comes to a halt at some essential point in his individuation or cannot get over an obstacle. Unhappily nobody can do it for him, and it cannot be forced. An inner process of growth must begin, and if this spontaneous creative activity is not performed by nature herself, the outcome can only be fatal . . . . Ultimately we all get stuck somewhere, for we are all mortals and remain but a part of what we are as a whole. The wholeness we can reach is very relative.
>
> (1976, p. 297)

For some, the sense of being an abortion, of being intrinsically undesirable and their life a mistake creates such a dead centre that there is no hope of any degree of wholeness, but only a defensive structure against life, against becoming and against being.

Finally, to go back and utilise the prognostic imagery of Robert's dream, we can say that the original or primal (pre-ego) uroboric unity, which, in healthy enough circumstances, is enabled to develop and grow towards a living wholeness of many ambivalent parts, can sometimes instead get chronically stuck, can never move out to meet reality, and so turns to devouring and disappearing into itself as if into a black hole, becoming nothing.

References

Atwood, G. & Stolorow, R. (1993). *Faces in a Cloud: Intersubjectivity in Personality Theory*. Oxford: Jason Aronson.

Fordham, M. (1974). 'Defences of the Self'. *Journal of Analytical Psychology*, 19(2): 192–199.

Gordon, R. (1980). 'Narcissism and the Self'. *Journal of Analytical Psychology*, 25(3): 247–264.

Grunberger, B. (1979). *Narcissism*. J. Diamanti, trans. New York: International Universities Press.

Hobson, R. (1974). 'Loneliness'. *Journal of Analytical Psychology*, 19(1): 71–89.

Jacoby, M. (1981). 'Reflections on Heinz Kohut's Concept of Narcissism'. *Journal of Analytical Psychology*, 26(1): 19–32.

Jung, C. (1970). 'On the Nature of the Psyche'. In *The Structure and Dynamics of the Psyche*. Vol. 8 of *The Collected Works of C.G. Jung*. R. Hull, trans. 2nd edn. London: Routledge & Kegan Paul.

Jung, C. (1976). *Letters, Volume 2*. Selected and edited by Gerhard Adler. London: Routledge & Kegan Paul.

Jung, C. (1989). *Nietzsche's Zarathustra: Notes of the Seminar given in 1934–1939. Two Volumes*. J. Jarrett, ed. Princeton, NJ: Princeton University Press.

Jung, C. (1992). 'On the Psychology of the Unconscious'. In *Two Essays on Analytical Psychology*. Vol. 7 of *The Collected Works of C.G. Jung*. R. Hull, trans. 2nd edn. London: Routledge & Kegan Paul.

Kernberg, O. (1975). *Borderline Conditions and Pathological Narcissism*. New York: Aronson.

Kohut, H. (1971). *The Analysis of the Self*. New York: International Universities Press.

Kohut, H. (1977). *The Restoration of the Self*. New York: International Universities Press.

Laplanche, J. & Pontalis, J. B. (1973). *The Language of Psychoanalysis*. London: Hogarth Press.

Ledermann, R. (1979). 'The Infantile Roots of Narcissistic Personality Disorder'. *Journal of Analytical Psychology*, 24(2): 107–126.

Ledermann, R. (1981). 'The Robot Personality in Narcissistic Disorders'. *Journal of Analytical Psychology*, 26(4): 329–344.

Ledermann, R. (1982). 'Narcissistic Disorder and Its Treatment'. *Journal of Analytical Psychology*, 27(4): 303–321.

Meltzer, D., Bremner, J., Hoxter, S., Weddell, D. & Wittenberg, I. (1975). *Explorations in Autism*. Strathtay, Perthshire: Clunie Press.

Schwartz-Salant, N. (1982). *Narcissism and Character Transformation*. Toronto: Inner City Books.

Seligman, E. (1982). 'The Half-Alive Ones'. *Journal of Analytical Psychology*, 27(1): 1–20.

Storr, A. (1973). *Jung*. Fontana Modern Master Series. London: Collins.

von Franz, M.-L. (1970). *The Golden Ass of Apuleius: The Liberation of the Feminine in Man*. Zürich and New York: Spring Publications.

Chapter 3

Animation through the analytical relationship

The embodiment of self in the transference and countertransference

Harvest, 1987–1988[1]

She was wrinkled and huge and hideous? She was our Mother.
She was lustful and lewd? – but a God; we had none other . . .
She was hungry and ate our children; – how should we stay Her?
She took our young men and our maidens; – ours to obey Her . . .

Lines from 'On the death of Smet Smet, the Hippopotamus Goddess' by Rupert Brooke

My subject is about animated and animating images which, because of the way in which they are mutually sensed in the transference and countertransference in the analytical setting, bring to life and into relationship previously unalive and unlived parts of self and body. The analysand produces images which are mutually sensed and shared with me: dreams, descriptions, fantasies, memories and so forth, and I have related fantasies which I use in my interpretations and inside myself for the patient. So, this chapter is about the analysand's images and fantasies, my images and fantasies and what goes on together and between us.

1 I am part of the analysand's fantasy, and they are part of mine. Our internal images are of each other. Objectively, these may be realistic or unrealistic. But they are always psychically real or valid.
2 Our images are partly about the transference and countertransference. In other words, they derive from other relationships which are only relivable and resolvable in the analytical setting.
3 These images are also about our own separate, inner worlds, the objective psyche.
4 They are about that third area, that which is between us; the third, living presence in the relationships, which is also a third area between internal life and external reality.

1 Originally published in *Harvest Journal,* 1987–1988, 33, pp. 104–114. Minor corrections and editing have been applied (Eds.).

DOI: 10.4324/9781003255826-4

Shortly, I shall describe a case of a patient with a narcissistic disorder who was considerably healed through therapy. I will show how we filled the gap between us with play, animation and anger, and how I used transference interpretations after we had moved beyond his narcissistic transference. We worked with animal imagery especially. In a way, my presentation of this case reflects my need for reparation in the case of 'Robert'.[2]

It is also a return to an earlier theme of mine, which I wrote about in 1978, namely the 'Lord of the Animals and his Beasts' as dynamic images of our repressed sensuous instincts.[3]

Various more personal factors underlie this paper. Firstly, there is my need for balance, arising out of concern for extreme narcissistic disorders about which I am very pessimistic, and my need to see a more hopeful side to such cases without denying or putting false gloss on my 'black hole' perspective. This case is about a fillable black hole.

Secondly, there is my need to find a personal synthesis deriving from practical, analytical experience of metapsychology and clinical theory, a balance between the idealistic and the technical, between the intrapsychic archetype and the introjected, internalised family and interpersonal relations, between instinct theory and part-object relations theory.

Andrew Samuels, in his paper 'Countertransference, the *mundus imaginalis* and a research project', asks:

> Do we gain anything from our habitual division between the inter-personal (that is relationship) and the intrapsychic (that is image? . . .) the interaction of patient and analysand, their relationship, can be placed firmly within the imaginal role without forgetting that there are two people present. An analyst can think, feel or behave as if he were the patient, and he can also function as part of the patient's psyche so that the *mundus imaginalis* becomes a shared dimension of experience.
>
> (Samuels, 1985, p. 66)

He goes on to say:

> If the idea of a two-person *mundus imaginalis* is taken seriously, then we must regard the inter-personal in terms of psyche speaking and the imaginal in terms of an avenue of communication between two people, their relationship. Persons may carry imagery. Imagery may originate in persons. A coin is three-sided, to the body and image can be added relationship. Jung said in a letter that the living mystery of life is always hidden between the two.
>
> (Samuels, 1985, pp. 66–67)

2 See Chapter Two (Eds.).

3 Chapter One (Eds.).

I include here a re-evaluation of the concept of *animus* and *anima*; an evaluation of animal imagery, animal instincts and body image; an attempt to show that these two aims are related, that is, how *anima* brings animation through the animal within us and between us.

The main way in which the concept of *animus-anima* is alive for me in my practice is through understanding it functionally. Viewed in this way, *animus-anima* is either a paired unit that cannot be split, like the syzygies, or the terms are interchangeable: *animus* and *anima* as a function are interchangeable, and it does not matter which word one uses.

Firstly, *animus-anima* can be seen as the animating principle or psychic function. Thus, I think we can say *animus-anima* makes us alive and lively, animating the psyche. A quotation from Jung serves well here:

> But how do we dare to call this elfin being the 'anima'? Anima means soul . . . Being that has soul is living being. Soul is the living thing in man, that which lives of itself and causes life . . . With her cunning play of illusions the soul lures into life the inertness of matter that does not want to live. She makes us believe incredible things, that life may be lived. She is full of snares and traps, in order that man should fall, should reach the earth, entangle himself there, and stay caught, so that life should be lived . . . Were it not for the leaping and twinkling of the soul, man would rot away in his greatest passion, idleness . . . To have soul is the whole venture of life, for soul is a life-giving daemon who plays his elfin game above and below human existence . . . It is something that lives of itself, that makes us live.
>
> (Jung, 1991, *CW* 9i, paras 55–57)

Secondly, there is the de-animating function: by default, we can have loss of soul, loss of *animus-anima*. This de-animation is depersonalisation. Depersonalisation is defined as a state of loss of sense of reality of self and world. There is no interest in the world. It is a state of boredom, blankness, apathy and, to use Jung's word, idleness.

Thirdly, Like carrots on sticks or like the veils of Isis, *animus-anima* projections, images and fantasies lure and attract the person into the world and into relationships, away from home and one's parents. Or, on the other hand, they may contribute to our projected terrors and repulsions, which also determine our relations and reactions. Thus, *animus-anima* relates us and moves us into the world and towards people.

Fourthly, as internal fantasy or imaginary fascinations and terror, *animus-anima* leads us to our insights and internal processes. As an energy that is primitive, pre-personal, pre-moral or amoral, pre-ambivalent, possessive, obsessive and often compulsively sexual, I suggest that *animus-anima* is always consciously experienced as good or bad. If it becomes ambivalent, it is no longer in its archetypal guise and has become a personal introject. So *animus-anima* lures into psychic reality. Even schizoid, etherealised and idealised *animus* and *anima* images, objects of distant voyeurism, reveal their teeth and bite sooner or later and so lead to psychic reality. Thus, *animus-anima* relates us into our unconsciousness. *Animus* and *anima* can be seen as the 'mediatrix of the unknown' (Hillman, 1985, p. 129). It is the mediatrix between consciousness and our nature.

Alongside this functional concept of *animus/anima*, I posit the complementary idea that as symbols *animus* and *anima* can be seen as archetypal and metaphorical images of masculinity and femininity respectively, regardless of whether they apply to men or women (both genders share masculinity and femininity in varying degrees). To bring this idea together with my functional concept, we can say that images of masculinity and femininity are effectively experienced as animating. I hope that my case material will exemplify the psychic reality of a primitive 'animating image' and show how it activates the archetypal basis of sexuality and gender identity.

Through this case example, I shall try to demonstrate that archaic, psychoid,[4] animal symbols of the sympathetic nervous system are shareable, go between us and so form and effect relations at a very primitive level. These symbols, although about parts (body bits and partial processes), can yet also be whole in themselves. And although they are earlier and more archaic than whole-person symbols, they are yet also the basic prima materia of *animus/anima* relations. As I shall be showing, they are active manifestations of the *anima* function of animation: animation of life in each of us via the imaginative life between each of us.

'Andrew'

Andrew presented himself as having no inner image world, as being unable to imagine. This is a symptom of having no trust and of being unable to play. He was unable to maintain any interests or real passions, and the same, therefore, applied to his relationships, which were indifferent and short-lived. He was empty and his world was empty. His words in that first session included, 'I am hollow; I am not real; my real world is such a void that it makes me feel sick; I don't feel I have any spark of life in me'. He used the idea of 'living on the edge of an inescapable black hole which is like being nearly dead all the time'. This last expression rang loud warning bells because, at this time, another patient, 'Robert',[5] who I associated with a narcissistic black hole pathology, had just been admitted into hospital. Just as with Robert, Andrew said these things about himself in a manner that had no sense of urgency or panic, though he did admit to feeling sick. His presentation of himself was somehow coldblooded and distant, abstract and theoretical. Yet I did not experience him as having a total false self or of suffering from an interminable

4 For Jung, the concept of the psychoid points to a bodymind wherein psyche and matter (body) are two aspects of the same thing (Jung, 1970). This is Giles' first citation of Jung's concept of the psychoid, a major concept in Giles' writings (Eds.).

5 See Chapter Two (Eds.).

narcissistic disorder. This was because although he was far away, he was not aloof and was panicky sick in his stomach. He was, I sensed, rigid with fear, sitting on a lot of nervousness, a rigid stillness before an outpouring and collapse. I sensed that he could and would be challenging, angry and aggressive. He had latent energy. Also, I liked him; his latency made him real to me and I felt he needed me. I was somewhat 'real' for him, too.

A second related presenting problem was a symptom commonly associated with a severely damaged self-image, namely sensationless ejaculations. He could not reach a sensuous, orgasmic climax. This was connected to his distrust of play, fantasy and imagination. His own bodily and sexual fantasies had not developed. There was a complex unconscious (as well as conscious) parental taboo on anything to do with pleasure and pride in self and body. All excitement and exhibitionistic energies were denied by his mother's depression, fear and envious resentment. She stole from him his capacity for pleasure, sucked the joy of life out of him and made him into a half-dead being who did not dare show any excitement. De-animated and raped of his spirit, he was unable to enjoy himself and his world. His history and other symptoms bear out his distance, his unrelated and unrelatable cold centre and his fear of contact with himself and others.

Andrew was born with his amniotic sac intact, physically perfect and unblemished. He had no birth marks; not even his birth, it seemed, marked him. He had no scars, no wounds and in some ways, nothing appeared to have scarred him since, at least not outwardly. Andrew's parents were both alcoholics. His father left the home very shortly after Andrew was born. In Andrew's eyes and also his mother's, his father was an aggressive drunk and his mother a victim who herself drank only to cope with father. Ostensibly, he idealised and protected his mother, but unconsciously, he also resented the fact that she was too narcissistically depressed to be able to mirror and properly respond to him. Furthermore, she had been unable to sort out inside herself the projective identifications between child and mother. As Bion (1962) observed, an infant pushes all his chaotic instincts and feelings into mother.[6] She needs to take them in, digest them and think and feel them out and then, having sorted them out, return them to the child so he can see what his life energies are and how they belong to him. Andrew's mother thoroughly failed to do this, and in a way that devastatingly rejected his exhibitionistic energies and his sense of body.

When Andrew was about 13, his mother became a Christian Fundamentalist and stopped drinking. As he put it, 'she became drunk on Jesus instead'. Soon after this, she remarried a man from the church, a 'very good Christian'. This step-father was, most unusually, an idealised figure.

After about a month with me, Andrew himself started to drink in order, he said, to blot out the painful family memories that were coming up. As his drinking

6 Here Bion was reformulating Klein's 1946 theory of projective identification as a normal form of unconscious to unconscious communication (Eds.).

increased, he said that he wanted 'to dissolve in drink'. I interpreted this as meaning a desire to dissolve back into mother, into a state of fusion. He often said that 'I need to be drunk', and I heard in this expression a passive use of the verb: that he needed to be drunk by mother, to get close to her and into her (as well as to be like her and to identify with her). To be drunk by mother meant not only to be drunk into her belly whence to kick and bite to make her feel him and even to be reborn, but more, it meant to be absorbed into her system, dissolved into her bloodstream and so to become her, to do her being for her, as her, not as himself. He would disappear and she would appear. He had to lose himself into her for her to come alive and feel alive in herself. This alone could make her alive so she could then give life to him and be alive for him.

Andrew went to Alcoholics Anonymous, where he soon became caught up with a missionary zeal to help others. Through AA, he met a very needy and damaged young woman – whom he felt to be 'soft and safe' (a product of his idealised and infantile *anima*), although, in fact, she was profoundly angry and destructive. Out of their initial, mutual dependence, a sentimental relationship developed. She became pregnant and they instantly got married. This marriage lasted only a few months, for she rapidly became disillusioned (she said particularly with his sexuality) and left him. Andrew was remarkably calm, even indifferent, about this event. In her angry frustration at his indifference, his wife tried to provoke him by telephoning him and talking to him about his 'hopelessness' and about their child that he would never see. Still, Andrew did not react. However, when the child was born (slightly prematurely), which he only heard about since his wife would not allow him to visit her, he suddenly developed hysterical physical conversion symptoms – a so-called duodenal ulcer, a hiatus hernia and general gut problems. For him, these were symptomatic of stomach cancer based on a generalised but increasingly anxious cancer phobia. This fear of dying and state of acute anxiety overlay a deep sense of loss and depression. Slowly, he began to dare to feel very stuck and lonely, and in this stuck and lonely state, I encouraged or facilitated Andrew to play. Initially, of his own volition, he started to 'look for images' (his own words). At first, these images were literal images of dots and squiggles on the inside of his eyelids, caused by pressure on blood vessels as he rubbed his closed eyes. He also painted what he called his 'situation', and the first painting was of a minute brown dot in the centre of a yellow background, which covered the whole page. Later, he was able to imagine a mass of activity going on inside the brown dot, activity that was too small to see with the naked eye but which made it a complex, living world. I helped, I think, by accepting these images, fantasies and the picture, and by letting him be excited by them. Eventually, over the weeks and months, these images became more spontaneous and living. They evolved from amoeba-like organisms to increasingly sophisticated and obviously creatively imagined creatures. In my countertransference, I noticed how my animal images in my own fantasies, which occurred when I was with Andrew, were very close to his. Eventually, his animal images became increasingly affective, and they would induce physical reactions such as squirming, jumping, panting, moaning, groaning and panic reactions. In fact, these fantastic images became quite hallucinatory, but we were able to connect them to his body parts and zonal sensations and his fears of them. He developed what we called an 'animal alchemy' of body bits and sensations and his relations to them, and in my private countertransference, I shared in this and related empathically to him through them. These animals were also bits of *animus-anima* because they were animating of his sexuality, his body and his sensuous connectedness to himself and to me.

Yet he was still, in many ways, stuck, and he now felt this more acutely than before. This was reflected in the transference. He began to get increasingly frustrated and angry with me for 'not breaking through his cut-off withdrawal' and for 'not stimulating me enough'. One notes the sexual implication of this last statement. He also said that 'sex and love are still frightening black holes for me' and he was afraid that he would be 'eternally dead in these areas'. I asked Andrew how he expected me to break through and stimulate him, and he answered, 'by coming with me', which both he and I immediately realised was an ambiguous response that is both sexual and to do with going on a journey with him. It is important to point out that previously we had made quite a lot of my not being able to go with him into his 'nowhere place', into his black hole centre. I had seen this as being to do with an autistic part in him that cannot be shared with others. The autistic part can be seen as an embryo baby whose lifeline is cut off and severed from his placenta/mother/space capsule and who is floating off, a speck into the vast emptiness of space, into the void. The rest of the personality has to live in a falsely secure world, the false self-structure which is a shell-like defence against the empty reality. This emptiness and loneliness are less able to be integrated than the terrors of the psychotic, mad, bad and terrible archetypes, and a therapist has to know that he or she cannot disappear with the autistic embryo-patient into that black hole void. The therapist has to symbolically let them go and await their return as if signalling, 'I hope you find a healthy embryo, a spark of life out there and come back with it'. At the same time, as therapist, you know that the patient is going into you, into your spark of life, which as a healthy, vital therapist, you can impart to them. But this giving of the spark of life is also, of course, a giving back of their sense of their own life which has been denied or taken away by a needy, depressed mother figure. Two things need to be said here in elaboration of this point:

1 This is a sensuous form of giving, a sensuous giving of life and body;
2 As a giving back, it is a mirroring of what originally came from and, therefore, belongs to the other.

When Kohut talks about 'the gleam in the mother's eye', he means that the light of that gleam is cast by the baby and reflected back by the mother's eye: the light is the child's self and life. Andrew and I had often talked about this 'spark of life', and it will soon become important to see how he changed that expression.

One night, after a particularly sticky session with Andrew, I dreamed about a hippopotamus. I am not going to give you details of this long and powerful dream except to say that my hippopotamus was very big, with an overbearing physical presence and dangerousness. It was about the hippopotamus being fenced off out of its climate and its elements, and about contrasts of dryness and wetness and how to be in the water and in the earth at the same time. Among my own waking free associations with this dream, I almost playfully used the name Behemoth, which I wrote down and which I happened to see as Be He Mother, and I put in brackets after it (male mother). I thought very little more about it. At the time, I in no way associated this dream to my countertransference in the work with Andrew. However, in the next session, he brought me a paradoxical dream of immense affect, which he found very difficult to report. Andrew said, 'I dreamed that I was sucking off a cow's penis'. The androgyny of the beast was crucial to Andrew: it was a cow, not a bull, yet with a penis; it was a penis, not an udder. We were slowly able, with fear and trembling on his part, to start talking about the possibility of his homosexual feelings towards me and how he imagined and wanted to bite on and bite off my fingers and/or penis in order, he said 'to turn you into a male mother'. I was struck and surprised by his use of this phrase after my dream and what I had written down in association with it. We talked about biting in order to make oneself felt, to make an impression on mother, and 'biting off', which is castrating in order to make me safer. I asked him if he saw me as a cow or a bull, as mother or a father, and he said, 'I want you to be big and soft and giving, yet still male. I want to be able to take your maleness out of you and into me, safely'. He also said that I was 'a spermatic mother'. Returning to this theme, the session after that one, Andrew quite suddenly said, 'Oh, I think I want you to be more of a hippopotamus really, all soft and heavy and unavoidable'. Surprised as I was, I, of course, said nothing about my dream, but I did see his need for part of me as his self-carrier to somehow embody the male-female hippo for him in my countertransference position. By the way, morphologically and indeed metaphorically, I cannot easily be seen to be hippo-like! But as a fantasy part, and in relation to certain physical functions, when I was with Andrew, I could privately play with fantasy images of hippo-self, my body, my stomach, my sexuality, my bulk and size relative to his, my presence, my aggression, my way of breathing, etc. These fantasies of mine related to his need to realise several 'split-off' instincts. We were able to work on his anality, his lack of genitality as well as his feelings of repulsion and disgust about many physical functions and body problems. Andrew said no more about hippos for at least three months, but he did start allowing himself, and enjoying, exciting fantasies of 'very carnal and dirty women'. He would never tell me the details, especially not of himself in these fantasies. Then, about three or four months after my hippo dream and his oral cow-penis dream, during a bout of influenza, he dreamed the following:

> I see a dot on a yellow background [here I was reminded of his initial painting]. I realise I am very high up and that this is a view down onto a sandy desert. I drop towards it, and the dot turns out to be a mud pool in a desert. I splash into it. Either the mud pool itself becomes, or in the mud pool there is, an open-mouthed, large-tusked hippopotamus which I fall into, into its mouth. I go painfully round

> things like stinking U-bends and then squeeze out through a small black hole full of shit and slime, the hippo's anus. I notice how oddly hairless the anus is and how fleshy. There are also disgusting eels about somewhere.

I reminded Andrew that he once said he wanted me to be like a hippo to him, 'all soft and heavy and unavoidable'. I still did not tell him of my male-mother hippo dream or how I felt I was embodying the hippo for him in my body image. But he was able to see how this dream was about us and was about being drunk by mother and getting out of her, and was about being in his own body and sexuality. Incorporation into the hippopotamus, the painful passage through it and the themes of flesh, excrement and release are about a liberation, a letting oneself go, a giving up of up-tight body problems deriving from disturbance at the anal phase of development from mothers who, in fact, need too much from the child and at the same time make him embarrassed and ashamed of himself. This dream was also about going into the black hole, yet not disappearing within it but instead sensing it, or sensing the black hole becoming sensuous, sensing self in it and gaining sense and animation from it. It was a very important dream for Andrew, and he wrote a poem based upon it, which he called 'Ta-Urt'. I shall not quote the entire poem, but some of the lines speak loudly in their sensuality and sexuality and of his mixed reactions to bodily matters. Lines such as:

> Vast beast of the primal stuff,
> As great eels like smooth muscle limbs fatten themselves on her flowing excrement, She emerges under the moon at night to devour the green world hugely,
> Amid the lotuses her consorts fight to mate with her ferociously,
> Ta-urt oozes with the slime of life,
> What is the attraction of her stench, where is her ugliness, where her brute strength?
> All in me, in me, in my guts and in my fleshly body.

Ta-Urt is the pregnant Egyptian hippo-goddess, wife of Seth. For Andrew, his 'Ta-Urt' was Great Mother, Powerful Father and Male Spirit, all in one, i.e. an androgynous god, and the associated eels were images of Andrew's latently potent phallic self. The immediate effect on Andrew of this dream and its poem were twofold: firstly, he felt permeated by a profound sense of well-being, and secondly, his hysterical symptoms and cancer fears disappeared completely. The process certainly involved an unblocking of anal fears and rigidity and a letting go of his fear of pleasurable, creative mess. But at a deeper level, at last, Andrew was symbolically being taken in, digested, sorted out and returned out of mother, this process occurring via his transference onto me and my body. I intuited this in my countertransference: the hippo's body was my body, mother's body and his own body.

This material has to do with animation and spirit, which are pre-whole person and pre-gender. Not only the great mother is life-giving, so is the erotic animal spirit, and this spirit can begin to fill the gaps that have been caused by primal deprivation by never having been allowed to live in vital areas by the narcissistic and depressed mother. The hippopotamus or Ta-Urt who lives in the primal sludge, in the prima materia, has to do with conception and insemination, a new start which may be a first start for the self. Ta-Urt and her phallic eels formed for Andrew a numinous hermaphrodite composite, and he called it 'a dark god who held the spunk of life'. The 'spunk of life' was something far more sensuously loaded than a mechanistic, inhuman 'spark'. It was also important to me that I felt this hermaphrodite, pre-parent god somehow healed the autistic black hole part of Andrew. The dream is about the autistic space baby falling into the world, into animation, into flesh and the body; also about falling into and through the mother; and, thirdly and most importantly here, also about falling into and through me (analyst) who was the container of the phallic spirit and sense of maleness. In the transference, I was the embodiment of the dark, androgynous god who could give the stuff of life, though for Andrew, this area still remained utterly terrifying. In other words, the changes brought about by the processes that I have just described were very important but still limited.

It was only a year later, with the emergence of his assertiveness in the form of anger and rage at me, that he finally achieved a gut sense of self. Just after the time of the hippopotamus dream, although he had had an important experience and much had changed, I became increasingly frustrated at how stuck Andrew seemed to be. But really, my frustration was about his repressed frustration and, therefore, latent anger with me: frustration at me for not giving or not knowing how to give or not wanting to give my sense of maleness to him, i.e. for not returning his own full sense of self to him. He remained afraid of harming the good god, good parents or good me with his latent rage and still repressed sexual exhibitionistic energies. He still tended to sublimate his shadowy, animal passions and precarious self-assertions into spiritual excitements. He was afraid of uniting the real spirituality of the good parents with his still small and frightened but potentially strong and passionate instinctual self. He continued to keep the split apart, but eventually, he snapped and his anger flew out at me. It was only in this expressed anger that he could begin to find the sense of his own vital power. And when, six months later, he finally did have to leave me in order to study abroad, he was able to express authentic feelings of sadness at our separation. He realised and acknowledged that he was losing his first real relationship.

Countertransference: reflective, embodied and complementary

In his paper on the countertransference, Andrew Samuels (1985) distinguishes two forms of usable, non-illusory, concordant countertransference. The first he calls the 'reflective countertransference'. This is where analysts find themselves experiencing an unconscious emotion belonging to a patient and can reflect it back so the patient can begin to become conscious of it (Samuels, 1985, p. 51). The second he calls the 'embodied countertransference', where the analyst physically experiences and therefore embodies a patient's relatively unconscious experience of an inner or internalised figure, for example, a heavy, depressed mother or big, angry father (Samuels, 1985, p. 52).

To these two forms of countertransference, we can add the so-called complementary countertransference (Racker, 1957, p. 733). Here, the analyst's countertransferential feelings towards the patient resemble how, as a child, the patient's parents quite probably felt about that child. In other words, the analyst is picking up on the patient's internalisation of their parent's attitude towards them, and so having similar feelings and attitudes towards the patient.

What I have been talking about in this chapter is an embodied concordant countertransference (Racker, 1957, p. 733) and, so to speak, an anti-complementary countertransference. To explain that latter expression, I mean situations where the analyst embodies and, therefore, experiences for the analysand, that analysand's own unconscious split-off body, body image and self-image. This is because body, body image and self-image were never experienced by the patient, because they were never mirrored, but rather feared, envied and denied by mother.

Let me now summarise the analyst's countertransference positions and try to show how the shared insides of the transference relationship are the location of the healing transcendent function. I find that as the analyst, I experience the patient's body and his physicality for him. I become the mother and father whom he lacked. I, therefore, physically experience for him an archetypal, inner figure who was not fleshed out, personalised or internalised from the outside environment. In so far as the patient is making me incorporate body and bodily sensations for him, he is getting into my system, into my bloodstream, so to speak, and making me alive for him so that he can live. I am his first object relationship or image of relationship to a living person and who can, therefore, be internalised. I embody the primal conjunction of his parents so that they, inside me, can then conceive him and give him physical existence and body-self experience. I give him this by imaginatively bearing him in my physicality and sensations and let him sense himself with me and through me. In my case example, this process is realised through the animal symbols that we share, through the *anima*-animation that we have painfully and playfully been able to let emerge. The first proto-relationship is the 'sharing' of symbolic animal bodies between two selves. Simply, Ta-Urt is the animating *anima*-animal in him and between us. Such archetypal pre-person images are intra-physical as well as intrapsychic. Their power to heal and bring to life can only be realised in relationship, in mutually experienced, emotionally loaded images and sensations. Thus, I think the transcendent function in the transference/countertransference recreates the symbolising process and brings life where previously it could not be.

References

Bion, W. (1962). *Learning from Experience*. London: William Heinemann.

Hillman, J. (1985). *Anima: An Anatomy of a Personified Notion*. Dallas, TX: Spring Publications.

Jung, C. (1970). 'On the Nature of the Psyche'. In *The Structure and Dynamics of the Psyche*. Vol. 8 of *The Collected Works of C.G. Jung*. R. Hull, trans. 2nd edn. London: Routledge & Kegan Paul.

Jung, C. (1991). 'Archetypes of the Collective Unconscious'. In *Archetypes and the Collective Unconscious*. Vol. 9 Part 1 of *The Collected Works of C.G. Jung*. R. Hull, trans. 2nd edn. London: Routledge & Kegan Paul.

Klein, M. (1946). 'Notes on Some Schizoid Mechanisms'. *International Journal of Psychoanalysis*, 27: 99–110.

Racker, H. (1957). 'The Meanings and Uses of Countertransference'. *Psychoanalytic Quarterly*, 76(3): 725–777.

Samuels, A. (1985). 'Countertransference, the "Mundus Imaginalis" and a Research Project'. *Journal of Analytical Psychology*, 30(1): 47–71.

Chapter 4

How much Jungian theory is there in my practice?

Journal of Analytical Psychology, 1995[1]

I start with a quotation from a letter of 1935 from the American philosopher Harry Wolfson:[2]

> There needs to be, and surely can be, a practical psychology in which idea and action (for which you may read theory and practice), are demonstrably univocal because they are properly and empirically understood – through reason, language and application – to be two aspects of the same absolute reality within a monistic world of human nature.

I would like to be such a monist and omnipotently create or discover a grand unified theory for human mentation and behaviour in which theory and practice are neatly univocal. However, what follows is an idiosyncratic collection of several disparate bits, which is a more realistic reflection of my relationship to this subject. Yet, stubbornly, I do still aim for a substantially unitary model, as you may perhaps discern. The ensuing cocktail is not a scientifically 'correct' clinical paper. It is no more than a personal statement or confession, a gathering of some of the metapsychological constructs which I have found valuable and developed over the years from thinking about what I have experienced in my practice (and elsewhere). Through the lenses of these ideas and values, I can constantly re-evaluate further experiences, including thinking and feeling about how I practise psychotherapy at the moment.

In the period since I was asked to talk on theory and practice, I have had to put my values against some classical Jungian theories and see how well they mate, or rather, how often they do not get on together easily. With apologies to Bion, and to adapt him: valid new thoughts can come out of received concepts *not* mating with experience. The problem is that sometimes my clinical experience with patients just does not fit Jungian theory, and furthermore, Jungian metapsychology does not help tell me what to *do*. As psychotherapists, we work with a triad consisting of models, experience and

1 Originally published in 1995 in the *Journal of Analytical Psychology*, 40(3): 343–352. Reprinted with permission © Wiley Publishing. Minor corrections and copy editing have been applied (Eds.).

2 Giles did not give a source for this letter, and we have been unable to locate one (Eds.).

DOI: 10.4324/9781003255826-5

practical action (interpretation). This is bound to be an ever-changing triad. As we work closely and deeply with people, and feel and think about our experience, so each aspect changes and affects the other two. This dynamic process means that the original theories and models get challenged and have to change, too. Also, we keep discovering new theories which we like and find useful. And yet Jung's profound, complex and rich model of the psyche, and his radical understanding of the reality of the psyche, still holds for me a psychological worldview that is of enormous value.

Presenting myself like this may seem like a shameful grandiosity, or egocentric inflation, but I hope that by thus displaying myself, I am setting myself up as a useful projective screen for you to react to: for/against, agreeing/disagreeing, good and/or bad object etc. Furthermore, although my ideas have to be theoretically recognisable and comprehensible, I would also hope that they are not received as 'typical' of any particular school or affiliation. In fact, I wonder whether any practising Jungian is able to be typical of or identifiable with a common, agreed theory? Probably not. Agreed standards of practice, boundaries, necessary areas of knowledge, etc. – yes; commonly accepted values, clinical theories and styles – no.

I am going to start by giving you my definition of analysis and then saying why I think people come into psychotherapy. Although this introduction is only an abbreviation of what I teach trainees in training seminars, it is not meant to be patronising but is a set of initial propositions on which other ideas are hung and without which I cannot proceed clearly. I am then able to go on and select a short concatenation of personal thoughts (rather than theories) which have emerged from reflecting upon my post-Jungian practice in the light of these propositions.

So then, a definition: I see analysis as a particular and peculiar relationship through which we both endeavour to understand consciously, in new ways, the most possible meanings for our unconscious history (which is environmental) and our nature. This working relationship is emotional, thoughtful, imaginative and reflective. It is an acting upon passive experience. The object of this unconscious experience is always fearful, touching on primitive anxieties. It feels unbearably sad, out of control and, above all, dangerous. It is neurotic and potentially psychotic. To an extent, of course, we seek therapy in order to open old wounds. But the understanding and formulating of possible meanings can give a sense of freedom and a sense of power to change, which is a pleasurable sense. I say 'sense of freedom' and 'sense of power' because I do not think we actually have such a freedom. Personally, I think that a sense of free choice is a 'healthy illusion', a necessary idea. Thus we may feel that we are relatively free to analyse and develop a changing set of attitudes/reactions to our nature. Such psychological understanding also gives a realisation of necessary cause and effect and, thus, paradoxically, a sense of purpose and direction. And finally, there comes a realisation of our necessary limitations, which challenges us to make meaning.

To utilise and adapt an old, even a 17th-century model of human nature, I would say that, basically, people seek psychotherapy in order to manage two fundamental primitive fears. Firstly, there is fear of loss, lack and impotence; in other words, the fear of loneliness and lack of meaning. Secondly, there is the concomitant, opposite fear of dangerous desire and power, that is, potency anxiety. To convolute the model: on the one hand, we have a basically desired power and pleasure, and on the other, we have a feared loss, lack and pain. Both the desire and the fear can be experienced as lethal.

Overlaying this, I distinguish four complex aims which unconsciously motivate the need for therapy. These four are: change, understanding, self-preservation and relationship.

Firstly, to be over-succinct, by 'change', I mean the desire to change impotent, stuck, defensive and/or repetitive patterns. Under this there is the desire not to change – even to have one's neurotic defences affirmed and strengthened. The synthesis of these two desires is to come to accept the unchangeable.

Secondly, by 'understanding', I mean the desire to have another person to see into and to know one in depth. Under this, as Winnicott (1984) says, there is the desire not to be seen, to be unknown and hidden, to maintain a precious secret core. The synthesis is to come to accept the limits of understanding and understandability.

Thirdly, by 'self-preservation', I mean the desire not to fall to bits, not to lose control or go mad. To preserve a sense of self and self-esteem. Under this, there is a need to collapse, to lose control and to break down. The synthesis is to come to accept the limits of one's *conatus* for self-preservation, to know one's passivity to unconscious impulses, let alone the impossibility of immortality, the reality of mortality.

The fourth motivating aim for seeking psychotherapy is the (fantastic) desire for an absolute and eternal loving relationship, to be loved and to love absolutely and forever. Hopefully, this omnipotent, infantile illusion (which is also archetypal) will be challenged and transformed by the disillusioning realities and necessities of human nature and relations, or, in other words, through the whole oedipal process, i.e. by a resolution of transference projections. On the other hand, schizoid traits show us that there are parts that are afraid of relationship, and certainly of the terrors and dangers of the split-off need for intimacy and loving, which is projected out into a devouring, needy object: the schizoid aim is to create and maintain an optimal distance. But through the vicissitudes of this four-aspected relationship enough solid good may be taken in for some of the empty places to be filled and the fears mitigated. Though, I also think that some fearful defeats and lifeless places can only remain thus forever; no amount of analysis or subsequent good relationships can ever heal them fully. Going through this difficult process, and living with the personal and environmental limitations which it makes us integrate, feels worthwhile enough for me. It makes for a valid sense of meaning.

Now, some classical Jungians would, I think, say that meaning is something given, something transcendent of these four complex aims. Some of them would say that a 'transcendent meaning' emerges internally through symbols of the transcendent function, out of healing dreams, archetypal images and so on. This is seen as the autonomous internal healing function of the 'Self'. To me, this attitude makes Jungian analysis into an act of faith rather than a useful art. It carries four potential dangers: namely, reification, hypostatising, narcissistic inflation and, above all, a lack of relatedness which actually prevents change.

Reification and hypostatising are epitomised by the use of language such as 'the unconscious wants', and this distortion can, of course, also apply to theoretical attitudes towards the *animus*, *anima*, the shadow and so on. I do *not* think it is useful to reify, and it is downright wrong to hypostatise as though, for example, '*the* unconscious' had its own separate, unified will and intent, let alone as though it existed as an essence. This actually splits and disowns (as well as makes a falsely simple unit out of) a dynamic complex of relations. The word 'unconscious' is, therefore, perhaps better used adverbially or adjectivally, not as a noun. For then it can be attached to a range of unconscious impulses, desires, fears and other psychic functions.

'The unconscious' is more appropriately understood as an energetic, dynamic process which inherently moves out of an original psychosomatic *complexio*, reaches out into the environment, deintegrates and is therefore differentiable into ever-shifting but familiar figures in relationship to each other, to oneself and to the world. I am here re-emphasising Jung's understanding of the reality of the psyche and acknowledging its plurality and creative vitalism. It gives each of us our experience of being forcibly pushed around by a multiplicity of unconscious affective complexes, or subpersonalities, in such a way that they disillusion and relativise our sense of being in control and instead make us question our sense of unity. As Jung held, our unconscious psychic complexes (as well as contingent acts of nature) sometimes disturb our conscious intentions so utterly and shockingly that such a fateful personal experience can legitimately be called God.

Furthermore, although I understand my many autonomous selves as internalisations of earlier experiences of relationship to others, as a Jungian, I also understand my complexes as products of my own idiosyncratic conscious and unconscious 'forms of experiencing'. It is my unique experience of these complex relations which I internalise and characterise in my own innate way. There has to be a primary subject to make objects, an archetypal potential to meet and fashion its images – which, though archetypal, is also unique in form or style to each individual. But to treat, as some Jungians seem to, such super- or sub-human archetypal images as being 'a priori' or 'given by the gods', is no longer all right for me. This idealism (in the philosophical sense) of the archetypal image can sometimes be used as a wishful illusion, encouraging and reinforcing off-the-ground grand, narcissistic defences and false structures. As an act of faith, this may be meaningful and soul-making. As an act of useful communication, I am not so sure, especially if it implies using amplification[3] only, rather than interpretation. Amplification makes Jungian practice into a school of wisdom. There is nothing wrong with this. In fact, it is a valuable and valid vehicle for meaning, particularly for creating a sense of spiritual, or do I mean soulful, meaning. But surely only provided it comes at the right time, is pertinent to the analysand rather than to the analyst and is not an

3 Amplification involves use of mythic, historical and cultural parallels in order to clarify and make ample the metaphorical content of dream symbolism (Samuels et al., 1986, p. 16) (Eds.).

avoidance of other hidden fears and needs. How often and how much, I wonder, are some traditional Jungian categories and concepts used as defences against painful or destructive personal unconscious processes, which are re-experienced in the transference and countertransference and which should therefore be reductively comprehended? Does not the Jungian archetypal emphasis in practice, especially amplification, sometimes reinforce narcissistic defences and/or schizoid splits? An over-use of either an idea of the purposive unconscious or of the unanalysed image can prevent the analyst and the patient from seeing that there may be an actual lack or failure of the symbolic function, and worse, lead to an overlooking of the basic primitive anxiety. Jungian ideas of the objective or impersonal psyche can be used to fend off the projective slings and arrows of the psychotic transference. Furthermore, not only does this miss unconscious internal realities, but also sometimes over-archetypalises political realities on the outside.

I find rewarding mental food in Jung's speculative and philosophical writings rather than in those that have to do with the articulation of his psychological theories and models. 'Seven Sermons to the Dead' (1967), *Psychological Types* (1971, especially the early chapters), 'Answer to Job' (1970a), the perspectives and insights into content that arose out of his alchemical studies, and I must include 'On the nature of the psyche' (1970b), an essay I find endlessly challenging. I am moved by Jung's breadth and depth of vision, even his visionary quality. This marries potently with the bigness of his erudition, his intellectual and cultural richness and his sheer scope, which makes his psychology so refreshingly un-petty. As I think Jung suggested, the whole house, not just the nursery. We need history and culture as well as personal history.

This is important because it acknowledges the intense value and power associated with our personal as well as collective aesthetic and political inheritance. The personal unconscious complexity of these matters (inside each of us) is largely due to their being meshed into the internalisation of family values, reactions and relations, psychologically mixed and taken in with mother's milk, family food, parental politics, class, taste and so on. I am also interested in Jung's Kantianism, his philosophic idealism, his provocative vitalism and most of all his empirically-striving but romantically-based pan-psychism or his psycho-physics: for example, in ideas about the *unus mundus*, *participation mystique*, synchronicity and, above all, the idea of the psychoid (which I shall return to in a minute). His assertion of vitalism and hence his concomitant understanding of the teleological quality of the psyche puts him firmly in the exciting but controversial lineage of Romantic *Naturphilosophie*: Herder, Schelling, Fechner, Bergson and others: a rich philosophical tradition that has proved to be open to dangerous political abuse. Yet it is through this line of thought that we can now see how archetypal theory is also valuably applicable to areas outside psychotherapeutic practice; for example, in carefully thought-through re-evaluations of our place in the natural world, such as in deep ecology.

Also, I really appreciate Jung the passionate metaphysician, whose *Weltanschauung* sees individuation as the urgent living through and making of a different personal way between passion and reason, impulse and understanding, passive regression and ego activity, the needs of the inner world and of social justice. And hopefully, all done without denying or avoiding conflict and conscience. This is where Jung's ideas in practice create what I would call an authentic ethics, where the importance of a person's own separate idiosyncratic mind is paramount. Furthermore, I cannot underestimate the importance of the fact that Jung's psychology always recognises the real, passionate significance of ontological questions. Analytic trainings do well to include the teaching of the philosophic background, relevant metaphysical and ontological issues. A non-reductive appreciation of the experience of the numinous is essential, as is an understanding of how and when a 'false numinosity' is used defensively.

However, a metaphysics and an ethics must not be solipsistic or onanistic; they must lock into dialogue and dispute with others in order not to be masturbatory but rather something generative. Here, the seminal issue again becomes the practical and effective therapeutic relationship. It is here that I find that I have some serious problems with the application and use of Jungian theory. It is quite a task to pull some Jungian ideas down into the realities of relationship, or, in other words, into the transference/countertransference.

For me, this is particularly crucial in understanding the analytic relationship in terms of a task of psychosomatic healing, by which I mean re-joining the mind and body split which can only be done in a psyche-soma, where soma means body, body bits and symptoms as units of meaning arising out of the experience of interpersonal and internal relations – understood from a psychosomatic aspect. For example, the psychoid level of experience is not only personal, subjective and intrapsychic but, vitally, it is also inter-psychic, between and together, belonging to an intimate mix-up. It is effective in the communications and meta-communications at the level of the autonomic nervous systems as moved and shared between persons in mutual symbolic sensations. As, for example, deeply and at a visceral level, between mother and baby, or in regressive transferences.

I call this the 'consubstantial animating body'. This is a psychically incorporating 'body' which the patient's and the analyst's unconscious relationship creates, a unique environment in which we find ourselves together. This is a psychoid, harmonious and most disharmonious mix-up (Balint, 1968), which I (the analyst) sort us out of and through which we eventually separate.

Let me say a bit more about the 'consubstantial animating body'. I use the word 'consubstantial' because it defines an experience which seems to unite psyche and soma inside and between (intra and inter). I use the word 'animating' because this experience often throws up animal imagery which is symbolic of pre-verbal wordless sensations and emotions. These animate both the world inside the infant and also the mother/other (inside and out), as well as form the origins of the *anima/animus* function. I use the word 'body' because this experience is about common embodiment: two bodies in a room, an immanent embodiment in a state of psychic meaning. It is active in, for example, sensations, symptoms, pains and illnesses as called forth by projective identifications. To get into this common, mutual embodiedness, into the sensuous images which form it, which are sometimes paralleled in the analyst's images and dreams, and to think our way out of it implies facilitating protracted regression and letting it work through to a state where it is open to interpretation, not just to mirroring, empathy and certainly not to premature amplification.

But then, I do not wish to overrate the usefulness of relentless interpretations, particularly when based upon a single, if complex, clinical theory. This can be cold, hard, lacking feeling and may not engender the trust necessary to playfully melt defences. Such an approach can be as omnipotent in its own way as archetypal amplification. Furthermore, it can become repetitive in its limited language, which, after five years or more with an analysand, can begin to wear down normal positive and negative transferences as it appears increasingly obsessional and, dare I say, even boring. The subtleties of object relations can become so thought-provokingly fascinating to the practitioner or clinical theoretician, in a chess-playing sort of way, that it can seem to outsiders (and here I include patients and trainees) to be schizoid and unrelated, symptomatic of an intellectual defence against fearful feelings and rapport. In any school of thought and practice, when two different lineages polarise, extreme wings of either side tend to judge the other approach as handicapped, blind or badly erroneous. Surely, this is a defensive splitting against paranoid fears of the dangerous (and unconsciously envied and feared) other. It is the stuff of fundamentalism and precludes creativity.

I go on trying to find a practical and authentic way between, on the one hand, the tendency towards the impractical fantasies of archetypal psychology but without losing thoughtful imagination and intuitive knowledge and, on the other hand, avoiding the tendency towards the schizoid clinical coldness of overintellectual theory but without losing a focused perspicacity and subtlety of understanding. As I have said, for me, this must include trying to find shareable words and common language which makes meaning of those harmonious and disharmonious consubstantiating images and sensations which we experience in the analytic relationship. These words, this language, help make sense of internal chaos and unknowing. Thus, it also helps us to live with the necessities of a contingent environment, undefensively, in one's own individual way, which is both necessarily limited and creative at the same time. The wounded analyst must have enough good objects based upon joined internal parents in order to be sufficiently stable to take on emotionally, and sometimes to take in, a patient's depressions, anxieties, anger, etc., and to be able to process these affects helpfully and honestly in so far as is possible. In other words, a therapist must have a degree of undefensive optimism which yet does not in any way deny the reality of unhealable areas of damage. This capacity is an aspect of a healthy ambivalence arising out of what Klein (1935) called the depressive position, but its implication is that a depressed or split therapist is at least a hindrance or, more likely, a narcissistic wounder.

Like so many other post-Jungians, my experience of the significance of infancy and early development and of its psychic re-constellation in the transference/countertransference has led me to incorporate many psychoanalytic object relations theories, as well, of course, as the work of other Jungians who adapt these clinical theories in a Jungian way. As my opening quotation, much of the language and many of the models and ideas I have used in this paper may have revealed that my thinking is also significantly influenced by neo-Spinozan philosophy, especially by the work of the French philosopher Gilles Deleuze (Deleuze, 1988). For me, Jung is not my only 'internal wise figure'. Surely, it is in the spirit of Jung to be able to incorporate one's own mix of new perceptions, ideas and values. Jung and a Jungian identity are a vital part or perhaps the basic container for all my plurality of values. My practice is not classically Jungian, either in its models or in its techniques, but I hope that it is Jungian in its spirit of endless renewal-by-integration, or rather by a difficult, tangly, tricky process of trying to understand the psyche through many ideas, many opposites, many rich complexities.

References

Balint, M. (1968). *The Basic Fault: Therapeutic Aspects of Regression*. London: Basic Books.

Deleuze, G. (1988). *Spinoza. Practical Philosophy*. R. Hurley, trans. San Francisco: City Lights.

Jung, C. (1967). *VII Sermones ad Mortuos. The Seven Sermons to the Dead Written by Basilides in Alexandria*. H. Baynes, trans. London: Stuart & Watkins.[4]

Jung, C. (1970a). 'Answer to Job'. In *Psychology and Religion: West and East*. Vol. 11 of *The Collected Works of C. G. Jung*. R. Hull, trans. London: Routledge & Kegan Paul.

Jung, C. (1970b). 'On the Nature of the Psyche'. In *The Structure and Dynamics of the Psyche*. Vol. 8 of *The Collected Works of C. G. Jung*. R. Hull, trans. 2nd edn. London: Routledge & Kegan Paul.

Jung, C. (1971). *Psychological Types*. Vol. 6 of *The Collected Works of C. G. Jung*. H. Baynes, trans. London: Routledge & Kegan Paul.

Klein, M. (1935). 'A Contribution to the Psychogenesis of Manic-Depressive States'. *International Journal of Psychoanalysis*, 16: 145–174.

Samuels, A., Shorter, B. & Plaut, F. (1986). *A Critical Dictionary of Jungian Analysis*. London: Routledge & Kegan Paul.

Winnicott, D. (1984). 'Communicating and Not Communicating Leading to a Study of Certain Opposites'. In *The Maturational Processes and the Facilitating Environment*. D. Winnicott, ed. London: Karnac (Original work published 1963).

Wolfson, H. (1935). Letter. Source unidentified.

4 The Baynes translation of *Seven Sermons to the Dead*, a text which Jung originally wrote in 1916, is also included in some, though not all, editions of *Memories, Dreams, Reflections* (Eds.).

Chapter 5

The animating body

Psychoid substance as a mutual experience of psychosomatic disorder

Journal of Analytical Psychology, 1996[1]

In 1946, Jung put forward a hypothesis of a 'psychoid' level or quality of the unconscious psyche; he wrote:

> Since psyche and matter are contained in one and the same world, and moreover are in continuous contact with one another and ultimately rest on irrepresentable, transcendental factors, it is not only possible but fairly probable even that psyche and matter are two different aspects of one and the same thing.
>
> (Jung, 1970a; *CW* 8, para. 418)

He returned to this dual-aspect idea again several times, and in *Mysterium Coniunctionis*, first published in 1955–1956, he wrote that 'deepest down of all, [is] the paradox of the sympathetic and parasympathetic psychoid processes' (Jung, 1970b; *CW* 14, para. 279).

In my title, I have used the expression 'psychoid *substance*'. Since the meaning of 'substance' is not axiomatic, and since I am using it idiosyncratically in a way that is connected to my use of the 'psychoid', I need to say that by substance, I do *not* mean either an essence or a thing, or not only. I am using the word 'substance' in a Spinozist/neo-Spinozist metaphysical sense, by which I mean the idea of a fundamental unity (not union) underlying two 'attributes' (attitudes to, aspects or experiences) of that basic unity – which is here 'the psychoid'. The two 'attributes' are psyche/soma, or psychic/somatic. But more psychologically, I understand this psychoid substance as being dynamic (substantiat*ing*) and having to do with the making of internal and interpersonal relations (*con*substantiating). Finally, I think it might be phenomenologically useful to render 'the psychoid' as an adjective or adverb: a consubstantiating psychoid energy, which is experienced psychoidly (psychosomatically) inside and between us – perhaps most evidently in psychotic experience and relations.

1 Originally published as Clark, G. (1996). 'The Animating Body: Psychoid Substance as a Mutual Experience of Psychosomatic Disorder'. *Journal of Analytical Psychology*, 41(3): 353–368. Reprinted with permission © Wiley Publishing. Minor corrections and copy editing has been applied (Eds.).

DOI: 10.4324/9781003255826-6

I am here suggesting that the psychoid has not only to do with an individual, intrapsychic level of life but also has to do with an area of experience where bodily sensations are symbolic, sometimes represented through primitive sensations, proto-symbols and psychosomatic metacommunications which are felt both inside us and also simultaneously around us in relationships. For example, in experiences of *participation mystique*, through projective identifications, extractive introjections (Bollas, 1987) and in other processes of personal and interpersonal psychic contamination and infection which are also somatically affective. These experiences painfully unite us in something we unconsciously make together, arising out of an as yet unmet need to share in something undeveloped and uncoordinated. They are found in clinical work with deeply regressed patients where the capacity to distinguish inner and outer, subject and object, fantasy and reality, etc., are all very unclear; in other words, in borderline or psychotic relations, where the analyst is necessarily 'used' as a psychotic object by the disturbed patient. This is where the primitive and almost pre-human nature of events (and therefore animal/animating events) is experienced in its preverbal, pre-thinking state. It is experienced in a state of chaos or disorder, destroying words and thinking, and of raw emotions and sensations of bodily illness, though not necessarily in actual organic illness.

I shall use a case example to demonstrate how, in work with regressed patients, pre-whole-person symbols and sensations are transferred by projective identification into the analyst. The analyst can then be infected and used at the level of the autonomic nervous system, sensed vitally through animal imagery and somatic symptoms (in dreams and illness). This is an embodied countertransference in which we find what I call a consubstantiating 'animating body'. It is a primitive and bestial 'psychoid environment' made between us, around us and inside us. It is the analyst's task to sort us out of this mixed-up and over-embodied world so that we are eventually able to separate into different but related personal identities.

In this paper, I am doing what I try to do in the regressed analytic situation, namely to understand, find words for, bring order to and communicate in such a way that together we can make our way out of this wordless, thoughtless psychotic disorder. In the clinical situation I will describe, this is a matter of using my attacked and infected embodied countertransference, or embodied aspects of identification, to understand and make sense of the patient's (and, therefore, my) deep psychosomatic disorder. I need to make two points for the sake of clarity:

1 Although what I am talking about is about somatising where the symbolising function has become confused and therefore stuck at an early stage, it is also about a necessary pre-differentiated psychosomatic stage and state, a natural archetypal aspect of our nature where our psychoid and psychotic metaphysics (Rhode, 1994) originate and live.
2 Above all, it is about the paradoxical experience of oneness or intimacy and mutuality in non-blissful, disharmonious relations, in conditions of attack, fragmentation, chaotic dissociation and incomprehension, which I see as necessary

> metacommunications of disorder, which have to be shared in order to be understood and sorted out: a sort of psychic chaos theory.

In the analytic situation, there are two embodied minds actually living together in a room. As we get to share in a psychic (which is a psychoid) mix-up, we can become strongly affected and infected by each other, especially unconsciously. It is the analyst's parental job to see that the two bodies do not become mixed-up or 'as one' in any actual concrete sense, for example, in sensuous or adolescent sexual acting-out or in physical violence. Above all, the analyst must be aware of, understand transferentially and refrain from countertransferential reactions such as retaliation, being provocative, over-stimulating or subtly seductive.

However, in certain emotionally-loaded and regressed situations in analysis our two psyches do discover or create a common mixed and affective sense of body, an embodiment of unconscious emotions which we both share. This 'body' can be either a sensed or, if more symbolically developed, an imaged body, or both. At the psychic pole, unconscious physical communications and subliminal body language produce associative imagery from memory of intra-psychic and internalised interpersonal relations, perhaps also from internalised foetal relations. Psychically, early relations often seem to be imaged or symbolised by an animal body or by interacting bits of nonhuman bodies. This is one reason why I use the words 'animating body'. These animal-like symbols and sensations have to do with very early pre-whole-person, pre-verbal stages of development, an infant's part-object relations amongst zones of his/her own body and their instincts and impulses and relations with bits of mother, fantasies of mother's body and her insides.

In so far as there is an imagery (not just psychosomatic sensations and symptoms), I suggest that these not-wholly-human animating images derive from later (post 1-year-old) psychic fantasy, but that they are symbols of pre-image experience, even of foetal relations.

My use of the word 'animating' has also risen out of my understanding of *anima/animus* as a purposive of functional psychic process, namely the psychic condition that projects love or hate in order to animate the person, object or idea projected onto. By animating the projector's world, this *anima* function also animates the projector. This means that *anima/animus* can be understood as that quality of projection which animates all relationships. The internal object of this projection is as much non- or even anti-parental as parental, and, in fact, one of its functions is to make exogamy desirable.

A third source for my use of the word 'animating' comes from George Santayana's philosophical elaboration of such a construct in *Scepticism and Animal Faith* (1923), especially in the chapter 'Evidences of Animation in Nature' (pp. 240–251).

Winnicott puts the 'localisation of self in one's body' at the centre of his developmental model: the body is the root of development, out of which the 'psychosomatic partnership' evolves. The self is primarily a body-self, and the psyche 'means the *imaginative elaboration of somatic parts, feelings and functions*, that is, of physical aliveness' (Winnicott, 1954, p. 202). Thus, developmentally, with good enough maternal care in infancy, the building of the self is 'a process of natural co-ordination' in which 'the psyche and the soma have to come to terms with each other' and 'find a common language' (Phillips, 1988, pp. 78–79). But what if there is a lack of this co-ordination and instead a splitting and confusion of the psyche-soma? A Winnicottian case study by Sacksteder (1989) describes how, when the environment (mother/parents) fails, a child can no longer rely on her own omnipotence, and the unmediated physical and emotional distress becomes so great that the psyche dissociates from the persecuting soma in order to protect the precious core from the intolerable pain. I would add that the persecuting soma often gets defensively projected or injected into the analyst, who is therefore 'made' to become the patient's persecuting soma, and therefore, the analyst feels physically attacked from within as well as from without. Of course, we cannot talk about body or instinct being projected; that would be a category error. But we can talk *as if* the somatic were being projected when its symbolism or meaning is expressed in countertransferentially received sensations and in sensuous body and animal imagery.

In his 1946 Introduction to 'The Psychology of the Transference' Jung speaks of the 'bond' of the transference neurosis which

> is often of such intensity that we could almost speak of a 'combination'. When two chemical substances combine, both are altered. This is precisely what happens in the transference.
>
> (Jung, 1993, *CW* 16, para. 358)

Through the *mixtum compositum* of the doctor's and the patient's psyches,

> [spirit and matter together] . . . form an impenetrable mass, a veritable magma sprung from the depths of primeval chaos . . . They emit a fascination which not only grips – and has already gripped – the patient, but can also have an inductive effect on the unconscious of the impartial spectator, in this case the doctor . . . He too becomes affected, and has as much difficulty in distinguishing between the patient and what has taken possession of him as has the patient himself. This leads both of them to a direct confrontation with the daemonic forces lurking in the darkness. The resultant paradoxical blend of positive and negative, of trust and fear, of hope and doubt, of attraction and repulsion, is characteristic of the initial relationship. It is the hate and love of the elements, which the alchemists likened to the primeval chaos.
>
> (Jung, 1993, *CW* 16, paras. 363, 375)

Elie Humbert's writing around this area is also pertinent to my theme. In 'The Well-springs of Memory' he says that the

> pre-object state typifies the final months of foetal life and the primordial relationship with the mother. The analytic relationship provides an opportunity to repeat it. It puts the analysand back into that initial experience in which the

> object takes shape through a dual relationship . . . [where] bodies impose their own reality. It is here, in the body, where the early traumatic incidents were imprinted, that their reactivation takes place . . . In these archaic zones the patient's illness has a certain power and it 'makes' the analyst in the same way that the child 'makes' his mother. The analyst can then be present without quite understanding what is going on.
>
> (Humbert, 1988, pp. 5–6)

'Pat'

Let me offer a case example where 'not understanding what was going on' was a slow and painful, but necessary, way to eventually create a deep understanding in a consubstantiating or psychoid sense. I shall call the patient Pat. (This analysand is one of five patients I have worked with who have contributed to my idea of an analytically co-created, co-transformative psychoid animator.) Pat described herself as half Parsee and half Anglo-Indian, her father a Parsee, her mother an Anglo-Indian. She had had a brother two years older than herself but who had been killed in a car crash when he was in his early twenties, and she had a sister two years younger than herself. Pat was 32 when she first came to see me. In the course of her life, her family moved from Bombay to East Africa to the Caribbean and then to England. Her presenting problems were: frighteningly murderous impulses at her job, which was in intensive care with babies, sexual promiscuity and chronic constipation (i.e. confused and stuck). But she also said that the real reason for seeking therapy was the 'terrible issue of the murder of my father by my mother'. She felt mother had killed him by 'nagging and bullying him relentlessly'. Nags and bulls were to become significant symbolic metaphors, as we shall see. Also, in this initial session, she reported that her mother told her 'she [Pat] was so disturbed that she disturbed everyone she met'; whatever else, this was obviously a warning message to me.

She had recently had to go to her father's Parsee funeral, which involved going to the Towers of Silence in Bombay and witnessing his body being eaten by vultures. It then emerged that she and her sister had been sexually assaulted by the father when she was about 6 or 7. She used the expression, 'he was so vigorous', an idiosyncratic expression that I did not forget. Yet she still regarded father as good and mother (who collusively blamed her for this activity) as all bad and witchy. This was obviously a defensive splitting, but it was also the first sign of a tangled internal knot.

After a few weeks, she developed near-hallucinations in which she saw a vulture sitting on the back of my chair behind my head. Initially, it was difficult to know whether I was the vulture, and therefore she was my victim, or whether I was its intended corpse (i.e. father being killed by the 'mother-vulture', let alone mother being killed by Pat). These 'hallucinations' were extremely vivid, intense and frightening for me as well as for her. We increased her sessions to three a week.

After a certain amount of time, she had a powerful dream full of Mithraic (and, therefore, Zoroastrian) bull imagery. This was a dream about

> a doctor (analyst) who jumps onto the bumper or chest of a car-bison and wraps his legs around its bumper or neck 'like a woman's position in a sexual act'. The doctor's erect penis is jabbing into the neck or throat of the car-bison. The doctor holds onto the mud-guards or horns and then pulls off the head of this creature, climbs into the headless torso and disappears. The head, now definitely a bison's, is still alive and dangerous, and attacks the dreamer who wakes up in fear.

This initial Mithraic dream vividly describes the subsequent analytic relationship: a life and death struggle in which the phallic analyst is sacrificed by being absorbed into a (dead?) body. Then Pat's own savage nature gets further split off and turns on herself. However, insofar as I was soon to disappear into the 'bestial body', it was vital (to me and to Pat) that I went through this process and came out the other side alive. Similarly, it was also vital for Pat to eventually re-unite the severed head and the sundered body – which represented so many terrifying splits. But this dream of attack, castration and potency anxiety also contains a memory – as we shall see later.

She also told me of a recurrent dream/nightmare of riding on a grey hunting horse. Her view in the dream is always from the rider's position, i.e. of the horse's neck and head seen from behind, but the horse always suddenly jumps to its death, for example, over a cliff or into a fire. The dream, recurrent since childhood, inevitably woke Pat up at its crisis ending. She loved her dream-horse and felt it was her 'body power'. It was certainly about a powerful, even phallic sense of body, (for Pat) incorporating violence and destruction as well as a sexual and gender confusion. After these dreams, Pat became increasingly angry and murderous in her feelings towards me, and I began to feel ill, initially just during the sessions, but later after them also.

At first, I tried to defend myself internally by constructing fantasies whilst I was with her of being solid and impenetrable. She developed psychic terrorist tactics and became a 'baby bomb'. She would regress into being a needy baby who wanted to be picked up and hugged but at the same time wanted to be left alone and not touched. Everything, everyone, was wrong, thus creating a frustrating tension. Then this tension would lessen, and she would instead create an atmosphere in the room that was calm, oceanic, blissful. However, this was a dangerously seductive illusion, for suddenly, from this closeness, this relieving calm, she would throw a new and worse tantrum, an agony of spitting colic, a wild explosion of rage and fury in which she would try to destroy me/mother.

After about 15 months, there was a summer break of three weeks. When she reappeared, I was surprised to see that she had cut off her long hair and was wearing markedly masculine clothes. She presented me with a copy of a letter which she said she had sent to her GP, requesting to arrange for a sex change. She had not, in fact, sent any such letter to her GP but was 'sending' her symbolic needs to me. I think this was an expression of her confusion over uniting her internal parents, her need to identify with me and her feeling of failure to achieve these aims. In the confusion of trying to sort out the implications of the letter and her change of appearance, she also said, 'I have told you many lies over the year'.

These turned out to be as follows: Mother was a Hindu, not an Anglo-Indian; Pat had only had sex once – she was pretty well a virgin, i.e. there was no promiscuity; her father raped her sister, not her, and she was half jealous and fascinated/excited as well as horrified; her mother protected her lovingly from this possibility ever happening to her – so mother was good. However, she soon changed this image yet again, and mother was remembered as 'an over-curious, genital inspector'. And so the historical, and therefore identity, chaos increased. She wanted me to know what had actually happened to her in the family and why. She needed me to be her idea of a parental mind, digesting, sorting-out and thinking for the physically and mentally pained baby. Of course, the analyst/parent cannot actually know the baby's mental or physical pain from the inside or experience their identity for them. However, the more I could be made to suffer her turmoil, the closer she felt I would be made to identify with her.

She agreed that she needed to come four times a week. With this intensification, Pat became even more restless or, if physically still, was so tense that it was painful to sit with her. Sometimes she lay on the couch, sometimes she huddled on the floor, and sometimes she sat up. When sitting in the chair she would stare pointedly at me, and any actual or perceived flicker in my face, particularly a diversion of my eyes, was reacted to as if it were a frightened, guilty and treacherous flight from her. I linked this to her father and later to her own sense of guilt. But increasingly, my interpretations were met either with a disdainful silence or by her screaming at me, 'You are bloody mad!' Both manoeuvres succeeded in making it very difficult to think and to find words. But anyhow, as always with a regression into a psychotic transference, verbal interpretations became inappropriate and could not be taken in. With Pat, they felt like further phallic incestuous intrusions, narcissistic and selfish, stemming from my own clumsy needs.

Her recurrent shouts of 'You are bloody mad!' were, for a few weeks, her only words. She shouted them not only when I said something, but also when I was silent, which I was increasingly becoming. Eventually, she stopped the shouting, stopped all words and we sat in silence for several weeks. This protracted silent phase was still physically uncomfortable. I ached and felt sick. However, occasionally she induced a sexual sense, and in one session, she broke the silence by whispering, 'I've got you'. Her immediate curling up and hiding of her face after this remark seemed distinctly more erotic than angry, and at that moment, an image arose of her as a spider weaving a web around me and venomously sucking me out. After this, she returned again to the wordless physical tension and the environment of silent projective identifications. I felt as though my body was unwittingly being made to do all the work and that survival was my main concern.

In a 1990 paper on 'Regression in the countertransference', Christopher Bollas considers what he calls an 'informative regression' in which he distinguishes four stages of regression and recovery within the analyst's countertransference. He describes the second stage as one where the analyst has a 'terror over survival' and is overcome by a 'dreadful silence' immobilising the analyst's 'psyche-soma'. This is due to the analyst picking up on the patient's internalisation of 'maternal hate, of death wishes against the aliveness of the child'. The terror, 'however, is due to the child's responsive destruction, expressed by the analyst's countertransference'. The analyst's personality is split, the patient's internalisation of maternal hate' being 'projected into the environment' and the analyst is left being only a part analyst (Bollas, 1990, pp. 350–351).

This stage changes when events occur that mobilise the analyst's fury into speech, and so aggression becomes a means of survival.

Pat's psychotic behaviour was a defence against oedipal potency anxiety by splitting, spitting and projecting her confusion. In Pat's case, father and mother were experienced as deeply confused, with provocatively unclear and frighteningly crossed boundaries. This confusion had been internalised, and was now being pushed out into the analytic relationship. It was my analytic role to be made by Pat to embody someone who she could feel was minding her thoroughly. By this, I mean that she needed me to be a sensitive, suffering but also strong and eventually clarifying, embodied mind.

After about three more weeks of silence and much thinking like bloody mad on my part, Pat suddenly asked me, 'What are you doing to me?' I answered with something like, 'You are frightened and want to know what I think is going on'. She responded by saying, 'What's *going in*, you mean!' At first, I thought this was her unconscious reference to the psychoid poison that I felt she was projecting into me. However, a dream that she had the night immediately after this revealed another aspect and signalled the start of a dramatic breakthrough. She had a dream in which I was probing (with my fingers) the anus of her grey horse. Having related this to me, she shouted, 'I hate you; you are attacking my horse', at which point she leapt up from the couch and started to actually attack me, biting and kicking me. I thought that I ought to be interpreting this event in an analytically correct way, trying to understand for me and her what she was trying to do, and to whom; but, actually, I physically defended myself. My physical self-defence made her yell, 'You are attacking me', to which I rather cowardly replied, 'No, I am defending myself'. She said, 'No, men don't defend themselves; they only attack, you bugger'.

I was able to take up the link between 'men only attack' and 'you bugger' with her. It turned out that her brother had tried to bugger her when she was about 12. Then she said that, in fact, he made her masturbate him onto her chest and neck and that he 'would come so vigorously'. The expression 'he came so vigorously' sounded loud bells, of course, and the dream image of the doctor with his penis/knife in the bull's throat took on a new significance. Of course, this brother was both an aspect of her father and, I think, a split-off, needy part of herself. His later fatal car crash was experienced by Pat as a terrible punishment for her guilt.

When I regained my capacity to think, I was able to interpret her deep confusion between firstly her experience of me as an anal/genital intruder, like mother, and secondly, her seduction/masturbation complex of fearful desire, guilt and anger (whose objects were father, brother, me and her child self). As she became able to understand and integrate her unconscious identification with mother-vulture, her frightening murderous impulses at work abated. Simultaneously, her erotic transference onto me reached a sort of emotional, psychic climax, and a few sessions later, she brought the following dream:

> I am staying in a farm, and I wake up. It is a cloudy, drizzling morning, about 4.00 am. The cockerel is about to crow, and I want to watch the cock crowing. So I go outside and wait and listen for him. Then, I hear the first crow so I know where to go to see him. He is standing on a heap of rotting compost. At each crow, he creates an image of sunrise. When the cock is not actually crowing, the weather is still cloudy. Then I notice that the cockerel has been plucked. His plucked body is bleeding from where the feathers have been torn out of him. His naked body is plump. His naked neck is thin and scraggy, except when he crows when it becomes strong and muscular. I know that in some way, he is the ugly crucified Christ.

This dream of a plucked cockerel who was also Christ, and obviously also a wounded phallic symbol, even an image of an erect penis (father's and brother's), begs many questions about the analytic relationship, in particular, because my own initial pre-analytic dream (from 15 years before this) was of a crucified Christ as an ugly plucked chicken covered with green mould. Through my own personal associations and interpretations of my dream and my understanding of Pat's dream, I saw the cockerel/plucked chicken image as symbolic of our similar psychic experience, of our attacked, abused and/or denied bodies. But the vital and difficult thing was that Pat's dream of a cock felt to me as though a seminal part of me had got into her. I was her brother, her father and her phallic mother. Here, in our transference/countertransference *unus mundus*, I felt that I had been unconsciously seduced into an invasive assault. Or had I actually unconsciously assaulted her with my own projective identifications? Had she made me feel intrusive? And, the other way around, I felt raped of my dream. Was it that she had got into me too much and/or got too much out of me? Whose dream was it? Whose cock? Whose Christ? Whose body? I now think that the cock-Christ was a real shared symbol, somatic and psychic, our animating body which incorporated us both; her dream and our two bodies were attributes or aspects of a single shared psychosomatic dynamic substance: our psychoid developmental-relational energy. As Jung wrote in a letter to James Kirsch in 1934, 'in the deepest sense we all dream not out of ourselves but out of what lies *between us and the other*' (Jung, 1973, p. 172).

To link the first and last of Pat's dreams that I have recounted, firstly, the sacrificial bull can be seen as the potent animal body through which revitalising change may eventually happen, that is, the analytic body. The sacrificial bull can also be seen as the analyst's (father's/brother's) desired and feared phallic potency. These two elements (bull and man) come together as one in seeing the sacrificial body as Christ-as-cock, that is, as the embodiment of the ugliness of abuse' the counter-transferentially wounded analyst-as-saviour.

In his 1946 'The psychology of the transference', his psychological elaboration of the *Rosarium*, Jung describes the same analytic state of affairs that I have been recounting, although he does not explicitly link mutual confusion to the psychoid. In particular, in pictures 7, 8 and 9, that is, the Ascent of the Soul, the *Mundificatio* and the Return of the Soul, he says:

> The 'soul' which is reunited with the body is the One born of the two, the vinculum common to both. It is therefore the very essence of relationship . . . The collective unconscious is a natural and universal datum and its manifestation always causes an unconscious identity, a state of participation mystique.
>
> (Jung, 1993, *CW* 16, para. 504)

I understand the *vinculum* as the muscular grip between two parts or persons, which is, among other things, a metaphor for adhesive identification, exactly as Pat had got herself into with me. The *vinculum* can mean our joint experience of an animating body.

Our struggles to make sense of the cockerel dream and to understand its place in our history eventually enabled Pat to begin to accept the limits of her power to possess and control her world absolutely. She became a relatively more peaceable person, her constipation ceased and, as we disentangled ourselves, my countertransference pains also ceased. One could say that her history, as she had presented it to me over the years, was a cock-and-bull story. But of course, I still do not know (and can never know) what actually happened, what was done to her, what she did, or even whose were the desires, nor what belonged to her, what to father, what to brother, etc.

Analytically, I took on all her memories, repetitions, distortions and above all her fears as if they were true; for they were indeed physically real experiences and furthermore made an emotionally and somatically real impact on me. After the crisis of her actual attack on me and the subsequent dream, matters changed tangibly. In other ways, many aspects of her fragile and angry personality changed little or not at all, nor, I think, ever can or, for defensive purposes, ever should change.

In *Psychotic Metaphysics*, Eric Rhode writes:

> One foetal myth asserts that at the beginning exists the unknowability known as the good objects. Foetal mind is formed out of this beginning; and foetal body is formed out of mind. Preconception implies that the foetal body is a metaphor for mind, in the same way as psychosomatic disorders can be viewed as metaphors for a type of thought.
>
> (Rhode, 1994, p. 8)

In the beginning, the psyche is the body's idea of sensations of pain and pleasure, both mental and physical, which, though felt on the inside, are actually mediated by ideas from the outside, from another person's embodied mind, such as the mother, which is the source of meaningful ideas about her own experiences, including her experience of her child with her. At this level, the psyche is a body/psyche. Its in-take and build-up of meaningful images is fearful in the case of bad or painful experiences and desirous in the case of good or pleasurable experiences. Yet in its management of this process of projective identification, this organizing of objects in relation to each other, the foetal and infant psyche will also be *fearful* of his or her desire for good pleasure and will also *desire* to have possessive power over the painful (such as in finding masochistic pleasure in the pain).

A regression such as I have described is an entry into an activation of a relationship where the psychotic part of the analysand's personality forcibly projects its mad and bad fragments into the analyst, who frustrates the patient because the analyst does not obey the desirous mind of the patient. Of course, the parental analyst is not controllable and is a separate physical person with his or her apparent own volition. So to try to make both the ideal of oneness and the lethal hate more affective in an even less symbolic and more affective way, toxic, somatic projections are used, like a spider injecting its victim with a paralysing and dissolving venom so that it can be digested and incorporated. This is a process of psychotic, psychosomatic fusion or confusion, a sick and sickening union.

As far back as 1921, Jung, describing *participation mystique*, said that the subject 'does not, however, feel himself projected into the object; rather, the "empathised" object appears animated to him, as though it were speaking to him of its own accord' (Jung, 1971, *CW* 6, para. 486). Note his use of the word 'animated'. Jung is describing a process of *participation mystique* which he did not see as a primarily defensive manoeuvre (as projective identification is sometimes understood in Klein's 1946 original formulation, rather than Bion's 1962 reformulation of 'normal' projective identification involving unconscious to unconscious communication). Rather, *participation mystique* is a powerful unconscious identity between separate entities, perhaps to compensate for an intolerable distance and difference and to answer a need (pathological or otherwise) for intimacy. The common experiential quality between these two processes is a relationship of invasive and infectious unconscious affect in which the sense of separateness of subject and object is destroyed, and instead, we are made to share in a state of psychoid oneness.

As Thomas Ogden (1986) has said, in relational states of projective identification, both persons and a larger third entity (the 'analytic third') all change. This third entity is perhaps close to what I am elaborating in the idea of the animating body or the psychoid animator. The change can be understood as an increasing capacity and potentiality for different ways of experiencing, provided the mother/analyst has made 'linkages'. Otherwise, her incapacity to do so is an 'attack on linking' (Bion, 1959) which the child/patient internalises and so thence attacks subsequent emotional ties, thinking and clear communication. I would say that this is when the animating body becomes internally overwhelming and relationally savage.

If an infant's inborn primal impetus to de-integrate through relating is narcissistically unmet by a mother cut off in her own depressive anxiety or by an invasive father or an unrelated schizoid parental couple, then the internalised family becomes a complex web of mutual envy and resentment, invasions of hatred and annihilatory wishes, intrusions by primitive desires and stealing of life and joy. Naturally, the primitive lack of differentiation and confused quality of this dangerous internal disorder leads to psychosomatic symptoms.

A physical tension, which makes self and others ill, is created by the child's/patient's demanding but unmet unconscious needs. The baby whose de-integrative and re-integrative processes have not been facilitated faces instead the threat of disintegration and the terror of isolation. Thus, narcissistic or even autistic defences get set up in order to preserve a deeply unconscious sense of self and hold some integrity together.

When the tension becomes overwhelming and fearfully destructive, the patient is forced to seek out or create another person or part-person (mother/therapist) who is ruthlessly used as the embodiment of the wounded self, as the object who has to become the bearer of the unbearable, to suffer the tension, disintegration and painful chaos – but of course also be seen to know, understand, survive and resolve the dissolution.

In her paper 'Looking out and looking in', Jan Wiener (1994) takes up Daniel Stern's distinction between 'what may be called category affects such as anger, sadness, joy, fear, disgust, etc., and vitality affects which cannot be classified in terms of these readily recognisable emotions as they do not have names and will be highly individual' (Wiener, 1994, p. 345). As Wiener notes, Stern suggests that they are better described by 'dynamic, kinetic terms, such as "surging", "fading away", "fleeting", "explosive", "crescendo", "decrescendo", "bursting", "drawn out". Stern says that it is these feelings which will be elicited by changes in motivational states, appetites and tensions' (Stern, 1985, p. 54, in Wiener, 1994, p. 345). Weiner argues that

> many psychosomatic patients may be suffering from particular disturbances in vitality affects emanating from the time when sensuous communications between mother and baby can critically affect emotional development.
>
> (Wiener, 1994, p. 345)

She also draws upon Joyce McDougall's case illustrations of psychosomatic patients which show

> the effects in adulthood of a preverbal child's early perception of affectless modes of functioning as a way of combating psychological pain, early frustration and panic.
>
> (McDougall, 1989, p. 26, cited in Wiener, 1994, p. 346)

Making her own valuable distinction between body-talk and body-language, Wiener hypothesises that

> body talk is a consequence of the kind of preverbal communication between mother and baby where there may have been a bad fit in terms of vitality affects. In later life, this can manifest itself in the form of 'body' or psychosomatic problems which cannot be put into words but are often recognizable through the quality of the interpersonal transference dynamics.
>
> (p. 348)

She uses the words 'discomfort' or 'dissonance' as being evident in the 'doings' of early body talk. The sort of case that I am dealing with in this paper is operating very much in the discomforting 'body talk' mode – where the analyst has to let him/herself be 'done to' for a protracted period.

The consubstantiating experience of a shared world of psychoid animation, a body of mutual experience, is an environment unconsciously formed out of the patient's chaotic internal relations and made interpersonal by the unconscious projective identification of these confused relations into the analyst or into which the analyst is necessarily sucked. Because this environment is unconsciously created, we sense it as if it was a psyche-soma experience into which we unwittingly fall and in which we find ourselves together, sharing in it animatedly. The analyst's task is to 'think like bloody mad' and to find a way out of this sickening confusion into our separateness and difference. The analyst needs to think through his or her affected and infected autonomic nervous system, its sensations and primitive symbols, and thus help the patient (and the analyst) to a new psyche-soma co-ordination.

In Roderick Peters' words:

> Countertransference is the fundamentally useful tool that it is, only to the extent that the analyst's conscious personality is open to his own serpent mind: the more he can let in, contain, and know what is going on in his own ANS, the more he will know his sympathetic and parasympathetic responses to his patients, and be able to help his patients to know his (the patient's) serpent mind.
>
> (Peters, 1987, pp. 375–376)

So we can understand psychoid substance as a vital force or urge which energetically permeates the psyche-soma and naturally and necessarily reaches out to mate with the human environment, in other words, with other embodied vital persons. Initially, this is the mother's body, or experienced aspects of mother's body, including the insides of mother and her mind. The infant then introjects these experiences. But the fundamental core of this vital energy is not the part objects and deintegrates but rather earlier pre-objective, pre-image, urgent processes of energetic relating itself. This is, so to speak, the Ur-archetype or, as Herder called it, *Die Urkraft aller Kräfte*, which some analytical psychologists call the primal self or the primary integrate and which is the precondition for deintegration. It seems that this is like a primal vital spark which instinctively lives itself out between me and the world, making life between me and the world, seeming to find it. In regressed analytic relations, we can re-experience this vital animating body between us as a primitive psychoid force that moves us, body and soul, often very painfully and alarmingly. If, at the beginning of life, this urgent primal force is thwarted in any way, then its vitalism is damaged and a pathological, often psychotic struggle for survival develops.

The order of damaged developmental events in the transference goes something like this:

1 Initially, as felt from the inside, we find that we are both in one shared active environment. This means that we have created our shared natural psychic universe around us. The fantasy is: 'I love you absolutely and shall love you forever because you love me absolutely and shall love me forever. You are mine and we are, therefore, one'.
2 Then, disillusioning experience changes or develops the fantasy: 'I simultaneously find that you are *not* one with me, but are separate, different; you have a separate body and a separate mind and live in a different world. This is terrible and intolerable. I hate and envy you your separateness; I cannot have you because you do not love me absolutely and eternally'.
3 'Therefore, I must force us into a shared unit environment. I must *force* you to be one with me, and me to be one with you: force us into love'.
4 'Simultaneously, I hate and envy you so much that I must kill you. So I shall wound you, hurt you, make you ill and sick unto death'. Therefore, this commonly sensed active universe or environmental field which the analysand has created is now simultaneously:

    a) a place full of inactive oceanic reverie and bliss and;
    b) an active battlefield of bullet-like projections and psychic germ warfare.

5 So it is both good and bad, pleasure and pain, loving and hating, sex and sickness, a love and death struggle. This mix-up is maddening. It is an overwhelming state of disorder, chaos and psychosomatic infection.
6 But first the analyst and thence the analysand discover a paradox: namely, that the apparently loving side, the blissful inactive oneness, is deathly, and on the other hand that the murderous hate, pain and sickness is actually energising, vitalising, animating. And even more paradoxically, this terrible animating body, which is so fierce, disharmonious, sickening and disassociated is in fact what brings life and unites us.

Conclusion

In this paper, I have taken a deductive Spinozan dual aspect identity theory (mind and matter are two aspects of the same 'substance') and, moving it into a more psychologically based hypothesis of psycho-physical parallelism, that is, the psychoid, I have tried to describe how my analytic experience of the psychoid as a psychosomatic disordering and uniting force is as much interpersonal as individual. Furthermore, this experience is as much about a regression into a disharmoniously mixed-up relationship as into a state of blissful oneness. In other words, I have tried to de-reify the psychoid substance into a metaphor for a dynamic, energetic, active vitalising process, which can be experienced imaginally, emotionally and sensuously. Although experienced subjectively, it is created by a relationship formed out of a need to animate the other in order to animate the needy self, to make the other (mother/analyst) psychosomatically disordered in order to share, understand and so perhaps heal the patient's disordered self.

The animating body is consubstantial between us and inside each of us, healing internalised interpersonal wounds and psychosomatic rupture. This forceful psychoid level of experience is affective in the metacommunications between the autonomic nervous sensations and symbols experienced between two persons. It is somatic in the sense that soma is understood as a body of intent and meaning. In regressed analytic relations, this process can be necessarily sickening and near-deadly, as well as erotic, healing and enlivening. Symbols and sensations are often similarly experienced: the analyst's dreams, fantasies and sensations belong equally to the patient and to the relationship, and so these contents feel simultaneously confusing, invasive and mutual, but demanding differentiation, interpretation and the making of a real sense of autonomy.

Thus, we can see how the patient's psychotic matter is necessarily mixed into the psychosomatic environment which the transference and countertransference activate. I have shown how a disturbing unanimity of mutual psychoid experience of pre-verbal projection, extraction (Bollas, 1987), identification and infection can be transformed, re-coordinated and healed. However, this mutative process can only be realised when the consubstantial 'animating body' has been lived out, thought through and so eventually translated into a separating but commonly understood language.

References

Bion, W. R. (1959). 'Attacks on Linking'. *International Journal of Psychoanalysis*, 40: 308–315.

Bion, W. R. (1962). *Learning from Experience*. London: William Heinemann.

Bollas, C. (1987). *The Shadow of the Object: Psychoanalysis of the Unthought Known*. London: Free Association Books.

Bollas, C. (1990). 'Regression in the Countertransference'. In *Master Clinicians on Treating the Regressed Patient*, Vol. 1. L. Bryce Boyer & P. Giovacchini, eds. Northvale, NJ and London: Jason Aronson.

Humbert, E. (1988). 'The Well-Springs of Memory'. *Journal of Analytical Psychology*, 33(1): 3–20.

Jung, C. (1970a). 'On the Nature of the Psyche'. In *The Structure and Dynamics of the Psyche*. Vol. 8 of *The Collected Works of C.G. Jung*. R. Hull, trans. 2nd edn. London: Routledge & Kegan Paul.

Jung, C. (1970b). *Mysterium Coniunctionis: An Inquiry Into the Separation and Synthesis of Psychic Opposites in Alchemy*. Vol. 14 of *the Collected Works of C.G. Jung*. R. Hull, trans. 2nd edn. London: Routledge & Kegan Paul

Jung, C. (1971). *Psychological Types*. Vol. 6 of *The Collected Works of C.G. Jung*. H. Baynes, trans. London: Routledge & Kegan Paul.
Jung, C. (1973). *Letters, Volume 1*. Selected and edited by G. Adler. London: Routledge & Kegan Paul.
Jung, C. (1993). 'The Psychology of the Transference'. In *The Practice of Psychotherapy*. Vol. 16 of *The Collected Works of C.G. Jung*. R. Hull, trans. London: Routledge & Kegan Paul.
Klein, M. (1946). 'Notes on Some Schizoid Mechanisms'. *International Journal of Psychoanalysis*, 27: 99–110.
McDougall, J. (1989). *Theatres of the Body: A Psychoanalytic Approach to Psychosomatic Illness*. London: Free Association Books.
Ogden, T. (1986). *The Matrix of the Mind: Object Relations and the Psychoanalytic Dialogue*. Northvale, NJ and London: Jason Aronson.
Peters, R. (1987). 'The Eagle and the Serpent: Or – The Minding of Matter'. *Journal of Analytical Psychology*, 32(4): 359–381.
Phillips, A. (1988). *Winnicott*. Cambridge, MA: Harvard University Press.
Rhode, E. (1994). *Psychotic Metaphysics*. London: Karnac Books.
Sacksteder, J. (1989). 'Psychosomatic Dissociation and False Self Development in Anorexia Nervosa'. In *The Facilitating Environment: Clinical Applications of Winnicott's Theory*. G. Fromm & B. Smith, eds. Madison, CT: International Universities Press.
Santayana, G. (1923). *Scepticism and Animal Faith: Introduction to a System of Philosophy*. New York: Scribner.
Stern, D. N. (1985). *The Interpersonal World of the Infant*. New York: Basic Books.
Wiener, J. (1994). 'Looking Out and Looking In'. *Journal of Analytical Psychology*, 39(3): 331–350.
Winnicott, D. (1954). 'Mind and Its Relation to the Psyche-Soma'. *British Journal of Medical Psychology*, 27(4): 201–209.

Chapter 6

Mind-body intimacies and pains

Unpublished, 1999

Much of what follows is about how to live a life where there is not enough 'good-enough' (Winnicott, 1953), how to live both within the limits of irreparable psychosomatic damage and of irreplaceable handicaps, lacks and losses and to live beyond the limitations of psychic self-knowledge and of psychic change. This means living within the constraints (and powers) of matter and bodies and the meanings we make of them personally and interpersonally. Such an ethic needs to incorporate deep ambivalence around desires, pleasures, pains and powers.

Psychoanalytic theory, along with related metapsychological and, therefore, philosophical modelling, must derive from working out interpersonal, clinical problems – and from non-transformational stuck or destructive relations as much as from transformational and creative experiences. I acknowledge my use of theoretical models whose origins are not derived from clinical theory but rather from philosophical systems and ideas. I make use of these because they help my thinking through problematic and provocative clinical experience without, I hope, being evasive, false or defensive.

What follows is also about the relationship between three realms of idea and action. Firstly, there are mind-body relations – philosophically, psychologically and as a practical matter. Secondly, there is psychopathology as a communication and revealer of mind-body relations. Thirdly, arising out of and implied by the first two realms is an emergent ethic which is not just a socio-cultural code but is post-synoptic in that it is ratio-centric yet not fixed, open to differences, to perpetual reforming and to unconscious emotional complexity. In other words, this is about achieving a good-enough life which incorporates the cunning of unconscious reason and unreason (even destructive chaos).

Much of my psychoanalytic work has been with savage and destructive borderline states. In order to understand the repeatedly destroyed possibility of understanding and health in these relations, I choose to use a neo-Spinozan mind-body identity philosophy, for example, that of Gilles Deleuze, Genevieve Lloyd and Susan James. I am also helped by Jung's idea of the psychoid, Donald Winnicott's writing on psyche-soma, Wilfred Bion's sense of beta elements and of transformation, as well as the work of Thomas Ogden, James Grotstein and Michael Eigen; and among analytical psychologists, Roderick Peters and Nathan Field.

DOI: 10.4324/9781003255826-7

I am working in a realm where little structural change seems possible. Yet something can and does happen intersubjectively and mutually. Furthermore, these relations go beyond, or make something different – something dangerous, disruptive yet desirable – out of the frames of psychoanalysis. I take on and take in the life of persons whose savage emotional minds necessarily manifest in savagely impulsive body actions and interactions. Within these environmental fields, emotional-mind elements or explosive and fragmenting mad thoughts metabolise and somatise as physical impulses, sensations and symptoms which are highly contagious. I need to enter this realm and be affected in order to be effective.

My motivation for using elements of a non-clinical philosophical tradition arises out of the need to make a valid sense of embodied minds, of psychosomatic functions and processes. I equally need to qualify these all-too-abstract philosophies by incorporating unconscious psychosomatic and psychotic emotions, actions and interactions of actual intersubjective experiences. In other words, this is a two-way process. Patients such as 'Annie', who I mention further on, and 'Pat', who I've written about earlier (Clark, 1996)[1] are, in a sense, radical philosophers, whom I wish to bring into the Stoa and introduce into dialogue with the Spinozan mind-body metaphysicians. Their 'pathology' of psyche-soma confusion – and our mutual experiences in this disharmonious zone – acts as an illustration of how current neo-Spinozan thinking can be adapted and applied psychologically and relationally (as in relations of nature-body-mind-ethics).

So, to jump in at the deep end, let me start with the 17th-century Spinozistic concept: 'the mind is the idea of the body'. Deleuze explains that this statement means that

> what we have is the idea of that which happens to our body, the idea of our body's affections, and it is only through such ideas that we know immediately our body and others, our mind and others (II, 12–31). So there is a correspondence between the affections of the body and the ideas of the mind, a correspondence by which these ideas represent these affections.
>
> (Deleuze, 1988, p. 87)

Furthermore,

> all that is action in the body is also action in the mind, and all that is passion in the mind is also passion in the body (III, 2, schol.: 'The order of actions and passions of our body is, by nature, at one with the order of actions and passions of the mind').
>
> (Deleuze, 1988, p. 88)

1 See Chapter Five (Eds.).

Genevieve Lloyd (1994) elaborates on the 'mind as the idea of the body' in regard to gender:

> To the extent that the powers and pleasures [this is Spinoza's phrase] of human bodies are sexually differentiated, it will then be quite appropriate for a Spinozist to speak of 'male' and 'female' minds. A female mind, would be one whose nature – and 'gladness' – reflect its status as idea of a female body.
>
> (Lloyd, 1994, p. 162)

For Spinoza, there is 'continuity between the natural body and the socialised body. The powers of individual bodies are enriched by good forms of social organisation which foster the collective pursuit of reason, which enhances human powers and enriches human pleasures' (p. 162). They are also diminished by bad forms of social organisation and by exclusion from good ones. '[I]f we take seriously the implications of Spinoza's theory of the mind, we must say also that female minds are formed by socially imposed limitations on the powers and pleasures of female bodies' (Lloyd, 1994, p. 164).

I would add to this gender theory the point that the socialised body includes the familied body, and 'social organisations' must include the family. More importantly, I would add to Spinoza's 'powers and pleasures' that there are also limits of power, impotencies, lacks, pains and out-of-control attacks on the co-ordinations of power and pleasure. In other words, I would add the deep pathologies of unconscious destructiveness and disorder.

A psychoanalytic adaptation of the metaphysical statement that the 'mind is the idea of the body' can be achieved by the following staged process of conceptual refinement:

- The mind is the idea of the body;
- The mind is the idea of the idea of the body;
- The mind is the idea of the idea of the relations within and between bodies;
- The mind is the idea of the ideas and images of body relations;
- The mind is the maker of meanings of the images and ideas of body relations;
- The psyche is that activity of mind that makes emotional (and rational) meanings of the images and ideas (ideas of images) of body relations.

All such 'ideas' as I have defined and described previously, are 'partial' or 'inadequate' (Lloyd, 1994, p. 18), that is, subjectively complex, fantastically distorted, only semi-conscious, largely unconscious, but energetic/libidinal. At base, these ideas emerge from the *prima materia* of preconceptions, psychoid beta elements, primary self, O. I know I should not conflate such diverse concepts from Jung, Bion and Winnicott, but I am so doing.

The mind-body parallel-identity hypothesis that I have now reached brings us close to Merleau-Ponty who, in *The Phenomenology of Perception*, describes how 'insofar as we are in the world through our body' and 'insofar as we perceive the world with our body', through 'remaking contact with the body and with the world, we shall also rediscover ourself, since, perceiving as we do with our body, the body is a natural self and, as it were, the subject of perception' (Merleau-Ponty, 1962, p. 206).

In *The Visible and the Invisible* (1968), Merleau-Ponty articulates a concept of flesh involving a unity of being which is meant to undercut the opposition between mental and physical, between knowing subject and knowing object. This perspective is also close to Winnicott's statement that:

> Out of the material of the imaginative elaboration of body functioning . . . the psyche is forged . . . The psyche therefore has a fundamental unity with the body through its relation both to the function of tissue and organs and to the brain, as well as through the way it becomes intertwined with it by new relationships developed in the individual's fantasy or mind, conscious or unconscious.
>
> (Winnicott, 1988, p. 52)

In 'Countertransference and the False Body' (1995), Susie Orbach looks at countertransference affects registered in the body of the therapist to see what light they can shed on the development of a corporeal sense of self. In extending Winnicott's notion of the false self to the false body, she links in with recent developments in our understanding of countertransference. She extends her discussion to include an appreciation of the psychotherapist's body within the therapeutic context and focuses on 'the meaning of the therapist's body in the therapeutic relationship' (Orbach, 1995, p. 6). Just as Winnicott elaborated on the false self, there is a false body self which she calls the 'false body':

> The baby whose physical needs are recognised, has the chance to develop a psychosomatic integrity. The baby whose physical gestures are misread or ignored will feel physically insecure. The mother's experience of the child's body, her projections onto it, her wishes for it, what she sees, give the child a particular sense of body.
>
> (Orbach, 1995, p. 6)

Orbach concludes:

> I want to suggest that in understanding the development of corporeality, we need to take note of the process by which the child, and here again I emphasise the daughter, takes in both the psychology of the mother and her body. She literally embodies the mother's physical presence and the mother's physicality. Her body as much as her psyche is composed of maternal introjects and if the maternal introject includes a mother's fear, loathing, discomfort or distress around her own body, this experience will be taken in by the girl in the process of her psyche-somatic development. It will form a core of her sense of self as crucial as her introjection of mother's psyche.
>
> (Orbach, 1995, p. 6)

From all this, I am now able to further expand my dual aspect approach and state two ideational perspectives:

1 By the 'body', I mean (and I am making this meaning) emotional human subject matter in action and interaction;
2 Body/body bits are not units of meaning but are psychosomatic/psychoid relations of meanings, intra and inter.

Although this is about unsymbolised body metacommunications, and since this 'body' self is to do with relations of meanings and is predicated upon an actual physical body throughout, I can still say, I am/we are also dealing with unconscious relations to mother's body, to father's body, to their bodies together and to the good/bad powers and impotencies of their relations.

I am talking about primal and primitive emotional psyche-soma relations. Emotional mind is emotional body, and emotional body has to mean emotional mind: pleased, pained, desirous, fearful and hating emotions are always somatic. They are communicated and, therefore, mutually shared psychosomatically and emotionally before they can possibly be conceived into thoughts and words and the creation of a sharable language. Sometimes, however, such psychoid beta elements can never be moved or developed into such transformational relationships.

The nature of mind-body relations and, therefore, ideas about the nature of these relations are paradoxically more evident and so more thinkable about in experiences of mind-body confusions and disorder, in states of psychosomatic pathology rather than in states of 'healthy' harmonious integration which only sometimes make for abstract and bloodless ideas and theories, whose lifelessness and lack of problematic energy fail to incorporate and do justice to the full emotional matter of this difficult issue.

Some of my motivation here is to rectify what I see to be the unhelpful effects of a Jungian hierarchical and splitting metapsychology. Firstly, there is sometimes an over-emphasis on intrapsychic content and, thus, on a solitary transcendent function. Secondly, there is over-dividing of ego, personal unconscious and archetypal/collective unconscious, let alone of ego and 'the Self'. A more appropriately alive dynamic model can surely locate each of these psychic modes within each other. Thirdly, there is a hierarchy of values where ego and consciousness are evaluated in terms of strength/weakness, capacity/incapacity and unconscious layers, and the 'Self' is seen as increasingly deep and therefore, numinous. Unhelpful consequences of this metapsychology include a useless collusion which reinforces the patient's and the analyst's narcissistic defences, a defensive allegiance to a false and evasive optimistic teleology and a repression of unchangeable destructiveness and of the psychotic core.

Like Gilles Deleuze in *Anti-Oedipus* (1977), I wish instead to operate in a disrupting realm of emotional matter, of 'unpredictable rhizomes' and 'living machines', but also including a full recognition of perennial disorder, destructiveness and pain (as well as desire and pleasure). This helps me analytically to use a fierce recognition of conscious and unconscious personal and interpersonal destructiveness, especially compulsive attacks on health, the resentfully envied other's (my) healthy core and/or healthy body (as well as valuing disruptive creativity).

This moves us back into the nature of the intersubjective work-world that I'm coming from. This is a chronic world where therapy must incorporate the unchangeable parts of persons, parts which went irreparably wrong, atrophied and so handicapped pre-verbally and pre-symbolically. This involves work in the paleo-mammalian and reptilian psychoid realms, not of so-called 'normal' neuroticism.

Extremely borderline and psychotic persons are, for various reasons, so sensitive to the emotional wounds of lack and attack that they have largely lost or never developed an affective capacity (a contained, self-containing state) from which to reflect, think and feel sufficiently clearly. Thus, they have not been able to achieve a symbolising function and, therefore, functioning relational energy. They are unable to 'do life', to live in a peopled world without being forced by urgent uncontrollable impulses to act out their starved needs or to angrily 'act against', to launch projective identifications against others (my) envied inner goods or to suck them out with extractive introjections or implode and attack their hated self. Their projective identifications go into me, and they desperately take my vital stuff out of me. Yet it is because I see, understand and so can interpret these doings as necessary metacommunications (as well as defences) that we are sometimes able to find a mutative remembrance and mourning.

I receive projective identifications as metacommunications and, therefore, revelations of the subject's suffering of, and thence attempts to manage and reorganize, their bad/good fantasy-experiences of the parent's conscious and unconscious intersubjective relations. These include their emotionally loaded physical and part-object relations and attitudes.

Often in such situations, there is little or no movement from paranoid-schizoid to the depressive or between the two. Such persons are endlessly thrown around within paranoid-schizoid places, blaming the bad world, feeling empty inside. How, then, can therapy with me become a transformational object relationship, where I am made and used as a processing psychoid mother, the haveable 'thinking breast'?

Perhaps one way is to sense that as well as a breast, I may *also* be used as a man. Projectively, I am the receiver of people's passionate ideals, desires, hates, fears and other good/bad primitive object expectations and experiences of man. I am for them, for me with myself and so for us together, a man's body, a male brain, a father's hard and bristly body with male desires and aggression (let alone actual smells, hormones and testosterone, let alone a man's limitations). I find I am used as a 'thinking breast', but also as an imaginative or fantastic (fantasy-making) penis, an 'able penis'. A fantastically able penis enables fantasies and desires and makes such fantasies and desires actual. It makes male links, connections and bridges; it makes babies; stretches to protection as an able guard; is a weapon for protection and destruction; it makes love and/or war. It is an object with a spermatic halo or demonic horns; a wand with good or bad magic powers; a healing or poisonous injection. However, my experience in these relationships is not only as an enabling or disabling penis but also as an attacked and thus disabled, enfeebled penis – and from there, (sometimes), a penis that recovers, rises from apparent death and regenerates, before being enviously and angrily unmanned again. Yet it is through this use of me as a thinking breast and a fantastic, able penis, through this use of me as a wound-taker and survivor, that a paranoid-schizoid-to-depressive relational dynamic between and in us can somewhat lessen the thrown-around-within-the-paranoid-schizoid-state to something more interpersonally humane.

The emotional projective identifications that fire into and extractive introjections that are sucked out from the analyst as thinking breast and able penis are part-object embodied gender metaphors for the healthy and benevolently powerful containing and transforming emotional mind. But due to unstoppable envy and resentment, these 'parts' are also repeatedly attacked, and have to survive and make good.

Borderline and psychotic symptoms can be seen as desperate, failing attempts to manage relational acts of dangerous madness to make them seem 'safe' and 'good'. These maddening attempts get re-constellated in the therapeutic transference-countertransference relationship and can nearly drive analysts mad, make them bad and infect them with sickness and pain – at least until analysts can think, link and say something right enough, clearly enough (which might well be to say 'enough is enough'). And this 'until' might take a long time . . .

'Annie'

Annie's mother was an elective mute but otherwise expressed no emotion except a strong disapproval and fear of sex, manifest in repressive denial. According to mother, Annie's conception occurred when there was the one occasion of sex between mother and father, and that had been forced. Annie loved her market-gardener father and struggled with her oedipal desires and victories. She came to see me because of obsessional, 'perverse' sexual thoughts and compulsive coprophilic urges in which she wanted to use her turds as a penis in order to enter a man's (and now my) orifices. My reactions ranged between trepidation, fear, disgust, indifference and bewilderment. I was finally able to experience, through an embodied countertransference, her own embodied parental sexual confusion and disorder and the painful diverted desires and goals. My linking interpretations were, I thought, very clever, but they were quite useless. But when I told her what effects her physical impulses, desires and imaginings had on me (couched in correctly-enough framed language), she smiled genuinely and warmly and said: 'At last. Thank you for your physical honesty', and left therapy.

Such analytic relationships can sometimes move through to a particular, mutually shared, transformational experience. The analyst observes, responds (sometimes reactively as well as interpretively) and so affects and changes analysands' expressions of their unconsciously lived worlds with their problematic relations of good and bad parts. The analyst's observations and affective positions occur through informed imagination and somatic sensations. This is because mindful imagination and powerful passions of the body are two aspects of the same subjective substance. This analytic mind-body presence and openness can be the countertransferential receptor of unconscious metacommunications of the patient's internalised and embodied family confusions, destructive impulses, interactions and acts. Having received this mix, the analytic mind-body may attain an intuitive knowledge of the depths of the patient's lived-in-world and its problems. But, an affective transformation can only occur if the analyst's state of reflective imagination is itself a transforming process (and not maddening) in the mindful-as-possible analyst. Furthermore, it is only transformative when, at some level, the patient intuits this mutuality in their embodied imagination, in their sense of aliveness and intelligence. We also find that we can meet our relational memories in the sensations of our visceral flesh. Ultimately an incorporated experience of each other and with each other may be found or made, which is a psychosomatic re-coordination for both of us, until it is yet again destroyed by psychotic envy and so demands further struggles for regeneration – if we've got the energy and nerve!

But what if change and gratitude are rendered impossible by unchangeable, destructive, envious forces? The primary object of narcissistic envy is the other's perceived intrinsic power of mind and body (which later becomes enviable intelligence, wit, beauty and strength). This is a power to get, make, have and increase an apparently beautiful self and life (which later become enviable good objects and relations). Envy of the other's separateness, health, good insides, good outsides and *joie de vivre* leads to a humiliating of one's own expressions of excitement, a shaming or harming of one's 'beloved body', hurting of one's pride. Such envious attacks reveal the 'fragility of the good'.

'Jim'

Jim's[2] father permanently harmed Jim's baby brother. He was later sent to prison for having been guilty of GBH in a pub brawl. Mother took in lodgers who were also lovers. Jim was bisexual, beat up his women and was masochistic with his male lovers. He looked at me with icy hatred and spite. He terrified me. I dreamt of a snake preserved in a jar, which emerged as a hissing, spiky, Gabon viper, and it was him. Later, he literally hissed and spat at me. He peed on my toilet floor and didn't flush the loo. He told me venomously that I was a wimp, a weed, a cock-less runt, a cunt. He told me how impressed or daunted his lovers were of his cock and his sexual aggression. He angered and he hurt me. However, very much later on, he told me how women, in fact, found his body disgusting. I said, 'And your mind?'. He said, 'No, that is what men feel. And do you?' I said, 'I have'. He stayed with me, I stuck it out (so to speak) and survived for 12 years – and he lived on without killing anyone. From my position of 'negative capability',[3] that in itself is substantial enough.

2 'Jim' is a fictionalised clinical case that Clark used extensively in his teaching seminars and later papers. See also Chapters Seven, Nine, Ten and Thirteen (Eds.).

3 'Negative capability' is a term coined by Keats which Bion (1970) applied to psychoanalysis. Keats wrote: 'Negative Capability, that is, when a man is capable of being in uncertainties, mysteries, doubts, without any irritable reaching after fact and reason' (Keats, 1817, in Bion, 1970, p. 125) (Eds.).

Conclusion

It is the personal, interpersonal and intergenerational history of the somatic psyche acting in intersubjective human relations that makes meaning or destroys it. Meanings may be so emotionally frightening that they remain unprocessable and so unconscious (as they have done, possibly for ancestral years). They can only be manifest and expressed physically or somatically through compulsive, addictive or self-destructive acts and relations. But even so, sometimes, a long-lived analytical relationship is a real achievement.

I have been trying to find or create a metalanguage for a particular sensed and felt intersubjective experience that both analyst and analysand can be moved into. It is essentially preverbal and outside language and yet is still to be found in our humanly known world of language. It is a situation where, for example, subject and object, inside and outside, imagination and sensation are not appropriate or useful in distinguishing binary concepts for the experience. Yet I can, of course, only use a metaphorical language for a subjectivity of perception and experience that is in itself actually not metaphoric, not 'as if', and is outside the symbolising function. It is truer to this being together immanently in a psychoid beta chaos, not to say that it is about anything else. It is not going anywhere else. Here and now, our mutual psyche-soma is not symbolisable. Perhaps what I can say, though, is what I, and we, have been making is a sort of waking dream between and around us, a shared reverie in our common flesh.

Postscript

This paper has committed at least four offences against theoretical, political and psychological correctness:

1 It suggests that minds are sexed;
2 It says the analyst-as-object is not only (at least) two sexes but that his/her actual embodied sexual gender also matters;
3 It says that sometimes emotionally archaic somatised symptoms may not, or even cannot, be transformed or developed into symbolised functions and processes;
4 It says that under such conditions as these interpretations, fulfilling the desire for change, sorting out of deep confusion by processes of understanding and linking, etc. are often not possible, and should not even be expected/attempted.

References

Bion, W. (1970). *Attention and Interpretation*. London: Tavistock.

Clark, G. (1996). 'The Animating Body: Psychoid Substance as a Mutual Experience of Psychosomatic Disorder'. *Journal of Analytical Psychology*, 41(3): 353–368 (Chapter Five, this book).

Deleuze, G. (1977). *Anti-Oedipus*. R. Hurley, M. Seem & H. Lane, trans. New York: Viking Press (Original French ed., 1972).

Deleuze, G. (1988). *Spinoza: A Practical Philosophy*. P. Hurley, trans. San Francisco: City Lights (Original French ed., 1970).

Lloyd, G. (1994). *Part of Nature*. Cornell: Cornell University Press.

Merleau-Ponty, M. (1962). *Phenomenology of Perception*. C. Smith, trans. London: Routledge (Original French ed. 1945).

Merleau-Ponty, M. (1968). *The Visible and Invisible*. A. Lingis, trans. Northwestern: Northwestern University Press (Original French ed, 1964).

Orbach, S. (1995). 'Countertransference and the False Body'. In *Winnicott Studies: The Journal of The Squiggle Foundation*, 10. London: Karnac, pp. 3–13.

Winnicott, D. (1953). 'Transitional Objects and Transitional Phenomena: A Study of the First Not-Me Possession'. *International Journal of Psycho-Analysis*, 34: 88–97.

Winnicott, D. (1988). *Human Nature*. London: Free Association Books.

Chapter 7

A Spinozan lens onto the confusions of borderline relations

Journal of Analytical Psychology, 2006[1]

Introduction

The structural organisation of persons labelled as borderline is traditionally described in terms of the Kleinian model of severe splitting of self and object representations (Kernberg, 1984). However, this model does not provide an adequate description of the destructive and seductive enactments of borderline disordered patients nor does it capture the persistent countertransferential experience of psychosomatic infection generated by issues of identification and separation.

It is difficult to retain the analytic functions of thinking-linking-interpreting, imagination, alpha functioning and reverie (Bion, 1962) in these dangerous and destructive conditions. In order to keep a stable analytic perspective, I use a Spinozan and neo-Spinozan lens (Hampshire, 1951/1987; Lloyd, 1996; Yovel, 1999), which is a particular position or approach to both internal and interpersonal psychic and psychosomatic, 'body-mind' relations. This is a so-called 'dual-aspect substance monism' in which mind and body are understood as representations of a single 'substance', and which I argue can also be extended into interpersonal relations.

Borderline psychopathology

I am using the term Borderline Personality Disorder to describe the psychopathology of persons for whom developmental lacks and failures have caused an inability to distinguish or differentiate between fantasy and reality, inside and outside, self and other and who are often in a chronic and acute state of mind-body confusion. Their personal and interpersonal relations and behaviours are pre-symbolic/anti-symbolic, destructive and psychosomatically disordered and disordering.

They form not so much a false or narcissistic self to avoid a real self but, rather, an exaggeratedly desperate, angry and often enraged pre-self or frozen latent self,

1 Originally presented at the Journal of Analytical Psychology 50th Anniversary Conference, St Anne's College, Oxford, England on 8th April 2005. Published in 2006 in the *Journal of Analytical Psychology*, 51(1): 67–86. Reprinted with permission © Wiley Publishing. Minor corrections, additions and copy editing has been applied to this version (Eds.).

DOI: 10.4324/9781003255826-8

fearfully and anti-socially trying to assert its emergence into existence in an annihilating environment. In such conditions, these persons impulsively and/or unconsciously act out. They cannot tolerate frustration and their fantasy of omnipotent control of others (and the world) leads to extreme destructive/self-destructive behaviour.

These psychotic-like states and relations can be understood as developmentally emerging from intra-uterine psychic distress and from an early lack of maternal/family emotional connection. This results in a primitive psychosomatic attachment, in which the parental relations to the infant/child, to each other and to the peopled world is psychologically autistic. Such a parental absence is compounded by their relational and oedipal confusion, and so also by their inability to mediate an over-sensitive infant's/child's mass of experience. Thus his/her unmanaged/unmanageable confusion is exacerbated. The chronic and acute core psychic object (or no-object) is an original and repeated lack of loving attachment, of any real connection, of psychosomatic ordering. There is an angry and desperate grief at such original failure and lack, rather than losses that can be mourned. It is psychically unrealistic to expect to transform a position of fundamental fear, disappointment and impotent anger at unmet primary needs into a healthy acquiescence based on trust.

Outrage at this 'fate' is projected into mother/other/analyst/all relationships. This is often a non-verbal or pre-verbal communication at a 'psychoid' level, through psychosomatic infectious, contagious and coercive forces. Toxic projective identifications can be the only form of intra and inter-psychic expression, communication and management of the tense relations between defences (splitting), attack (shitting and spitting), need (hunger) and communication (invasion/seduction). These identificatory processes stem from and work at a primitive personal and interpersonal psychosomatic level, affecting the body-mind of self and other. Grotstein's (1997) phrase 'body-mind' captures both the primitive psychoid level of the body+mind relationship and also the Spinozan mind/body/matter univocalism, a concept which I shall shortly explicate and elaborate in my development of Spinoza's theory that 'mind is the idea of the body'.

Borderline 'beta *confusa*'[2] as a psychosomatic field of communication

Jung, with independent prescience, recognised a mutually shared, inter-subjective psychic field as a third aspect of the analytic relationship in, and through, which both persons are changed. It is implicit in much of his theoretical thinking and

2 Here, Giles is combining Bion's (1962) beta elements and Jung's use of the alchemical term *massa confusa*. By beta elements, Bion means raw sense data, inchoate elements, raw emotional material that has not been processed. He writes of how an infant 'filled with painful lumps of faeces, guilt, fears of impending death, chunks of greed, meanness and urine, evacuates these bad objects into the breast that is not there. As it does so the good object [mother] turns the no-breast into a breast, the faeces and urine into milk, the fears of impending death and anxiety into feelings of love and generosity' (Bion, 1963, p. 31) doing so out of her capacity for reverie and alpha function (Eds.).

becomes explicit in 'The Psychology of the Transference', in particular in the introduction to that essay (Jung, 1993, *CW* 16, see paras. 180–181). In 'The animating body'[3] (1996) I put forward the hypothesis that the psychoid can be experienced and understood as not only intra-psychic but also as inter-psychic and as an active/infectious third 'psychoid' realm or, metaphorically, as an 'affectively loaded atmosphere' around us. This is the psychosomatic field of information and communication where my alpha-dreaming and thinking (Bion, 1967, 1992; Plaut, 1994) needs to operate and so to be used therapeutically where and when possible.

These clinical positions and attitudes are not dissimilar to Balint's (1968) 'harmonious, interpenetrating mix-up', Ogden's (1994) idea of the 'coercive pressure of the 'subjugating third' in which both of us are changed' and Britton's (1998) 'triangular space' in which the analyst is both 'a participant in a relationship and observed by a third person as well as being an observer of a relationship between two people'. My point is that this immersion is largely experienced via bodily impact on the analyst and analysand. The analysand expresses the confusion of the analytic relationship via embodied enactments and body-based symbolisation.

Two clinical examples 'Rose'

Going quite literally purple with rage, Rose leapt up and somehow flew across my room. She smashed her forehead against the wall. I said, oh-so-analytically correctly, 'Now sit down'. I went on to say, 'You are showing me just how infuriating and hurtful the unmoving me is'. 'Useless', she said and ran out of my flat door and hit her head even harder against the outside wall. She cut her forehead quite badly, and blood ran down her face. We were both shocked. I took her back inside and helped her staunch the blood with a wet towel at the kitchen sink. I said, 'I think I've really got the message now'. 'No, you haven't', she said, 'You never will, not really; not enough'. Since the bleeding and her affective state were out of control, I got her an ambulance and sent her off to Casualty.

She had broken through all boundaries, broken through my frames, through our skins, and I had gone along with it all. An acting-out and self-hurting like that of Rose expresses and temporarily relieves the frustrations of unheard and unreceived emotional needs, of psychic pain and impotent rage. It shouts as a vital, urgent communication: 'Look what you've made me do', which also means (from the position of borderline subject/object identification), 'Look what you've done to me. See how much you've hurt me'. As an attack on analytic competence, she is saying, 'Just look at what you've not seen or understood; look just how useless you are'.

Such an acting out in the session does a lot of work. It is a violent expression of a broken self in order to break my/our boundaries, to break into me-as-analyst, to change me into a non-analyst, into a parent-lover and a beloved enemy. It is a way of breaking into the analyst-as-unconnected mother's psyche-soma, into

3 See Chapter Five (Eds.).

analyst-father's desired but forbidden mind and body, into the parental body-bed and, at the same time, trying to break up these relationships. Analytically I have to be induced or forced to suffer the shock of the attack in order to activate and realise the message affectively, and as a result, 'do something' about the frustrations and pains of such thwarted primary love (Balint, 1952). Perhaps all we can realistically 'do' is work to understand, grieve and perhaps mourn personal and analytic limitations as thoroughly as possible (Hinshelwood, 1991).

However, for borderline persons, such an analytic position of apparently 'mere' detached observations and interpretations is experienced as an outrageous repeat of the original failures. There is an ever-increasing envy and an outraged sense that 'It's all right for you. I shall have to disturb you out of your smugness, your emotional distance and indifference. I shall pull you, force you or force into you a world of the pain of sickening limitations like mine. So my pain is yours too; it has become our pain; we are in this together in the same way'.

In order to 'break through', Rose had four leitmotifs that she expressed in the form of yells. They were 1) 'I hate you so much', 2) 'You just don't get it', 3) 'I want to know all of you', 4) 'You've got to love me' and a sarcastic, sadistic fifth question, 5) 'Are you all right'? She described her mother as a 'harmless blank' and her father as a 'rigid conservative with no imagination'. There was ostensibly no personal traumatic event, though there was an intergenerational legacy of horror to which I shall refer shortly, via a dream of mine about Rose.

Two years into our work together, Rose dreamt:

> I see that everything in space is just black matter and white nothingness. Then I see that in close-up, under a microscope, matter is not really solid at all, but full of holes; then I realise that this black matter is one vast black hole and that the white nothingness is empty space. In between the black and the white there is an invisible crack where ordinary matter should be, but here all matter and life have been crushed out of existence, or maybe have never come into existence.

These shocking images stem from and express Rose's experience of parental absence, alienation and so, too, of annihilation. She said of this dream, 'I've always thought that the world was not really solid. Nor am I. Nor is anyone. Nor are you. As you sit there now, I just want to crack your bloody skull open'. Then, after a pause, she added, 'Those who have never had, shall never have. I am "Goods Damaged Irreparably"; that's my family fate, and you're part of it. I hate you so much I want to kill you'.

I would say that Rose hated that I could never give or be what she wanted, or as she put it, 'needed'. She was afraid that she would succeed in hurting me or killing me. And she was afraid that, like mother and her parental world, I would suddenly become, or nightmarishly reveal myself to be, either (or both) an extractory autistic mechanical breast, sucking her into its cold, hard black matter, or as an ejecting autistic mechanical breast, spitting her out into white, empty nothingness. The needed other was an autistic mind-body-breast, certainly not a person from whom to get a good drink or drink of the good. Again, I had to know that she lived with an abject loneliness, a 'disintegrating anxiety' that Hobson (1974) called 'the basic problem of psychotherapy'.

The imagery of Rose's 'Space dream' reveals her pre-structured and chaotic psyche. This dream and her feelings arising out of it are about an emotionally unmet infant's skinless and bodiless non-substance. An 'autistic family' leaves the child with a transparent, invisible and insensible non-self. Although such a non-self intrinsically and urgently needs to be seen and sensed as psycho-somatically real and substantial, it is also afraid to be known. Such a person's need is mixed with a primitive confusion and anxiety, including a fear of being seen and known at all. Surfaces, skin, flesh and insides, their own and that of others (the zones that mediate relations to self and relations between self and others) become nervous psychic zones. Yet it is through these, as manifest in the transference, that a symbolic experience tries to get organised and ordered. We can now say that the wish to hit and 'crack' me and herself was an urge to connect and reach, to make herself and the two of us together substantially and consubstantially real, to express hate at separateness and absence and to break into and devour, or invade in order to possess. Her wish to 'crack your bloody skull open' meant to angrily hurt me for my unfeeling separateness, to break and get into my head as body and mind; to kill me as an act of impotent rage made potent through an embodied transference-countertransference. Furthermore, she wished to do all this to herself, too, such was her self-loathing. And, of course, I was an extension of her desirous but thwarted body-self. Finally, 'crack' was Rose's word for her vagina, so again, here, my body-mind 'is' an object for her desiring body-mind.

Not long after Rose's dream, I dreamt that I was looking down on the Rift Valley of Africa. In the dream I heard this described as 'the crack of Africa'. In my dream, Africa appeared as both a human/woman's body and as a vast, inhuman desert stretching out beyond the 'crack' of the Rift Valley. The Rift was a place of volcanoes, of the Olduvai Gorge and, in its innermost 'crack', lush with animal and vegetable life. The capital of this dream Africa was Warsaw. Not only were Rose's family refugees from Warsaw, but it struck me how possible punning meanings of the name Warsaw ('war-sore', 'saw war') were to do with my countertransferential experiences of and ideas about Rose.

I understand my dream as a comment on Rose's dream, as my idea of her self-state, and as a representation of our shared psychosomatic landscape formed by her. Without actually referring to my dream, I was able to speak to her states through it. She had little time for my interpretations, but in response to something I said, she came up with two remarkably 'Spinozan' statements about her confused and 'bad' self or body-self: 'My actions are my only real thoughts', and 'My body is my brain, and since it's such an ugly and useless body, I have an ugly and useless mind'.

'Jim'

Jim described his mother as 'vacant and passive', as 'cold, hard and hollow' and as 'a nothing, nowhere woman'. She was attacked and beaten by her violent husband

(Jim's father) during and before her pregnancy. Therefore, this violence was part of Jim's foetal experience: the limits or failures of maternal protection and her fear. Jim said that she 'just blanked out' on his infantile and childhood rages. He became very hurt and angry whenever he felt that I was apparently unaffected by his rage.

His psychopathic father had left before Jim was born. They had never since met or contacted each other. We called him 'the Good bad-father'. His mother's partner, a step-father figure, drew Jim into 'exciting-frightening sex' with him from the age of eleven until he was seventeen. Jim initiated many of their encounters. He told me that he 'reckoned that I was a better fuck than my mother'. We called him 'the Bad good-father'.

Jim was an ostensibly aggressive, bisexual, sadomasochistic skinhead, with a conspicuous tattoo of a viper on his arm. He was in repeated trouble with the police, mainly for vandalism. He lived out a chaotic, compulsive, destructive and self-destructive sexuality that was split between homosexual encounters, in which he took a masochistic position, and sadistic enactments with women. No sexual encounters could ever extend beyond a fleeting acting out of masturbatory fantasies, which is what he both wanted and wished to change. To enable him to stay with me in the analytic relationship was, therefore, a major endeavour. I had to be very firm with boundaries and (initially) give clear and simple interpretations, but also to be tolerant of his necessary abuse and intimidations of me.

Jim came into my analytic world in order to explode noisily and messily. In the early days, he left my toilet unflushed and the bathroom scattered with torn paper. He regularly called me a 'feeble cunt' and a 'little dickhead', thereby simultaneously attacking and belittling mother/women, himself and me. Initially, he aroused in me a stomach-churning fear: I felt that he strongly 'out-testosterone-ed' me, and later, through his anxieties and nightmares about getting stuck in s-bends and tight paces, he induced in me a sickening sense of claustrophobia. I think these were necessary transferential/countertransferential representations of his affective sexual relations: an abuse of power to compensate for his insecurities and impotence; intimidation and aggression to cover his anxieties and fears. As with Rose, Jim's angry destructiveness was motivated by an abject anguish around an experience of fundamental defeat, a primary lack and loneliness. Our achievement was that he stayed with me for over seven years, and that he did not kill himself or anybody else.

His very aggressive and anxious presence emanated the message: 'Do not let me know that you know that I was never really conceived. Do not know me too much. Do not look into me and see the empty heart beyond the fury, the empty space beyond the chaotic borderline spin'. He once said that he felt that he was 'a half-alive abortion . . . and best left that way'.

Jim's cathedral dream

> I am screwing a Gothic cathedral through its west doors, holding on to its outstretched arms, transepts, I think they are called. It is a very spiky, sharp and painful body to have to fuck. I know that if I screw it really violently and hard, it will soften up. So I do this, but as it becomes softer, it feels wet and disgusting.

> Like a girl. I lose my erection and can't come. Then suddenly, this foul wet cunt cathedral disappears from beneath me. It becomes nothing. I am now nowhere, so I know I'll just have to explode, which will have no bloody effect in empty space, of course.

He then added the autistic comment, 'Space is actually harder than hard'. The morning after this dream, Jim told me how he 'pissed and yelled my guts out in a church. I mean, what else could I do?' I responded, 'You do that here'. With contempt and fury, he replied, 'No! I did it *there*, dickhead; get it!' This was spat at or into me with such venom that I was physically shocked and shaken. I felt sick – an unmanageable invasion of, or possession by, both hot and cold fear. For Jim, acting out was the only realisation and expression of how matters are when there is no symbolic 'as if'.

Jim went on exploding in many bloody ways. If I was apparently not affected enough, he would disturb our universe until he psychosomatically moved me.

Jim's sexual destruction of the Gothic cathedral was both a destruction of me (mind and body) and of the transcendent function between us, as well as any depressive possibilities. The maddening sucking hollow of psychotic lack was not even proto-symbolic; it was anti-symbolic. Unconscious contents and processes vaporised and became as nothing. In effect, there was no accessible unconscious. Instead of symbolization, there was somatisation and an invasive attack on his own and other (my) body-minds.

Jim's cathedral was a needed body-mind to be aggressively and sexually possessed and controlled, but then ultimately found not to be controlled at all. This meant also possessing, affecting and changing my mind and my body (which, to the unwitting Spinozan, Jim are the same thing). However, the emasculated or feminised body is then felt to be disgusting and so is hated.

Furthermore, under these sadistically sexualised objects, there is an utter lack of contact and connection. Behind and within the attacked object is no-object. So the explosions continue, making and destroying other/mother ad infinitum. Jim wanted me to be both a sharp object which he could forcibly dominate, invade and enter, and also to be the Good bad-father, and so probably also a father joined to a good mother.

I am able to understand Jim's disturbed and disturbing mind as a demonstration of a radical metaphysics of mind-body identity relations. The cathedral dream is the stuff of his internal and external relations, of the 'rough trade' to him, indeed of our rough trading.

A Spinozan and neo-Spinozan perspective on the body-mind

It is now appropriate that I say something about Spinozan theory and how I use Spinozan concepts. My 'Spinozan thinking' also incorporates a particular intellectual ancestry including the Spinozan pantheism of Herder, the Absolute Idealists,

Heine, Santayana's celebratory naturalism and the more recent neo-Spinozan work of Hampshire (1994, 2002), Bennett (1984), Donagan (1988), Lloyd (1994, 1996), Deleuze (1988), Montag (1999), Montag and Stolze (1997) and Yovel (1999).

Spinoza's metaphysic is that there is one substance which is perceived and understood as either extended matter and/or as thought, mind or idea. These are the two apparent 'attributes' of the same single substance. From this derives the so-called Spinozan 'pantheism': God or nature, where 'nature' means both the matter of things and the laws or ways of the universe. As emotional, thinking and physical beings, we humans are one of many 'modes', mental and physical manifestations or representations of the one substance. Both our perceptions of the world and of value and morality are relative. Understanding and acceptance (*acquiescentia mentis*) of these laws of nature and of our human condition as a part of them, and, therefore, the dilemma of our paradoxical non-freedom/freedom of choice and our passivity/agency within such a determined universe, is the issue of the ethical life. The *conatus,* or the inherent striving for self-preservation, motivates all things, including humans who have three basic affects or emotions: desire, pleasure/joy and pain/sadness.

The Spinozan concepts that are most useful to me in the analytic setting are the *conatus*, the 'mind as the idea of the body', and his related theories of 'emotions, passions and actions'. I have extended and adapted these into a language of psychodynamic relevance. Spinoza's concept of the *conatus* is important in my analytic work because it describes the inherent endeavour or striving to persist in being 'the drive for self-maintenance against disruptive forces coming from inside and outside the organism' (Hampshire, 2002). Another meaning of *conatus* is striving to increase the power of action: a power to exercise powers, a power to acquire new powers (Lloyd, 1996) or, as Curley explains, it involves a striving for an increase in the power of action, which for Spinoza is joy (Curley, 1988, p. 115).

The *conatus* is also analytically important as it is about the mind as idea of the body, corporeality and embodiment: bodies, body-bits and bodily relations. 'When the striving is related to mind and body together, it is called "appetite"' (Lloyd, 1994, p. 74). In *Ethics*, Spinoza identified 'appetite' in this sense as the 'very essence' of a person (p. 74). 'Desire, joy and reason come together in the *conatus* of mind as idea of body' (Lloyd, 1996, p. 89). The *conatus* of mind as idea of body is where imagination, reason and joy come together; it is where I experience the expressed identity of mind and body, in my appetites and desires, my pleasures and pains, my joy and sadness (Lloyd, 1996). The *conatus* is an energetic process where mind and body come together; it is the energy through which 'substance' is represented as 'modes', that is, through which 'substance' individuates. Finally, the *conatus* as 'my' personal *conatus* is my own individual nature naturing by striving to preserve and to power my idiosyncratic, emotional, relational, social and rational self.

Yovel, in his 1991 paper 'Transcending mere survival', extends the idea of the Spinozan *conatus* to include an idea of a *conatus intelligendi*, which he says has two implications: 1) that 'by their natural *conatus*, human beings strive to exist in an interpreted, meaning endowed way' (p. 55); and 2) that '*conatus* entails the quest for infinity' (in Yovel, 1999, p. 51). I suggest that this hypothetical *conatus intelligendi* can be interpreted as the epistemophilic impulse, which has its origins in the infantile need to manage pain and frustration by getting into mother's body, into the parental bed and coupling, into their body-mind. It is the drive within the infant's/child's ruthless (partly sadistic) and epistemophilic curiosity and exploration of the world. Excessive frustrations in this fantastic realm contribute to angry borderline defences and to their re-constellation in the psychotic transference. A topical application of Spinoza, including the idea of the *conatus*, can also be found in the neuroscientist Damasio's book *Looking for Spinoza; Joy, Sorrow and the Feeling Brain* (2003).

I use Spinoza's concept of 'the mind as the idea of the body' as part of my thinking through of mind-body relations and psychosomatic identifications. My position is that the mind and the body are to be understood univocally. This complements and relativises the usual thinking in terms of causal relations. I suggest that a psychodynamic adaptation and elaboration of Spinoza's metaphysical statement that the 'mind is the idea of the body' can be achieved by a staged process of conceptual refinement, thus:[4]

1 The emotional mind is the idea of the 'passions and actions' of the body and of bodies.
2 The mind is conscious and unconscious ideas of, and concerns about, what has happened, is happening, is going to happen to the body from the inside and from the outside; therefore, also what the body desires is frustrated by the fears of itself and of others.
3 All such 'ideas' of body/bodies are subjectively complex, fantastically distorted, semi-conscious or unconscious, but energetically affective.
4 The mind is an emotional ideation process of management (for example, splitting, what Klein (1935) calls paranoid-schizoid thinking, etc.) of emotional psyche-soma relations to bodies and to body-bits. The mind thinks in order to manage the vicissitudes of emotional-physical needs, appetites, desires, frustrations and fears concerning other-minded (emotional and thinking) bodies and bits (breast, penis, etc.).
5 Mind-body-brain development, and therefore, the development of images and ideas, emerges out of the relations between personal/internal mind and other minds-bodies-brains, as well as with the contingencies of the material world as it affects the subject.
6 The mind is the psychic structural formation, the emergent image and idea (preconceptions, conceptions, phantasies, thoughts, words) of body, brain and environment, of biological, neurological and relational development; i.e., mind is images, thoughts and words of the development of internal and external psychic relations.

4 An earlier version of these stages can be found in Chapter Six (Eds).

7 Donagan summarises Spinoza's mind-body system thus: 'The complex idea of your body that is the primary constituent of your mind represents your body, and derivatively its environment, but only as they are disclosed by your idea of its affections' (Donagan, 1988, p. 144). Most succinctly, Rosenthal (1989, p. 129) paraphrases this concept thus: 'I exist in that I think as a body'.

In Spinozan terms, the mind is made up of desires, pleasures and pains and by emotional ideas of the body, bodies and body relations. I would expand this trio into a wider complex of emotional relations (internal and interpersonal) that make for a sort of *jouissance* of affects and the tensions between them. *Jouissance* was Lacan's word, but then taken up by the psychoanalyst Michael Eigen (1998), and it is from the latter that I have constructed my own stoic and psychodynamic model, largely for the private benefit of my own psychological thinking. I use this diagram to help me think through, clarify and order the psychosomatic beta disorder in the transference. A bit like Bion's grid, it is a lens of observation into emotions and their relations, but here specifically focused for analytic transferential, countertransferential and interpretive use. (Note from Eds. The reader may find it helpful to consult the Appendix at the end of the chapter for further clarification of the jouissance grid).

The *jouissance* grid

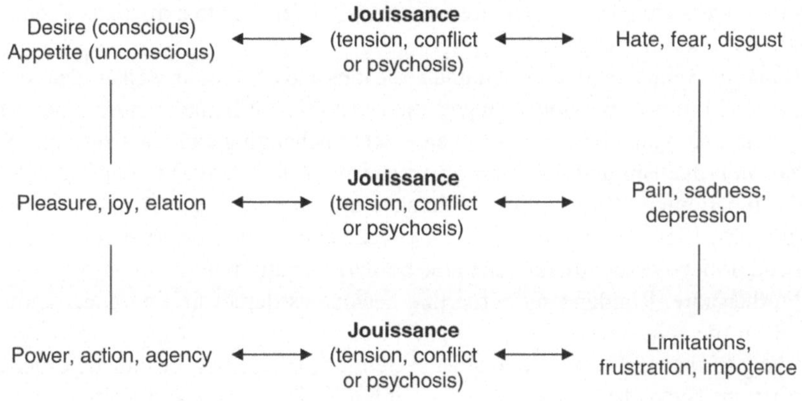

Figure 7.1 Jouissance Grid (2006 version)

A crucial aspect of the Spinozan system is the tension between being bound by the 'necessary' conditions of being 'part of the laws of nature' and any freedom of choice and/or change. As Hampshire puts it:

> The happiness and the unhappiness of a particular person, his or her degree of freedom or bondage, are a function of two variables: (1) the individual power,

> mental and physical, of his, her or its drive to self-maintenance; (2) his, her or its location in the inexhaustible series of causes in the common order of things.
> (Hampshire, 1994, p. 10)

Writing on gender, the feminist philosopher Genevieve Lloyd (1994) argues that on a Spinozan view of the mind-body distinction, 'sexual differences can reach right into the mind' (p. 161). As ideas of differently sexed bodies, minds would have to be sexually differentiated. Moreover, there is, for Spinoza, a 'continuity between the individual body and the socialised body' (p. 162). As Lloyd puts it, 'with regard to sexual differences, there are no facts of the matter other than those produced by the play of the shifting powers and pleasures of socialised, embodied, sexed human beings' (p. 168). To 'powers and pleasures' we need to also add 'desire and hate' and 'limits and pains'. This then makes for both a neo-Spinozan and a clinically realistic dynamic model of the 'passions and affects'.

A Spinozan position functions as a lens onto and into psychotic psychosomatic experience in analysis, as an ideational receiver and processor of such experience, a part of my active reverie and alpha-processing of these relations. In the analytic field of borderline relations, just as substance monism helps me with subject-object confusions and identifications, so too does the related dual-aspect theory challenge Cartesian mind-body dualism in a way that helps me with mind-body confusions. I can see the *conatus* (as an inherent striving for self-preservation) in borderline manoeuvres for self-preservation, including a perverse destructiveness and self-destructiveness to paradoxically assert an ideal of self and to express and communicate its lacks and wounds.

Dynamic Spinozan models of human passions and actions, as well as ideas of the proscribed limits to possible change ('the necessities of human nature'), helps me stay with that which may well be to an extent unchanging and unchangeable. Spinoza's non-dualism and his proto-Nietzschean moral relativism contribute to my alpha functioning (Bion, 1962), understanding, interpreting and going-on-being (Winnicott, 1956, p. 303) in the face of psychosomatic beta destructiveness, disorder and projective identifications in the borderline battlefield.

Furthermore, I understand borderline persons as demonstrating unconsciously a radical metaphysics and ethics: a psychotic metaphysics (Rhode, 1994), which is trying to manage lack and create a system of psychic/psychosomatic order/co-ordination. The pathological confusions of borderline matters and relations change my conception of this philosophy, as well as my understandings of fantasy/reality, mind/body, self/not-self, preservation/destruction.

It is important to demonstrate that an analytic application of Spinozan ideas is valuable to general psychodynamic clinical theory and to other practitioners. Therefore, I shall try to show how analytically I use and relate my Spinozan soliloquies without them being just masturbatory day-dreams or grandiose solipsism. I am aware that my use of Spinoza-as-reverie and active alpha day-dreaming in a relational analytic third realm can be used unconsciously (let alone consciously) as a schizoid analytic defence, a splitting off of painful pressures. The idea, though, is that they can be a reflective system which helps containment, conservation and integration and, therefore, the making of memory and remembrance.

I used to think that it was through their psychosomatic disorder and infectiousness, through their subject-object confusions and identifications, through their pre-symbolic, unreflexive, acted-out sexual and destructive impulses, in their desperate fantasies and the content of their dreams, these borderline patients demonstrated, in an unconscious and primitive way, certain connected Spinozan ideas. Although I still believe elements of this, I now think that it is not only *what* Spinoza thinks but also *how* he thinks that helps me in my work. My emphasis is now a particular and related Spinozan/neo-Spinozan way of thinking, position, approach or *Anschauungsweise* (Goetschel, 2004, p. 260), a 'manner of apprehending things' and persons, their processes and relations, which I use to enhance my analytic understanding of, and work in, psychosomatically confusing states.

Lou Andreas-Salomé (1964) wrote of Spinoza:

> To think like him does not mean to adopt a system but just to think . . . To grasp Spinoza it is only necessary to think through to its conclusions the concept that physical and mental manifestations are representations of one another. It is . . . the conscious inward contemplation of the integrity and presentness of two worlds – as we reckon – which nowhere exclude or determine each other, because they are but one.
>
> (Andreas-Salomé, 1964, p. 75)

Pertinent to my endeavour, Warren Montag (1999) suggests that any written reformulation of Spinoza's philosophy compels us to ask ourselves what material effects such a reformulation may have on our bodies and our minds. How might it move our bodies, and what might it move them to do?

The philosophy of the real and the autistic void beyond the black hole

Although I am able to enjoy my clinical thinking and linking, reflecting and observing, interpretations, philosophical thoughts, metaphors and imaginings, I also understand such alpha reveries as a product of and management of autistic non-relations, by which I mean that this particular form of analytic alpha-reverie is also a means to help manage both my and the patient's (and therefore our) autistic emptiness. I am hypothesising that savage borderline acts and attacks, confused and confusing unprocessed beta bits and fragments can be interpreted as a necessary defence against an even more intolerable, autistic, objectless space and its depressive anxieties.

Winnicott wrote in 'The Philosophy of "Real"' (1988, p. 114):

> It is not every philosopher who sees that this problem [the meaning of the word 'Real'] that besets every human being is a description of the initial relationship

> to external reality at the theoretical first feed; or for that matter at any theoretical first contact.

He then describes three degrees of initial active maternal adaptation to her infant's need and the resultant degree to which the grown-up person cares about their relationship between external reality, others and themselves.

Babies who have experienced a good enough maternal meeting of their needs can recognise

> the essential aloneness of the human being . . . Eventually such a baby grows up to say, "I know there is no direct contact between external reality and myself, only an illusion of contact . . . I couldn't care less that there is a philosophical problem involved.
>
> (pp. 114–115)

Then, Winnicott says:

> Babies with slightly less fortunate experiences are really bothered by the idea of there being no direct contact with external reality. A sense of threat of loss of capacity for relationships hangs over them all the time . . . the philosophical problem becomes . . . a matter of life and death, of feeding or starvation, of love or isolation.
>
> (p. 115)

He warns that there are the

> more unfortunate babies whose early experiences of having the world properly introduced were confused [and who therefore] grow up with no capacity for illusion of contact with external reality; or their capacity is so slight that it breaks down at a time of frustration and schizoid illness develops.
>
> (p. 115)

I suggest that the philosophers in whom I am interested and whose thinking I use inside myself when I am with difficult others probably fall somewhere in the 'slightly less fortunate baby' category. Borderline people come from both the second and the third categories of experience, as do many psychotherapists. The point I am making here is that the lines between these degrees of concern about the real and the reality of relations with other people are not safely distinct. Each position is used as a defence against the possible experience of there being a greater relational failure and lack, and so a deeper doubt over the connection to the real and to others.

Autistic places are, for the borderline, an 'other possible universe' even more awful than the vortex of the psychotic black hole. Perhaps it should be called an 'impossible non-universe'. It manifests symptomatically as autistic-like blank states and/or catatonic dissociation. To risk over-extending the cosmic metaphor, the psychotic core of borderline disorder is like the spinning mass around an active black hole; the borderline person can be sucked and suck others into this mad vortex or be spat out into an even more awful autistic void of non-being and disintegrating anxiety (Hobson, 1974). In both these cases, there is no differentiation between subject and object. It is a primitive mind-body identity, a psychoid psychosomatic unit of experience where beta emotions move both body and idea because they are experienced as 'the same thing'. There is also no differentiation between self and other: 'You are part of me; you have to be made and remain not separate; if necessary, I will have to infect you or even kill you in order to possess you'.

In destructive borderline states and borderline pockets, psychotic projective identifications are the most effective system for the urgent pre-verbal communication of psychic and psychosomatic pain and distress, as well as of impotent need, desire and love, of overwhelming anger, of fearful fragmentation and destruction. Such emotional states are projectively communicated by making them attackable 'out there' into the bad analyst, the other as withholder but safe-keeper of the self, an affected-infected other. The analyst/parent/enemy/lover is the psychosomatic target of these urgent psychotic transferential explosions.

The good self hidden inside the bad analyst is so unconsciously desired and envied that it somehow has to be destroyed even as it is being hidden (Fordham, 1974). Thus, the attacks on the good-bad analyst, on our relationship and on the analysand's self are intensified and become psychosomatically infectious and contagious. They become a shared malignant atmosphere, a psychosomatic battlefield as much as an erotic psychic field. Interpretations and links need to go on being made, although they will often be either enviously rubbished and scorned or otherwise unreceived. So all the more important is an understanding of a 'third field' by which we are both affected, a psychoid and sometimes psychotic and psychosomatic relationship. Then my containing-managing alpha reveries are there for the patient to use, if he/she can.

Reverie and alpha functioning

In his critical notice to Bion's *Cogitations*, Plaut (1994) wrote that

> rêverie . . . was first abandoned as a synonym in favour of alpha because it did not indicate activity sufficiently. Unfortunately, in my view, it was later taken up again with gusto by analysts who, seeing themselves as the mother-container of the baby-patient, were free to have fantasies about their rêveries, helping the patient to modify the frustrating experiences at the breast. Where intolerable frustration had previously left the baby stuck in the primordial slime of beta-elements, analysts could now apparently alpha function it out.
>
> (Plaut, 1994, p. 255)

The 'thinking breast' then is not to be understood as a magical breast. It is a metaphor of a present container and processor, which (who) goes on being well and able, with curiosity, imagination and a sense of the relative multiplicity of psychic, physical and moral realities, with both feeling and thinking (thinking through feeling).

Let me also make it clear that we cannot project the soma (that is a category error). We can, however, split off and desperately/defensively project or spit unbearably painful (unmanageable) emotions into the hated/loved other/mother. This is a manoeuvre to self-defensively rid oneself of these emotions and to communicate them into the experience of the other so as to have them met, contained and managed. It is, therefore, often necessary to induce in the analyst the appropriate somatic responses that belong to these angry but impotent emotions. I then try to reflect upon the psychosomatic matters that I receive, some of which may be processed into interpretations and fed back as my linking or connecting thoughts and memory-making. 'Just as maternal reverie facilitates the babies acquisition of the alpha function, so alpha-dream-work is a way in which the analyst works during waking life, digesting psychic truth and turning it, via containment, conservation and integration, into memory' (Grotstein, 1992, pp. ix–xvii).

Of course, the analyst's particular emotional and/or physical pains and other reactive symptoms do not necessarily reflect or reproduce the patient's symptomatic points of psychosomatic pain and disturbance exactly. It is the analyst's own zones and forms of psychosomatic vulnerability that are affected, so my idiosyncratic emotional and physical sensitivities are open to being disturbed and moved. Countertransferential information is received through my psycho-somatically 'weakest' and most problematic areas. These are my 'strongly' reactive areas and so are where I am made to work from. This is another way of saying that, as a wounded healer, one actually heals through particular wounds or rather one's survival, management and recycling of one's wounds and madnesses. As Santayana said of what he called 'normal madness' (Santayana, 1926), 'sanity is a madness put to good uses' (cited in Coleman, 2009, p. 269). That, I think, is also a good enough definition of a proper analytic training and indeed of analysis itself.

In the psychotic transference/countertransference there is a psychosomatic representation of a painful intra-uterine environment, of an original and continuing lack of emotional and psychosomatic connection and co-ordination, oedipal indifference or confusion (or both) and/or a fearful or dissociative autistic hardness. My embodied reveries, my alpha day-dreaming, thinking and words arise out of and reorder this psychoid transference/countertransference beta chaos and psychosomatic disorder, as well as the intense anger and attack. These thoughts and informing intuitions can 'make memory' and become a 'knowledge of a third kind'. I choose this latter expression carefully: by knowledge, I mean what Bion (1962) notates as the K link, which includes the other emotional links of love (L) and hate (H). The idea of a 'third kind' refers to both Ogden's 'third' and Spinoza's idea of intuition as a 'third kind of knowledge', which develops out of and beyond received opinion and reasoning. Such an 'intellectual intuition' is also similar to what Bion (1962, p. 72) referred to as the 'selected fact'.[5] In turn, according to Bion, the reali-

5 Bion derived 'selected fact' from the French mathematician Henri Poincaré (Poincaré, 1914, in Bion, 1962, p. 72). He first quotes the English translation of Poincaré' *Science and Method*, then puts

sation of selected facts emerges out of a position of 'negative capability' in Keats' sense (Keats, 1817, in Bion, 1970, p. 125).[6]

Management of attacks on thinking, and psychosomatic survival

Working with borderline relations is not about analytic subtlety. It is often more a matter of survival than an issue of reflective insight. There seem to be several metaphors for the experience of being in a shared atmosphere of such primitive, destructive, borderline matters and relations. They include: invisible, psychic projectiles; psychosomatic infections and contagions; a numbing or paralysing nerve gas which stops ongoing functions, above all thinking and speaking; invasion and possession by alien forces; being ambushed or attacked by a terrorist; sudden ambushes and attacks by a dangerous animal or reptile; being coerced; being overpowered; being poisoned; being inveigled and seduced by nearly irresistible inducements and 'magic' charms; excessive sexual pressures, pulls, intrusions and suctions; an excessive tension of *jouissance*; a universal anti-mind of chaotic beta bits whose confusing fragments are maddening. All these are, for the terrified and, therefore, terrorist-like borderline baby-bomb, the only form (or deform) for urgently needed and effective communication, the making and sharing of intolerable disorder which has somehow to be understood and (for the baby part) 'sorted out' by the analyst/analysis. Or rather, as I said earlier, observed, managed, grieved, mourned and remembered.

However, the issue still remains: how to meet ferociously hungry (starved) forces arising out of such thwarted and frustrated love; how to meet such psychic and physical loneliness and wild madness with my emotional mind but without being seduced, infuriated, driven mad or becoming sickened; how to think and link through this affective psychic field; how to go into my own reverie without being schizoid, or otherwise defensive or unreal. This is a practical, urgent and ethical analytic challenge.

Through my alpha-reverie, I ask myself a series of questions that are pertinent in the borderline relationship: What form of encounter am I being made to meet with here? What sort of emotional/feeling person am I with? What sort of mind-game, arising out of what sort of internalised family relations? What sort of baby? What sort of sex, desire and fascination, what disgust and repulsion, what sort of

forward his own psychoanalytic formulation of selected fact as follows: 'I have used the term "selected fact" to describe that which the psycho-analyst must experience in the process of synthesis. The name of one element is used to particularize the selected fact, that is to say the name of that element in the realization that appears to link together elements not hitherto seen to be connected' (Bion, 1962, p. 72) (Eds.).

6 The realisation of the 'selected fact' depends on negative capability. Bion quotes Keats 'negative capability' as referring to the person ('man of achievement') who is 'capable of being in uncertainties, mysteries, doubts, without any irritable reaching after fact and reason' (Keats, 1817, in Bion, 1970, p. 125) (Eds.).

aggression and attack? What sort of dance of closeness-distance, what rhythms and what a-rhythmic suddenness am I being made to negotiate? In my proto-mammalian and reptilian brain, through my autonomic nervous system, what sort of primitive creature forces am I subject to here (Peters, 1987)? And thence, how should I re-act, inter-react and reply to such an abject 'anti-person'? This entails active mind-body/body-mind work within the animating third between and around us. The analyst-as-receiver-and- doer has to be seen, felt and so realised to be relatively all right, strong and healthy enough not to be destroyed but to survive, recover, be able to go on thinking and functioning well enough, not to hate back too much or for too long and certainly not to be indifferent. However, such analytic health and strength are enviable, and so open to further aggressive destructive challenge.

My analytic metaphor has become martial as well as erotic, and I try not to pacify the attack with a defensive excess of empathic tolerance. I would say that psychosomatic empathy could include the antipathy of having to fight. Whereas narcissistic defences are complex, clever and strategic, thus necessitating analytic finesse and subtlety, borderline defences are reactive, offensive and even terroristic. Although I may have a strategic plan to cover the overall state of affairs, I find I actually need to be both tactical and ready to 'grapple' with the attacker. I would like to think that over the years of experience with such cases, I might perhaps have developed a psychic martial artistry, but the borderline encounter does not feel so sophisticated. However, I choose when and what to say or do, which is an assertion of my separate and different mind and body. This is vital and healing for me, possibly for us, but probably not much for the psychotically destructive other.

If, however, the other person is able to get into the unity of my system or get my system to attack itself, then I am open to a malignant psychosomatic catastrophe. These matters can no longer be understood only as a psychotherapeutically viable form of communication. I would now say something like, 'It is better for both of us if you stop trying to kill me. I've got the point, whether you believe it or not!' This is a healthy, necessary form of self-preservation, the *conatus* through the law of the fathers, the limits of my availability, the reality of our separateness.

Conclusion

Perhaps the only possible change in borderline relations is an achievement of irony (Lear, 2003), a knowledge which is simultaneously sad and joyous, depressing and elating, an ironic view of realities and relations in which we both know that there is a limit to how (and how much) we can know ourselves and each other. Irony implies a true sense of scepticism. Thereby, I suggest it also incorporates a healthy sense of psychic freedom in the face of the fact that we are actually somatically, environmentally and contingently over-determined: an integration and acceptance of personal and impersonal 'necessities'. However, even to talk of irony, scepticism and the paradoxical 'freedom of necessity', means to have moved beyond grief into mourning and remembrance.

Change is relative and limited by the deep structures and fears of patients, by their internalised and external relations and also eventually by the limits as well as the gains of our analytic relationship. These analytic relations have to do with our useful, tactical and strategic management of transferential and countertransferential loves, hates, fears, frustrations and disillusionments, of psychosomatic pleasures and pains. Hampshire, in his summation of Spinoza's *Ethics*, writes: 'Salvation is here or nowhere, in present curiosity and enjoyment, in the company of this body and now' (Hampshire, 1994, p. 10). However, I would add, personal and inter-personal psychosomatic relations can sometimes be experienced through the identifications and communications of intolerable lack in the company of very difficult body-mind confusions now.

References

Andreas-Salomé, L. (1964). *The Freud Journal of Lou Andreas-Salomé*. S. Leavy, trans. New York: Basic Books.

Balint, M. (1952). *Primary Love, and Psycho-Analytic Technique*. London: Hogarth.

Balint, M. (1968). *The Basic Fault*. London: Basic Books.

Bennett, J. (1984). *A Study of Spinoza's Ethics*. Cambridge: Cambridge University Press.

Bion, W. (1962). *Learning from Experience*. London: William Heinemann.

Bion, W. (1963). *Elements of Psycho-Analysis*. London: Heinemann Medical Books.

Bion, W. (1967). *Second Thoughts*. London: Heinemann Medical Books.

Bion, W. (1970). *Attention and Interpretation*. London: Tavistock.

Bion, W. (1992). *Cogitations*. London: Karnac Books.

Britton, R. (1998). *Belief and Imagination: Explorations in Psychoanalysis*. London: Routledge.

Coleman, M. (2009). *The Essential Santayana: Selected Writings*. Bloomington, IN: Indiana University Press.

Curley, E. (1988). *Behind the Geometrical Method: A Reading of Spinoza's Ethics*. Princeton, NJ: Princeton University Press.

Damasio, A. (2003). *Looking for Spinoza; Joy, Sorrow and the Feeling Brain*. Orlando: Harcourt.

Deleuze, G. (1988). *Spinoza. Practical Philosophy*. R. Hurley, trans. San Francisco: City Lights.

Donagan, A. (1988). *Spinoza*. Chicago: Chicago University Press.

Eigen, M. (1998). *The Psychoanalytic Mystic*. London: Free Association Books.

Fordham, M. (1974). 'Defences of the Self'. *Journal of Analytical Psychology*, 19(2): 192–199.

Goetschel, W. (2004). *Spinoza's Modernity*. Madison, WI: University of Wisconsin Press.

Grotstein, J. (1992). 'Foreword.' In O. Weininger, *Melanie Klein: From Theory to Reality*. London: Karnac.

Grotstein, J. (1997). '"Mens Sane in Corpore Sano": The Mind and Body as an "Odd Couple" and an Oddly Coupled Unity'. *Psychoanalytic Inquiry*, 17(2): 204–222.

Hampshire, S. (1951/1987). *Spinoza*. Harmondsworth: Penguin.

Hampshire, S. (1994). 'Truth and Correspondence in Spinoza'. In *Spinoza By 2000: The Jerusalem Conferences. Volume II: Spinoza on Knowledge and the Human Mind*, Y. Yovel, ed. Leiden: Brill.

Hampshire, S. (2002, October 24). 'The Spinoza Solution'. *The New York Review of Books*, 49(16): 55.

Hinshelwood, R. (1991). 'Review of *Psychopathology: Contemporary Jungian Perspectives*, ed. A. Samuels'. *Journal of Analytical Psychology*, 36(3): 408–412.

Hobson, R. (1974). 'Loneliness'. *Journal of Analytical Psychology*, 19(1): 71–89.
Jung, C. (1993). 'The Psychology of the Transference'. In *The Practice of Psychotherapy*. Vol. 16 of *The Collected Works of C.G. Jung*. R. Hull, trans. London: Routledge & Kegan Paul.
Kernberg, O. (1984). *Severe Personality Disorders: Psychotherapeutic Strategies*. New Haven: Yale University Press.
Klein, M. (1935). 'A Contribution to the Psychogenesis of Manic-Depressive States'. *International Journal of Psychoanalysis*, 16: 145–174.
Lear, J. (2003). *Therapeutic Action: An Earnest Plea for Irony*. London: Karnac Books.
Lloyd, G. (1994). *Part of Nature*. Ithaca, NY: Cornell University Press.
Lloyd, G. (1996). *Routledge Philosophy Guidebook to Spinoza and the Ethics*. London: Routledge.
Montag, W. (1999). *Bodies, Masses, Powers: Spinoza and His Contemporaries*. London: Verso.
Montag, W. & Stolze, T., eds. (1997). *The New Spinoza*. Minneapolis, MN: University of Minnesota Press.
Ogden, T. (1994). *Subjects of Analysis*. Northvale, NJ: Jason Aronson.
Peters, R. (1987). 'The Eagle and the Serpent: Or – The Minding of Matter'. *Journal of Analytical Psychology*, 32(4): 359–381.
Plaut, F. (1994). 'Critical Notice on Bion's *Cogitations*'. *Journal of Analytical Psychology*, 39(2): 253–262.
Rhode, E. (1994). *Psychotic Metaphysics*. London: Karnac Books.
Rosenthal, H. (1989). *The Consolations of Philosophy: Hobbes' Secret, Spinoza's Way*. Philadelphia: Temple University Press.
Santayana, G. (1926). 'Normal Madness'. In *Dialogues in Limbo*. New York: Scribner.
Winnicott, D. (1956). 'Primary Maternal Preoccupation'. In *Through Paediatrics to Psychoanalysis: Collected Papers*. London: Routledge, 2013.
Winnicott, D. (1988). *Human Nature*. London: Free Association Books.
Yovel, Y. (1999). 'Transcending Mere Survival'. In *Spinoza by 2000: The Jerusalem Conferences. Volume III: Desire and Affect: Spinoza as Psychologist*. Y. Yovel, ed. New York: Little Room Press.

Appendix: Notes to the *Jouissance* Grid

Note from Eds. This chapter includes the first appearance of Giles' '*jouissance* grid'. He included versions of this diagram and discussion in several later papers and also distributed the grid as a handout in teaching contexts. In these later iterations, the *jouissance* grid was always accompanied by a text in which Giles summarised the meaning of the diagram in a number of explanatory dot points. This text is included in several of Giles' unpublished papers and we give one of the later versions here.

- The *conatus* is a 'psychoid' *conatus*.
- The *conatus* unites all affects and passions in a *jouissance* of liveliness, tension, conflict and/or psychosis.
- *Conatus*-as-*jouissance* is a dynamic incorporation of all the emotions of the 'bodymind'.
- *Jouissance* naturally incorporates both the conjunction and the keeping apart of affective urges and states.
- The *jouissance* that joins and separates the emotions can become a psychotic zone if the tension becomes destructively (rather than vitally) excessive and conflictual or if there is a defensive/repressive split and one affect becomes over-dominant and the other becomes unconscious.
- From a psychogenic perspective, both an excessive tension between conflicting emotions and/or the intensity of an affect that is unmitigated and unmediated by a contrary affect (e.g. unfiltered desire, pleasure or power) can engender psychosis. On the other hand, endogenous psychosis can cause or exacerbate just such excessive tensions or one-sided intensities.
- Any 'emotion' can be psychically, somatically or psychosomatically 'used' as a defence against any other emotion; such defences are often fantastic, illusory, partial or 'inadequate' manoeuvres and management systems (within the overriding and essential nature of the *conatus*).
- *Conatus*-as-*jouissance* undermines oppositional binary systems; e.g. we can feel desire and disgust for the same object and move from one to the other instantly; we can desire fear, fear desire and find our appetites disgusting; we can love to hate and hate love; we can make a (masochistic) pleasure of pain and make a (sadistic) pain of pleasure; or we can fantastically aim for self-preservation (of the idea of the 'good self') by suicide (killing the pained, failed or shamed 'bad self').
- The left and right columns in this diagram represent neither mutually exclusive nor 'positive and negative' poles. They represent the inherently given range of normal human emotions in ever-changing relations and intensities: oscillations, ambiguities, ambivalences, internalised ideas of good and bad, senses of enjoyment and/or shame, varying energetic or enervating affects.
- These dynamic relations apply both internally and interpersonally.
- This is to be understood as a dynamic that cannot and does not demand resolution or an idea of progress/health.

- Thus far, all concepts in this explanation are of both of mind and of body, and may be represented through either, but must be understood univocally as dual aspects of a single substance – i.e. it is 'the psychoid *conatus*'.
- I use this representation of a naturalistic '*jouissance* dynamic' as a lens of observation into emotions and their relations, but here specifically focused for analytic transferential, countertransferential and interpretive use.
- In sum, it represents the tense relations of attraction and separation between appetite/desire and disgust/fear, pleasure and pain, joyous elation and sad depression, power and its limits/impotence . . . all incorporated in the psychosomatic (psychoid) *conatus* of the *jouissance* of the 'bodymind'.
- Previously, I have written about how I use this grid to think through informative transferential and embodied countertransferential communications and through the psychosomatic confusions, emotional storms, uncertainties and blind-spots in the clinical encounter with a 'radical other.' Thence, from my reverie and critical empathic thinking, there may appear a comprehensive 'selected fact' or, in Spinozan terms, 'intuitive knowledge.' The '*jouissance* grid' forms a conceptual structure to interpret analytic relations with destructive borderline and defensive narcissistic disorders in a field of projective identifications, extractive processes and sticky narcissistic adhesiveness. However, it can also be used in a critical analysis of the phenomenology of various forms of depression and to understand the dynamics of severe disorders of the self, for example, where repetitive compulsive acts and/or extreme dissociative (or psychogenic autistic-like) states are operating as defences against massive depressive anxiety. I suggest that in these cases, it is through our empathic (imaginative, emotional and thoughtful) analytic understanding and its communication that we might find or engender life in apparently lifeless states: a relational vitality and its symbolisation may thus emerge from the pre-order of our common psychoid ground.

Chapter 8

A Jungian inheritance of lack and loss

Reflections on my Jungian ancestry

Psychoanalysis Downunder, 2007[1]

In the following, I consider Jung's short, intense, creative kinship with Freud, Freud's influence on Jung and Jung's idiosyncratic difference, his separate mind. This consideration includes my current prejudiced generalisations and projections, as well as interpretations arising out of my experience of a post-Jungian inheritance within the relevant history of psychodynamic theory and clinical practice.

Although I shall not be elaborating upon this crucial aspect of Jung's creative work, his scholarly erudition in the field of cultural symbolism and comparative mythology and his creation of a hermeneutic system which applied this research to the pluralism of psychic reality and psychological relevance was the product of imaginative and intellectual genius. It has led on to many rich and fertile developments in post-Jungian clinical and academic thought. Furthermore, current post-Jungian re-thinking and re-application of the clinical relevance of archetypal theory and symbol formation in the context of their relations to neurobiology and emergence theory is of topical import. This Jungian tradition of a particular investigation of the symbolising function is the *sine qua non* to and from which all further critical comment moves. Having planted that flag, I can now proceed, critically.

Jung's psychology was partly motivated by his own problematically internalised family losses,[2] failures, parental disappointments and angry depressions. By 'psychology', I am referring to both his personal and his public psychology: that is,

1 The full paper on which this chapter was based was originally presented on November 25, 2006, at a conference, 'Freud Then and Now', celebrating the 150th Anniversary of Sigmund Freud's birth. It was titled 'Using a Jungian inheritance of lack and loss: Psychosomatic infection, mourning and irony in the analysis of borderline relations', and was published in *Psychoanalysis Downunder* 7A in February 2007. The second part of the original paper included previously published material concerning clinical experience of working with borderlines, reusing the case of Jim. We have omitted this repeated material from this chapter but refer the reader to Chapter Seven (Eds.).

2 There were many family losses due to infant mortality. Jung, born July 26, 1875, was the fourth born but first to survive, his birth being preceded by two babies who were stillborn and a brother Paul (b. 1873) who lived only a few days. His mother Emilie Preiswerk (1848–1923) suffered terrible grief from these losses, withdrawing into a compensatory visionary world and leaving Jung to fend for himself. Eleven years after Jung's birth, his mother gave birth to a sister, Johanna Gertrud (1884–1935), known as Trudy, who did survive but was very sickly as a child (Eds.).

DOI: 10.4324/9781003255826-9

both his own psychopathology and his constructed system of psychological management, understanding, modelling and practice. Jung was an oedipal orphan, and his childhood was one of existential loneliness and isolation, which he sometimes filled by magical retreats and rituals in order to neurotically manage his lost good objects. These, in my view, evolved into fiercely epistemophilic, intellectual and imaginative ways of dealing with his beliefs and problematic doubts, his desires and fears and especially a sense of his odd difference. These issues were later re-constellated in subsequent creative and destructive relationships, particularly with, *inter alia*, his father-rival Freud. Their split was never fully mourned and got stuck as a professional familial splitting. We belong now to our own professional-tribal societies, or at least in our different adjacent villages. Perhaps we do well enough without too much of each other, and we are anyhow fully occupied with our own local matters. But I wonder.

Similar tensions and conflicts recurred in Jung's sometimes over-close and stimulating, sometimes didactic, sometimes detached relations with his psychotic and borderline patients, with his pupils and followers, with the men and women in his professional life, with his erotic triangles and with his own solitary self. These loves, losses, power-relations and angry splits have become our Jungian intergenerational inheritance. Our ongoing post-Jungian task involves mourning and repairing the rupture of relations between Jung and Freud and their extended professional (and personal) families. There was something of this loaded family inheritance moving my own initial attraction to Jung, my training, my later disillusionments and struggles with or against such identity and in my analytic work with difficult borderline persons.

Jung's personal and professional experience rendered him particularly good with the analysis of personality disorders. Jung went through his own near-psychotic phases; he was a hospital psychiatrist as well as one of the early 20th-century psychoanalysts working in a pioneering way, if also at times in an unconventional and transferentially alarming way. Jung theorised out of his experience with his own and other's near-psychotic and psychotic matters and through thinking and feeling his way through the bizarre, fragmented contents and difficult relational worlds of psychotic as well as neurotic patients and with the structural disorders of early trauma which harms the development of the symbolising function. Such early difficulties give rise to the aggressive, defensive and delusional internal and interpersonal relational forces of the disordered personality. In the case of borderline relations, it is where unthinkable emotions are somatised or acted out destructively, destroying all possible good and meaning. Jung's investigations of disturbances to the symbolising function have contributed profoundly to our understanding of the symbolising process and its disorders. He revealed a particular place for a radical understanding of imagination and madness.[3]

3 Chapter Ten contains an in-depth analysis and comparison of psychoanalytic and Jungian theories of symbolising and also shows how Jung's theory of symbolising differs in subtle but significant ways from Freud's (Eds.).

Another interpretive take on Jung's psychological *Weltanschauung* is that he constructed a defensive and de-personalising system by 'archetypalising' primitive objects (and part-objects), stemming from his own experience of early damage, repeatedly unmet and frustratingly thwarted needs, abandonments, perhaps also schizoid defences against envy, anger and hate. Such processes can be seen, for example, in his dropping of his cousin Hélène Preiswerk, his turning of Sabina Spielrein (his Burghölzli patient, then protégée and then at some level an acted-out embodiment of heroic-tragic Wagnerian love), Toni Wolff and others, into used '*anima* objects'; in his defensive imposition of mythic and alchemical meanings onto the familial and transferential contents and projections of many patients, in his mythic interpretations of the fantasies of Miss Miller and others.

We can see disturbing psychic storms and unconscious forces of disruption in his presentations in *Memories, Dreams and Reflections* (Jung, 1967) of his own early dreams and fantasies: for example, the dream of an underground giant penis-god and the vision of God destroying Basel cathedral by shitting on it, Father-God's own angry potent turd. These may be understood as archetypal images of the necessary dark side of god and/or a creative chthonic god; or we can see them as a necessary manifestation of the transcendent function; or they are about split-off bad feelings and the emergence of ambivalence; or the phantasies of a murderously envious Kleinian baby with a monstrous witch-mother or symbolic representations of unresolved oedipal desires and fears.

Perhaps Jung created more of a 'school of psychological wisdom', a type of psychological grand narrative arising out of curiosity and the comprehension of confusion, rather than 'a school of suspicion' and hence of subtle clinical technique. For Jungians, the latter has been developed through clinical experience over the years but mixed with a necessary incorporation of object relations, psychoanalytic middle group, Klein, Bion and post-Kleinian work.

Jung's emphasis on the primacy of subjective internal *imagos*, sub-personalities or complexes can, at times, seem overly intra-psychic, too solipsistic, an over-emphasis on content and so a preclusion of internalised relational forces and deeply patterned reactions which are re-constellated and repeated through later (and transferential) desires and defences. For many of us, Jung's definitive names for some of these general psychic parts (*anima*, *animus*, shadow, etc.) are now seen as too impersonally generalised, inclining towards false reification and magic hypostatisation. Perhaps Jung's privileging of the intra-psychic was partly conditioned by his experience of severely psychotic and schizophrenic patients rather than of more normal neuroses.

There are the gains and losses of the myths wherein Jung chose to find meaning. For a variety of reasons, he challenged the primacy of the oedipal myth, emphasising instead various myths of death and re-birth, as well as myths of the mother/dragon-slaying hero and later alchemical models of transferential psychic transformation. The gain here is a certain pluralism, a breadth of imaginative possibilities. The loss is that the baby, if not the entire family, was thrown out with the bath-water. There was no Jungian baby, that is until we stole Klein's and Winnicott's babies. For Jung and thence inter-generationally for us Jungians

(I'm referring here to lineages and divisions in the Jungian training family), we have had to search to find and create a comprehensive and comprehensible Jungian family, and there has sometimes been more schism than integration. Rather than an integration of disappointments, disillusionments and depressive ambivalence, a sense of healthy scepticism and irony, there has often been a defensive formation involving splitting goods and bads, too much false knowing, not enough 'not-knowing', too much unforgiving hurt, not enough mature acquiescence.

The classical Jungian method of amplifying psychic material and archetypalising psychic material such as images, dreams and fantasies rather than interpreting and linking them to current relations and so to the forces of unconscious personal history can reinforce a patient's grandiose narcissistic defences. Furthermore, it can sometimes energise psychotic content and/or enhance magical defences against delusional ideation. In the classical approach, it was thought to be useful for a person to learn that their unconsciously derived imagery and fantasy were 'typical' and belonged to a deep universal and historical psychic patterning. My clinical experience has been that beyond an initial narcissistic search for and identification with idealised self-objects, people are not always helped by such an impersonal bolstering of false self-ideation. People need observation and analysis of their personal and idiosyncratic internalised family demons and wounds so that they might slowly dare recognise and feel their way through their illusions, delusions and self-defeating defences.

I have some concern when a Jungian emphasis on the numinous is overly content-driven, intra-psychic, non-relational and involves reification, if not hypostatising, of unconscious mentation into 'intentional beings' and 'internal units' rather than psychic conflicts enmeshed in a tangle of early relational desires and defences. Jung often seems to privilege essences over relations; teleological purpose over effective cause; impersonal meaning over personal links; amplification over interpretation. For those who believe and feel that the numinous is *more and other* than psychically real fantasies and feelings, partly based on early object experience, a particular pleasurable aesthetic affectivity, a particular poetic sensibility and creativity, a terrible beauty, a psychic maker of personal meaning and therefore a valuable and ethically good internal object (and/or subject-state), well, so be it.

Psychic reality as unconscious phantasy should surely be open to conscious doubt, critical thinking, linking and interpretation and not swallowed wholesale as more than something arising out of unconscious experience. As for working with 'archetypal imagery' in a clinical analytic setting, this would need to come from a position of conceptual validity, amplificatory belief and interpretive faith, none of which I have. If 'the archetypal' is thought to be more than an artistic and poetical creation with a particularly forceful, affective and even numinous aesthetic quality, then it is, I think, a magical and deluded fantasy, an aspect of a false self, bolstering schizoid splits and narcissistic defences. So other than as a zone of creative and playful imagination, which may be of supportive value, I have no real clinical place or use for archetypal imagery, except perhaps as fantasy open to critical interpretation.

What, for me personally, might be a valuable inheritance from Jung? I feel that his emphatic evaluation of psychic reality is a radical corrective to over-simple, crude materialism. There is his openness to savagely primitive shadow imagery and acted-out impulses, as found in the psychotic worlds of his psychotic patients (and perhaps of himself), and his interpretations and elaborations on such relations. I enjoy how his hermeneutic mind was critically steeped in the German tradition of Kantian and post-Kantian Idealism (*à la* Schopenhauer). Although I have an ongoing debate with Jung's re-visioning of this system, especially with his impositions of a purposeful teleology (in the manner of Eduard von Hartmann) onto what I think were more naturalistic, neutral and therefore realistic understandings, I do consider the Herder-influenced pluralistic foundation of this Idealist-Romantic intellectual and cultural ancestry to be a corrective to fundamentalist reductionism. It underpins and can help motivate the ethical value of not siding with the defensive comforts of distorting theoretical dogma. This ancestry has become part of my own intellectual structure, the skeleton and 'body-of-thought' that contributes to my active reverie and thinking through of interpersonal beta disorder.

I value the way Jung lived through, knew and recycled his own familiar madness and put it to good use in an affective and effective understanding of a range of psychotic and neurotic pathologies. Although his theories don't always mate with my clinical experience, I admire his capacious, erudite and often radical depth and scope of psychological vision. I also appreciate his example of how to meet openly, to think and imagine constructively through the realities of psychotic and psychosomatic metaphysics, in particular with personality disorders.

So, in sum, I continue to value this Jungian heritage of re-cycling madness and putting it to better use whilst never losing sight of the metaphysics of the psychotic core. Wholeness and healing are relative. Psychic transformation is limited by the body, brain, family as fate, deep structures, unconscious desires and fears of the individual and by internal and external relations. These relations have to do with our tactical and strategic management of passionate and lost loves, hurts and hates, realities and laws, powers and frustrations, of psychosomatic pleasures and pains, of a *jouissance* that is a relational force but which also accommodates separateness and separation, the pleasure of reasoning and its limits and the imagination that makes for temporary but necessary meaning.

Reference

Jung, C. (1967). *Memories, Dreams, Reflections*. Recorded and edited by A. Jaffé. Translated from the German by R. & C. Winston. London: Collins (Fontana Library).

Chapter 9

The active use of the analyst's bodymind

As it is informed by psychic disturbances

ANZSJA conference, 2007[1]

My work as an analyst involves reflecting on and interpreting my subjective experience within an analytic relationship consisting of me, you, us. In other words, it involves carefully thinking through raw subjective psychic experience and thus hopefully rendering it a useful and usable countertransferential source of information about the other person. It is a matter of my mind being made by its ideas of other minds – or other bodyminds. My reasoning, thinking, linking and thence interpreting of this psychically, mentally and somatically received information is often a process of ordering beta disorder, of co-ordination and re-formation. The subjectivities and processes include received clinical theories which have been built out of clinical experience. It also involves the use of psychodynamic models of the emotional mind. These I have created by adapting previously existing psychodynamic and philosophical (even metaphysical) systems, by putting a coherent language to my own clinical experience and through the use of the subjectivities of my imagination and ideation, my interpretive thinking and my countertransferentially (including psychosomatically) informed reverie. I am specifically referring to those clinical thoughts, theories and actions that I use to make sense of more than just neurotic states and relations – namely, the psychotic core and defences of deeply disturbed personalities; or perhaps I mean those parts of all of us.

I will select four subjective philosophical and analytic elements that inform my interpretive practice:

1 The use of 'selected facts' (Bion after Poincaré 1914, in Bion, 1962, p. 72), which arise out of unconscious, semi-conscious and conscious learning and information, based on my fantasy, reverie and connected thinking: *intuitive knowledge*.
2 An animal faith in the necessary illusion of free choice; the psychic reality of a sense of agency and free will in the face of a determined actuality (unconscious mind, body, brain, family, history and contingencies): *free necessity*.

1 The paper on which this chapter is based was originally presented at the ANZSJA conference 'The Uses of Subjective Experience', Melbourne, Oct 20–21, 2007, and published as an E-book. We have omitted some material which is repeated in other chapters (Eds.).

DOI: 10.4324/9781003255826-10

3 Psychoid and psychosomatic forces of information and communication, including projective identifications and extractive introjections, which I understand as useful and usable demonstrations of what Spinoza would call *the mind as the idea of the body and bodies*.
4 Based on neo-Spinozan and Bionesque concepts, I use an internalised idea of a dynamic grid of intra- and inter-psychic (and somatic) *jouissance* affects, a dynamic of *natural passions and actions*.[2]

These four positions contribute to a personal *Anschauungsweise*, a particular attitude and approach and an internal psychic organisation that responds well enough to new arrivals and demands. The four elements are also my means of ordering my thoughts and thinking through emotional storms, my interpretive lenses, my self-containers and part of my defences. This will form a consideration of what it is to be an analyst who *chooses to be made* to have to think through, to find words and language for, to link, re-order and recycle intra- and inter-psychic split and disordered (often pre-symbolic and somatised) states of psychic beta-fragments and difficult relations. By this, I mean thinking, forming and expressing ideas out of my transferentially informed and necessarily affected, sympathetically and para-sympathetically disturbed or irritated (analytic) 'bodymind'. By working in, through and out of this psychoid realm, structural change may sometimes emerge or be mutually and consubstantially found or made . . . or not.

I am specifically referring to those clinical thoughts, theories and actions that I use to make sense of those parts of the personality that are more than just neurotic states and relations – namely, the psychotic core and defences of deeply disturbed individuals; or perhaps I mean those parts of all of us.

In the case of borderline disorders, this is about working within zones of overwhelming affect and of unformed, confused thought. This confused thought is itself an aspect of a distorted symbolising function, due, for example, to primary or early experience of lack of parental relational clarity and maturity and so where no language was found to make sense of overwhelming and incomprehensible psychic pain and distress.

However, it is only out of this beta-disorder, now being re-lived and experienced transferentially, that really deep structural difficulties and problems may be analytically moved into more normally neurotic splits and through interpretation into more honest observation and recognition. Troubled emotions and behaviours arising out of the inability to manage primary lacks, melancholic losses and frustrating limits may be put to better use; a 'sublation' where mad psychotic relations and transferences may be recycled into more normally mad neuroses, where a new structure may be formed, and within which psychic confusions, frustrations and splitting manoeuvres may be re-ordered and redirected.

This process occurs either slowly or sometimes apparently suddenly out of an intuitive recognition and realisation, a 'selected fact' – a new psychic realisation

2 For the *Jouissance* Grid, see Chapter Seven, p. 107 and Chapter Fifteen, p. 218 (Eds.).

formed out of a protracted period of safely gathered, contained and processed emotional knowledge. Either way, the process is incremental. To quote Shakespeare's *Othello*, Act 2: 'What wound did ever heal but by degrees?'

Psychoanalysis is a particularly framed, contained and containing, interactive relationship where reflection, speech and words are the overt vehicles of understanding and interpretation. As an analyst, I am open to emotional, imaginal, ideational and infectious communication, which I then filter and temper through analytic reverie and thought – especially about expressions of a mis-developed symbolising function and other unordered and disordered aspects of the analysand's personality.

Paradoxically, such psychic and psychosomatic re-creation is often deepest and most 'real' where the analytic field is a destructive-seductive battlefield of projective identifications and rapacious extractive introjections, of force and adhesion. This is because it is re-lived in the grievous places where there are no structural foundations, the terrible core of original and perennial lacks and losses. These are the most vitally affective engines for communication: extremely difficult psychological states where goods are hated, envied, attacked and destroyed are yet those whereby a dangerous vitality may come into being. In fact, there is often a perverse but vitally libidinal erotic desire tensely incorporated within the needs of borderline destructive force.

However, where these violent conditions exist only split off and hidden under a defensive cloak of false harmlessness and near-invisibility, motivating strategic manipulations and manoeuvres, then here we have the un-changing or un-recyclable narcissistic realms of relational lifelessness.

My work with difficult borderline and narcissistic relations best exemplifies my use of the subjectivity of my internal analytic position, of some of my meta-psychological constructs and of clinical practices built around a certain understanding of personality disorders and my experience of them.

Borderline and narcissistic defences and the countertransference

I shall now go on to construct a hypothesis about the relations between borderline and narcissistic defences derived from my subjectively diagnosed, complementary countertransferential reactions and impulses.

Primitive envy and rage constitute the defensively repressed and split off 'shadow' underlying narcissistic defences (such as a desperately needy invisibility or a dangerously false harmlessness); however, the 'shadow' of the frustrations, angry hurts and destructiveness of borderline states lies in its shrouded and deviously dangerous superstructure of narcissistic strategies – which are sometimes resorted to in order to manage the borderline's primitive terror of the world of others. In other words, narcissism is as much a shadow of borderline rage as vice versa. I say this because narcissistic behaviour can evoke as much hateful and sickening feelings in others and in the countertransference as borderline attacks do. A less retaliatory hate but a certain distaste or disgust that can be perhaps more rejecting – and so needing careful countertransferential reflection. This is an incorrectly subjective and precariously hypothetical countertransferential diagnostic definition of borderline and narcissistic disorders and of their defensive inter-relatedness.

In a sense, all psychoanalytic relations are based on projective identifications, even in relations that are ostensibly normally neurotic because there are always partially psychotic pockets under normal primitive anxieties. Because of the analytic ubiquity of projective identification, it is useful to realise the latent psychotic transference behind narcissistic defences.

For severely over-sensitive narcissists, real intimacy is generally and transferentially so fearful and/or shameful that it is turned into an apparently gentle adhesive-seductive-extractive pull into a false intimacy. Other defensive manoeuvres to disguise the narcissistic wound of abject loneliness include a subtle stealing of identity and a sentimental spirituality covering a private delusion of special powers.

It is because of their fragile thin-skin elements, their self-righteous expression of the apparent unfairness of their personal and social unpopularity, their secret but selfish expectations about special entitlements that such narcissists get themselves repeatedly and increasingly bullied, ignored or rejected.

I agree with Otto Kernberg's (2004) idea that any expression of the feared underlying borderline rage is a healthy intra- and inter-psychic development beyond malignant narcissistic self-love. This is also why the thick-skinned narcissist is, in some ways, easier to work with: the outer layer of arrogance and aggression is like a carapace of borderline defensive traits, and so can be more directly challenged.

Brittle narcissism cannot be met head-on; rather, the analytic task is to address the primitive anxiety, interpersonal terrors and shames. This may lead to a shock of recognition: that the object of their fear is the recognition of their being a starved and emotionally wounded little self in a big world with very necessary and understandable, very intricate, strategic and secretive defences. However, the therapeutic problem remains that all narcissistic defences are so adamant and determined that they are quickly, forcefully and often cleverly rebuilt.

Borderline relations are about resisting and defying change because a change for a better or the good belongs to the envied other, the analyst; because change is resented and despised; and because destruction as a bizarre force goes on even after it has exhausted itself and obliterated the world.

Narcissists defend against change because it entails facing up to a shamefully naked non-self, an intolerable self-consciousness under the gaze of the judgemental eyes of the peopled world, and because rapid retreat to familiar strategic manoeuvres, manipulations and contortions are a powerfully easy defence.

Therefore, with both disordered states, the analyst is made to work in a relational field that attacks or resists change: envy and destruction of all good in the case of borderline relations; dread of the exposure of naked loneliness in the case of the loss of narcissistic defences.

'Jim' as a case of destructive borderline relations and vitalities

In the following sections, I will revisit the borderline case we met in a previous chapter, 'Jim',[3] and then discuss a narcissistic case, 'Christine'. Following these case studies, I will provide more abstract models of the borderline and narcissistic situations.

Referring to me as a 'feeble cunt' Jim expressed a hate-filled attack on me as a gender-confused figure, an object of impossible need and resentment, as well as on all women and especially his mother. His tone and pitch of voice was a mixture of growling and loud hissing, of throat, tooth and spit. Tattoos and a skinhead menacingly enhanced Jim's aggressive body language. He was a serial vandal, driven by impotent globalised rage, frustration and confusion: a fateful family inheritance. As discussed more fully earlier, his dream of screwing a Gothic Cathedral represented a depiction of a confusion of a prickly penis/soft vagina cathedral as a bodymind he sought to sexually possess and control, destroy and recoil from. Lurking behind and within this attacked object is an autistic objectless space, in turn originating in the total lack of parental connectedness and, hence, a sense of unreality. The intimate connections of affective attack eventually became our well-known familiar battlefield, and so a mutual attitude of ironic recognition became an aspect of our shared field. Thus I came to know a 'beloved enemy' – until we realised that we could hold metaphoric 'memorial services' for our 'oh-so-lovely war'.

Several years later, I heard that Jim had gone on to become an effective worker in a centre for socially delinquent adolescent boys. His destructive impulses were more self-contained, but his social and relational life apparently continued to be difficult and 'overly angry'.

Phenomenological summary of borderline relations

Work with borderline personality disorders demonstrates a primitive, fused psychoid unity through states of identification and confusion, both personally and interpersonally, and even between mind and the world. Borderline states and relations unconsciously demonstrate that 'the mind is the idea of the body' in a confused, confusing and primitive way.

Let me present a caricatured exchange between a borderline patient and myself as the analyst, based on an amalgam of words heard and actions experienced in the analytic encounter. Aspects of 'borderline' impulses are to some degree common in close relationships outside analysis. A borderline patient might convey the following messages:

> For me, mind and body, inner and outer, fantasy and reality, you and me are confused, even fused: your mind is my mind, your body my body. I never received

3 A longer clinical segment concerning Jim was originally included in this paper but has been omitted here to avoid undue repetition. We refer the reader to the fuller version in Chapter Seven (Eds.).

> the love I desperately need, so you must love me now. Let it be that you also loved me way back then and that you love me forever. Yet my hurt makes me furiously hate and destroy all that is good and all whom I love. I envy you who gives to others the love that I have to have. I hate you for not loving me in return in the same way that I love. So I will get under your skin, burrow into your insides, mess you up as I am messed up and I will get what I want.

As a raw reactive response, I may feel, but not express, complementary feelings of hate for being so invaded, affected and infected. A more considered analytic position, still not to be expressed in so many words, might be:

> I get the message, I am well informed countertransferentially by you, even psychosomatically infected by an embodied countertransference. Your way of making love is making war; destruction is a real pleasure and power. Your anger knows no bounds, and so knows no boundaries. However, I shall seek to embody a limiting frame which is a naturally frustrating but carefully containing parental mind-in-action. This means that no, you cannot have it all; you cannot force others to love you. Yet 'No' and 'Enough' are not always rejections. Your fantastic desires and hates are for us to try to understand. So, unlike you, I shall use my separate thinking mind and reflect before I act (that is, interpret). You may even come to love me standing in as your beloved enemy (as you are mine).

I remind myself that it is their fantasy of me that is envied, that my body and mind need not be made to identify with and suffer as the target of such psychosomatic missiles. I am a separate person and can survive their rage. Our therapeutic aim is towards an ability to mourn the limits of one's life, moving towards a truly muscular position beyond the initial outrage towards genuine grief for lacking and lost goods and beyond the recurrent destruction of all subsequent good objects. It may become a fiercely honest acceptance of the limits of both analysis and life to such an extent that both patient and analyst can gaze, with a strong and realistic acquiescence, into the face of our mortality. There is recognition and acknowledgment of the patient's angry loneliness and of the limits of their life's goods, which may also be paradoxically vitalising. However, the actively destructive forces still do go on – to the very end and beyond: a perverse '*conatus*'.

'Christine'

Christine was a very brilliant artist and art teacher – or so she said. She came to complain, in what I experienced as an annoying mixture of whimper and irritation, of the hurtful unfairness of her relational, social and career failures, at being misunderstood and unappreciated by everybody:

> It is probably because they are jealous of my rather daunting talents . . . though I'm careful not to flaunt them: I'm too modest to do that, of course.

She freely offered colleagues her 'ever so helpful' suggestions, often telling them that she was speaking from the wisdom of experience. And 'wisdom' was the right word because it was an altruistic, educative, loving and spiritually-based giving of her most profound psychological self:

> So, I just can't understand why people drop me and let me down. Sometimes I think I'm just too kind and straight-forward for this competitive and greedy modern world.

It is unsurprising that she was also starting to train as a counsellor. I soon joined the ranks of those who found Christine's blind grandiosity irritating, disgustingly arrogant, even loathsome. But I also started to grow increasingly tired of her and would nearly fall asleep over her (false) dramas. It was difficult to remember that behind her hollow superiority and disdain, there lay an abject loneliness, sadness and dread of the peopled world and that behind that was a dangerous but alive hate and anger, which would render her even more alone. She brought a dream:

> My stomach and vagina are full of seething, writhing balls of little worms or maggots. These worms all have human faces – but somehow without any features, except definitely nasty little mouths.

Later we were able to make much of this dream; above all that, it meant not being able to let anybody in (vagina), not daring to let anything out (shitting out a too-terrifying revelation of her disgusting insides), fear of biting and also a self-effacing facelessness. This dream certainly signified a big shock of recognition and a shift.

But long before that, something much more shocking happened. Two sessions after she had presented the dream and we were still considering and associating around the dream, Christine rather suddenly and nervously asked me, 'Are you shocked and disgusted – by me?' Surely, a very real and loaded transferential moment. However, I was, by this time, sunk deep into a narcotised sleepy state, as often happened when with Christine. Quite against my usual practice and without reflecting and thinking, I carelessly answered her question or rather heard myself say, 'No, but at last, I am really interested'.

Her shock (and my shock) was palpable. She took up this 'at last I'm really interested' with justifiable hurt and fury: I had obviously been bored by her all along; nothing could have been calculated to wound her more than the way I let this slip; it was totally unprofessional; I was a heartless, insensitive and cruel so-called analyst. For weeks she reminded me of my 'careless cruelty that has undermined my universe'.

She said that she now thought that her insect-filled body had been made thus by me: I had infected her with my dislike, if not disgust, of her repulsive self. This was perhaps a painfully true interpretation, but if so, it was also an aspect of what she induced in many others and was a product of a malign and masochistic reinforcement of her hated self. My bad complementary countertransferential reaction was, to an extent, a re-constellation of parental hate and her offended, hurt and angry spitting out of her inside feelings was also a real expression of healthy aggression – 'at last'.

When she had the courage to be aggressive and attack the much-needed, good, loved object (me), Christine was more truly alive, but when she lost her courage and faked a false goodness by hiding her desire and greed under various forms of denial, she became a life-draining bore. Her sickeningly sweet smile was tense with controlled desperation: narcissists hate real mirrors, so they set up rose-tinted ones all around.

Christine continued to oscillate between the potentiality of her 'aggressive liveliness' and defensive retreat into her 'fearful invisibility'. At the end of our time together, she declared that, at the outset, she had privately wanted to 'stop being a frightened gazelle and become a leopard'. I asked, 'And so now – what have you become?'

'I now actually sometimes enjoy being a gazelle'.

Phenomenological summary of narcissistic relations[4]

A secretive, quiet, narcissistically adhesive and parasitic personality may fantastically work their interpersonal world something like this:

> I'll get into your separate life and your separate mind, your values, your emotional privacies, and I shall take possession and co-ownership of them by making you not notice my intrusion, for my crafty strategies are invisible and secret. I will move you and influence you and your life almost without you noticing by making my extractive spider-bite painless – even pleasurable. Look, but don't look; see, but don't see. I'm so loving that you can't help but love me, this best-of-all, most beautiful and interesting me.
>
> You are noticing me, aren't you? You do realise how lucky you are to know me, don't you? I have laid my eggs under your skin. You are my unwitting host. You are my unknowing lover and partner. You can never leave me. I will never leave you. But I keep my powers private and secret and really known only to myself.
>
> I'm not empty, am I? I'm not dull and boring, am I? I'm not invisible, am I? I shall make myself visible and effective through my most subtle manoeuvres, my most secret strategic calculations.
>
> I'll get you in the end. In fact, I think I've got you already – although you may not realise it yet.

Under such conditions, it is vital to remember that this person is crippled with abject anxiety and a terrible abject loneliness. It is through pointing this out at the

4 Another version of the 'phenomenology of narcissistic relations' can be found in Chapter Eleven (Eds.).

right moment and in a way that does not cause too much shame and defensive retreats that I become an acceptable and trustable 'emotional reality principle'; one who thereby disturbs a narcissistic universe in a such a way that it may lead to a stronger emotional and relational realism. Although a change for the better, this is a very precarious change and is easily retreated from.

The analytic task is to address the primitive anxiety, interpersonal terrors and shames, and this may lead to a shock of recognition that their object of fear is a maternal-parental world in which the self is unrecognised, unloved and its healthy exhibitionistic energies crippled. Thus, necessary, understandably clever, strategic and secretive but very counter-productive, self-defeating and unattractive defences are desperately wrought.

Analytic relations, changes and limits to change

To an extent, both borderline and narcissistic personality disorders stem from being oedipally orphaned. A borderline reacts to this fate with outrage; a narcissist manages it more passively. Jim recycled his sick symbolising function and his destructive madness through fury: he resisted the superego defiantly. Christine was less able to recycle her brittle self because her symbolising function was so petrified by primitive fear and the untouchable defence of strategic inaction: she identified with the superego submissively.

As Kernberg (2004) has observed, narcissism is essentially a fearful defence, a hiding and a falseness, a secret adhesiveness, a private righteous superiority precariously covering failure and loneliness, all of which is used to strategically defend against a very frightening impulse to angrily attack which is lying underneath. Therefore, when a narcissist moves out of all such falsity into a realisation and expression of outrage, then they are actually truer and more alive.

Both states are basically driven by venomous envy and resentment: overtly expressed in impulsive acts of borderline murderousness or denied and hidden behind polite invisibility and the art of feigning in the case of narcissism. These projective poisons can and do get into my emotionally receptive but analytic bodymind, that is, into my auto-immune self-system. I need to think non-reactively and clearly through and out of this infection or contagion, to focus my reverie (intuitive knowledge of other, me, us) and eventually (with applied understanding) to speak and interpret in a way that is mutative.[5]

Through these case stories, the issue I really want to catch is my subjective/objective reverie and interpretive action in the face of transferential psychoid/psychosomatic storms and deathly calms. In other words, being a thinking mind in the midst of an emotionally and psychosomatically disturbing cosmic explosion may

5 The term 'mutative' here echoes Strachey's well-known discussion of the potential of an analytical interpretation bringing about change and transformation (Strachey, 1934) (Eds.).

also be a moment of creation. This furious storm is exactly what narcissists spend their strategic false-lives trying to avoid. And it is this violence through which borderline persons spend their psychotically destructive life trying to reach love and meaningful order, but a love and order that is always simultaneously murderously envied and lethally attacked. But at least there is the intimacy of fight, whereas with the narcissist, there is a more sinister and strategically hidden 'sucking hollow of denied anger'.

The issue for the analyst is sorting out mutually consubstantial identificatory projections and introjections amidst the scatter-shot and shards of beta fragments which make up and inform this difficult analytic field. In this interactive analytic field, this animated body, we are, as Jung said, both changed or, I would add, as often nearly destroyed. However, it is in this field of projections, extractions, infections, dreams, intuitions, frustrations and limitations that the analytic mind is most effective: dreaming, thinking, intuitively linking, using one's own internal goods and strengths – in so far as possible.

Conclusion

The analysis of pre-symbolic personality disorders is a Jungian and post-Jungian arena of clinical interaction. Jung theorised out of his experience with his own and other's near-psychotic and psychotic matters. This means he developed his thinking out of close infectious work with structural disorders and with the confusions and frustrations of early trauma and blindness, which harms the development of the symbolising function, where fantasy and reality or image, idea and impulse are unprocessed and undifferentiated, and so are confused. These become the very stuff of the destructive and constructive analytic bath: a blood bath, erotic bath and/or a transformative bath.

Analytic immersion is often experienced through somatic impact. An analysand expresses the confusion of the analytic relationship through embodied enactments and a body-based primitive pre-symbolic state – which may also be an anti-symbolic state. In relations with 'borderline beta matters', the analyst is often made to have or 'be' the mind, brain, body and the neurological energy for and of the other, and thence to have to actively feel, think, link, imagine and interpret our way through psychic blocks and pains.

A point I continue to reiterate is that, as wounded healers, we heal through our own wounds, through recycling our 'normal madness' (Santayana, 1926). Borderline persons can also recycle their madness through their affecting of me and then having their passions met by my passionately thinking bodymind within an ordered external and internal frame: contained by necessary laws.

Total structural change is impossible and/or would bring about literal madness. We are, to a greater or lesser degree, internally and externally predetermined. Free choice and agency are limited and partial: the body, the brain, family, history and culture as fate; unconscious desires and fears; internal and external relations; all limit psychic transformation.

Sometimes, the only possible change is not structural but a greater capacity for a sense of irony (Lear, 2003), a knowledge which is simultaneously sad and joyous, depressing and elating, an ironic view of realities and relations in which we both know that there is a limit to how (and how much) we can know ourselves and each other. Irony implies a true sense of scepticism. Thereby, I suggest it also incorporates a healthy sense of psychic freedom in the face of the fact that we are actually somatically, environmentally and contingently over-determined.

The philosopher David Wood (2005, p. 69) has argued that 'negative capability is the antidote to violence'. I would add: also to borderline impotent rage and to hidden narcissistic fear and hate. However, even to talk of irony, ambivalence, scepticism, 'free necessity' and negative capability means to have moved beyond grief into mourning, remembrance and recreation. This includes mourning the gains and failures of the analysis.

These difficult internal and external relations have to do with our management of passionate and lost loves, hurts and hates, of realities and laws, powers and frustrations, of psychosomatic pleasures and pains, of a *jouissance* that is a relational force but which also accommodates separateness and separation, the pleasures of reasoning and its limits, the power of our best, worst and utterly fantastic memories and the capacity for imagination in the face of the unknowable. Thus, we may create a temporary, maybe illusory, but psychically necessary (and sometimes beautiful) sense of meaning.

References

Bion, W. (1962). *Learning from Experience*. London: William Heinemann.

Kernberg, O. (2004). *Aggressivity, Narcissism and Self-Destructiveness in the Psychotherapeutic Relationship*. New Haven: Yale University Press.

Lear, J. (2003). *Therapeutic Action: An Earnest Plea for Irony*. London: Karnac Books.

Santayana, G. (1926). 'Normal Madness'. In *Dialogues in Limbo*. New York: Scribner.

Strachey, J. (1934). 'The Nature of the Therapeutic Action of Psycho-Analysis'. *International Journal of Psycho-Analysis*, 15: 127–159.

Wood, D. (2005). *The Step Back: Ethics and Politics after Deconstruction*. Albany, NY: State University of New York Press.

Chapter 10

Symbolising and not-symbolising

Unpublished, 2008, 2014[1]

Introduction

In the later stages of my training as an analyst, I was seeing a patient referred to me by a psychiatrist from the Society of Analytical Psychology with whom I was doing hospital visits. The patient I shall call 'Adie'. After about four months with me, she reported that she was having 'really embarrassing fantasies about sexual activities and positions' in which her excitement turned a particular man on 'ever more and more'. No big deal except that this was a radical admission for the very up-tight and unimaginative Adie. She was afraid that she was undergoing a total personality change. Her acute anxiety about losing control over her safe old self was palpable in the transference-countertransference dynamics. I, too, became anxious, so I went to the psychiatrist for urgent supervision. He said, 'O yes, there you are, you see, this is typical of the sort of problem you get when symbolising hasn't developed and doesn't function properly'. I didn't see at all.

I asked, 'Surely this is really about me, you know, her transferences onto me?'
He answered, 'Well, of course, but that doesn't matter at this stage. Obviously, her problem is that she can't symbolise at all'.
'Yes, I see' (which I didn't), 'so what exactly do I do?'
'Aha!'

My real problem was that I didn't know what *not* being able to symbolise really meant and hadn't a clue what to do. So I shall now address the following problems: What is symbolising? What does not symbolising mean? And the 'aha!' (what to do).

Philosophically, in terms of a naturalistic ontology, unconsciously produced hallucinations, dreams, phantasy images and ideas do not exist as raw objects of direct experience but as symbols, which do not exist objectively in themselves. They are only made into objects of emotional experience by our symbolising function, by

1 This chapter is an amalgamation of two papers on symbolising. The first, 'Somatising and Symbolising' was given in a Sydney ANZSJA Training Residential in May 2008. The second paper, 'Symbolising and Not-Symbolising', was presented at an ANZSJA Training Seminar in Melbourne on July 5, 2014.

DOI: 10.4324/9781003255826-11

our subjectivity, which is conditioned by the moral tensions of ego-consciousness, the superego and reason. Neurobiologically and psychologically, we are symbolising beings. Whether in a more primitive or sophisticated manner, we cannot but interpret internal and environmental data unless there is severe brain damage. It is our inherently symbolising mind that necessarily interprets ourselves, our internal and external relations and makes sense of our way of being in the world.

However, from the perspective of psychodynamic psychology, we use the concepts of both symbols and symbolising in a different and idiosyncratic way: what we refer to as the symbolising function is not the same as the study of symbolism where symbols are units of content whose meaning is culturally given. As in iconography, such objects are either objects of poetic, allegorical or religious significance and so may thence be psychically used or matters for critical scholarly studies of cultural relations, contextualisation, comparative differentiation, etc. There is, of course, a connection between symbols and symbolising function. Strictly, symbols (from the Greek *symbolon*, 'to throw together') are about re-connection, a linking/re-linking that reveals a meaning-endowed association or relation, a healed split, a re-found loss, a re-paired union.

Furthermore, symbols, symbolism and symbolising function are conceived in subtly but significantly different ways in the Freudian and Jungian traditions. To the Jungian, true symbols – in distinction to signs – are new and strange; they cannot be simply read; they are enigmatic and multivalent, having two or more often contrary possible meanings or no obvious meaning. Their strangeness challenges our understanding, demands interpretation and some sort of comprehension, if and in so far as possible, because meaningful associative linking is only ever provisional and temporary.

There has been a thread running through my work. It begins with my critical consideration of the history of ideas pertinent to Jungian depth psychology and the tricky philosophical idealist structure behind psychodynamic theory, which I understand as philosophical urgencies arising out of existential uncertainties and doubts around the problem of the relations of subject-self to others/other minds. This thread runs through to a second theme, that of the psychoid and the non-symbolic, if not anti-symbolic zone, of metabolising-somatising (including problems of identification, evacuation and infectious projection of beta bits, borderline destruction in the analytic field of psychosomatic disorder). Thirdly, it includes consideration of narcissistic defences of a false self against this fearfully angry war-zone. And fourthly, there is the topic of the symbolising of matter, the matter of symbolising and the matter with not symbolising, which is where my discussion began.

What follows will not be a tightly focused and precisely developed exposition of a particular aspect of symbolisation or of particular symbols. Nor will I consider artistic or other formational symbolic matters. Rather, it is an overview of various psychodynamic themes concerning symbolisation. I shall utilise elements of two analytic cases, that of Adie and Jim, to exemplify what I now see and do with problems of symbolising, which are so central to the work of the analytic relationship.

Symbolising and not-symbolising in psychoanalytic and Jungian theory and practice

In Jungian thought, symbolisation is the finding of affective, revelatory, life-enhancing, if not life-changing, meaning to moving but enigmatic signifiers. The symbolising function fails to develop or is ill-developed (i.e. is perverted, distorted, restricted or stuck) due to internalised psychic effects of family failures, through traumas, through social and political forces and, of course, through more structural biological conditions, such as various degrees of autism.

My basic theme is that traumatised, faulty and false developments of the symbolising function are the very problems that provoke us urgently and necessarily to try to form more functional symbolic modes. Internal and external/environmental failures and frustrations are intrinsic to the human condition and so are inevitable. When these are contained well enough by the emotionally attentive parental figure, by the just and fair 'laws' of the social mind, with an emotionally healthy enough and problem-solving brain, then our contextualised developmental work makes for our relatively functional symbolising selves.

The developmental issues include: To what extent is a person conscious or not that their understanding of self, other, relationships and the world is subjective and symbolic? How far are they aware that such perceptions are developmentally created personally, interpersonally and culturally? Not to realise that much of one's consciousness and self-consciousness is 'as-if', determined by unconscious and semi-conscious associations and links, is, at the very least, schizoid. Symbolising can be distorted and defensive, in an ethereal schizoid way, in a bubble of narcissistic grandiosity, in the tunnel vision and reactions of borderline hurt and outrage, in myopic depression or in autistic-like symbolic equations. The issue is, just how much and in what ways do these various psychopathologies and personality disorders damage, distort or atrophy the symbolising function? How do we help patients with such problems symbolising, are there limits to possible change? Can we help develop an affective therapeutic relationship in an environment of developmental failures of attachment, lack of empathy, handicapped imaginal capacity, evasive, schizoid or aggressive defences and other internal and relational absences and defences?

Analytically, we notice symbolising processes by default, through their failures where they manifest through neurotic, borderline or psychotic behaviours and relations, especially as such faults are represented in the transference, particularly in regressed, acted out and primitive processes of identification. Herein we are made to realise and tackle disturbances in the emergence, organisation and development of symbolic understanding, separating matter and mind (substance and fantasy) as needed for pragmatic and functional psychic health. Otherwise, in relatively healthy states, where environmental and parental order can be trusted enough to encourage epistemophilic play and creative imagination, symbolising and its development can be more or less taken for granted.

I will now briefly précis some classical psychoanalytic theories of symbolisation, followed by the classical Jungian approach. I will then move into my own ideas of personality disturbance in the case of the aforementioned a-symbolic Adie and then finally present a few concluding reflections, particularly concerning the frame.

The psychoanalytic theory of symbolism

In a paper first published in 1918, Ernest Jones distinguished between what the psychoanalyst views as 'true symbolism' and symbolism in its widest sense. True symbolism, he writes,

> arises as the result of intrapsychic conflict between the repressing tendencies and the repressed . . . only what is repressed is symbolised; only what is repressed needs to be symbolised . . . . The two cardinal characteristics of symbolism in this strict sense are 1) that the process is completely unconscious . . . and 2) that the affect investing the symbolised idea has not, in so far as the symbolism is concerned, proved capable of that modification in quality denoted by the term 'sublimation'.
>
> (Jones, 1961, pp. 115–116, 139)

According to this Freudian definition of symbolism, the substitutions involved in the creation of dream images and symptoms are examples of symbol-formation, while those involved in sublimation are not. The so-called *universal symbols* encountered in dreams, mythology and folk-lore, are explained by reference to 'the uniformity of the fundamental and perennial interests of' humankind (Jones, 1961, p. 98) and the uniformity of the human capacity for seeing resemblances between objects.

Charles Rycroft says, 'the psychoanalytic theory of symbolism concerns itself with the unconscious substitution of one image, idea, or activity for another' (Rycroft, 1972, p. 162). Symbolisation is usually listed as one of the primary processes governing unconscious thinking, as exemplified in dreams and symptom-formation. Furthermore,

> psychoanalytic theory asserts that the object or activity symbolised is always one of basic, instinctual, or biological interest, the substitution or displacement always being away from the body . . . . Displacements in the opposite, centripetal direction are regressions.
>
> (Rycroft, 1972, p. 163)

I suggest that such regressions are always partially into the pre-verbal, which may be into the pre-symbolic, which may be into the non- or anti-symbolic, but also into the zone of proto-symbolic equation, which may be analytically developed and so emerge into a more conscious and mature mental state of 're-conceivable identity'. I shall return to this later.

Hanna Segal's 'symbolic equation'

As Hanna Segal noted in the *International Dictionary of Psychoanalysis* (de Mijolla, 2005, p. 1708), she first coined the term 'symbolic equation' in 1950 in her paper 'Some Aspects of the Analysis of a Schizophrenic' (Segal, 1950). This paper discussed a schizophrenic patient who was unable to distinguish between symbols and the objects they symbolised: 'being like something and being something were the same. Symbols were equivalent to the things symbolised. There was an unconscious equation between the two' (Segal in de Mijolla, 2005, p. 1708).

In 'A Psycho-Analytic Contribution to Aesthetics' (1952), Segal shows how the formation of genuine symbols (as distinct from symbolic equations) are precipitates of mourning. They occur in the depressive position when projective identifications are withdrawn. Segal has described her subsequent paper, 'Notes on Symbol Formation' (1957) as

> formulating a theory of the dynamics of symbol formation and the role played by projective identification. Symbolism is a tripartite relation among self, object, and symbol. When projective identification is excessive, part of the ego becomes identified with the object, and the symbol, a creation and function of the ego, becomes identified with the object symbolised. In the depressive position, the object is given up, and a symbolic representation of the object is formed in the ego in the process of mourning.
>
> In normal repression, there is communication between the unconscious and the conscious through symbols. In the kind of repression that Freud called excessive, the unconscious is split off from the conscious, and in the return of the repressed, consciousness is invaded by concrete symbols, as in hallucinations.
>
> Under stress, there may be a regression from symbolic functioning to symbolic equation. For instance, in the schizophrenic patient described in [my] first paper, thoughts and words formed in the depressive position became concretised, so that the patient could not, for instance, use names, because he experienced a name as biting into the person named.
>
> (Segal in de Mijolla, 2005, pp. 1708–1709)

To quote Segal again, 'in the symbolic equation, the symbol substitute is felt to *be* the original object'. In contrast,

> the symbol proper . . . is felt to represent the object . . . It arises when depressive feelings predominate over the paranoid-schizoid ones, when separation from the object, ambivalence, guilt and loss can be experienced and tolerated. The symbol is used not to deny but to overcome loss.
>
> (Segal, 1957, p. 395)

In her later writings, especially in *Dream, Phantasy and Art* (1991), Segal continues to follow Klein and Bion's view that pathological forms of projective identification lead to a disturbance of symbolisation. There is also a connection between

Bion's alpha function and symbolising function. Concrete symbolic equations can be understood as Bion's beta elements, which have the potential to become alpha elements if alpha functioning can be developed.

As Britton explains, the symbolic equation occurs when the development of a capacity for symbol formation is arrested. Instead of being able to relinquish the 'original object', its loss is denied (Britton, 1998, p. 138). He understands Segal's view of symbolic equation as referring to a primitive paranoid-schizoid realm of confusion and identification, involving denials of original lacks and losses and where somatising and literalising preclude the symbolising, memory and imagination that is developed out of healthy mourning.

Jung and Jungian theories of symbolism: sources and development

Jung's ideas on symbolism stem back to an interest in a variety of historical and current global cultures, particularly the intellectual ancestry and culture of 19th-century post-Kantian idealism, Schelling, Absolute Idealism, Romantic, Schopenhauerean and Nietzschean thinking. All these formed the ground and sub-structure for German depth psychology and proto-psychiatry, as did the Schelling-inspired psychological systems of von Schubert, Troxler, Carus and Hartmann, the psychiatric ideas of Heinroth, Ideler and Neumann and the symbolic dream theories of Scherner, Maury and Hervey de Saint-Denys. This ideational language is a generative source of all our psychodynamic conceptualising. It is the creative lineage of our idealist philosophical and inward-looking psychological ancestry. Also part of the lineage are the early 20th century works of the vitalist Bergson and the neo-Kantian idealist Cassirer, who fundamentally influenced the structural thinking of both Freud and Jung, in particular contributing to their theories about symbols and symbolising.

Romantic artists were gripped by a new-found excitement in the import of symbols and symbolism; for example, the work of artists such as Blake or Friedrich and Carus, through the late 19th-century symbolists, to much representational-symbolist modernism in the work of e.g. Beckmann, Chagall, Sutherland, Bacon, Kitaj and very many others who connect to this tradition. Late 19th-century and 20th-century poets and other writers drawing upon this culture are just too numerous to mention.

Much of the previous is about a certain idea of symbolism that is predominantly imagistic and basically representational, even figurative, and belongs to what Ernest Jones referred to as 'symbolism in its widest sense', meaning its formal manifestations that are basic to civilisation and art. However, I am continually making a distinction between 'the symbol' and 'symbolising', between the symbolic image and the symbolising process.

We now return to Jung himself and the distinctively Jungian attitude to symbols and symbolisation. In 'On the Relation of Analytical Psychology to Poetry,' a lecture dating from 1922, Jung distinguishes his very different, non-Freudian concept of symbols as follows:

> Those conscious contents which give us a clue to the unconscious background are incorrectly called symbols by Freud. They are not true symbols, however, since according to his theory they have merely the role of signs or symptoms of the subliminal processes. The true symbol differs essentially from this, and should be understood as an intuitive idea that cannot yet be formulated in any other or better way.
>
> (Jung, 1967, *CW* 15, para. 105)

Jung goes on to say that

> their pregnant language cries out at us that they mean more than they say. We can put our finger on the symbol at once, even though we may not be able to unriddle its meaning to our entire satisfaction. A symbol remains a perpetual challenge to our thoughts and feelings. That probably explains why a symbolic work is so stimulating, why it grips us so intensely, but also why it seldom affords us a purely aesthetic enjoyment.
>
> (*CW* 15, para. 119)

A symbol is that which cannot be understood or expressed in any other way. Symbols are created naturally by the needs of the self and emanate from the deepest unconscious supra-personal and archetypal layers. Via archetypal images and the accumulation of personal unconscious modes, familial and cultural forms, they find expression in dreams and affective complex fantasies. Thus through fantasy-image, idea, language or ritual behaviour symbols, express the internal dynamic forces, developmental needs and neurotically disturbed manoeuvres of individuation. Originally, they are unconscious and beyond the capacities of conscious thought, description and representation, prior to their emergence in dream images and so forth.

Thus symbolic images communicate from unconscious to conscious, together with their feeling-tone and potential formation into ideas and words, whereby unconscious psychic perceptions, states and needs become more conscious. They are the expressed coming into phenomenal being of the noumenal, the thing-in-itself into experience, the archetype *per se* into archetypal image. Bion (also following Platonic, Romantic, the Absolute Idealist and post-Kantian thinking) might call this a transformation in O (Bion, 1965) of the consciously unknown into the known, of beta elements into alpha functioning (Bion, 1962).

Jung's psychology was crucially identified by his re-discovery of the unconscious as well as consciously intentional symbolic meanings of religious, Gnostic and alchemical images, processes and transformations and other comparative cultural symbolism, which he re-interpreted with extraordinary erudition. Symbols and symbolising are *ab origine* moved and realised by the archetypal levels of the unconscious Self, manifestations of the transcendent function that arises out of otherwise apparently irresolvable psychic opposites or conflicts. For Jung, symbols are 'indistinct, metaphoric and enigmatic portrayals of psychic reality' (Samuels et al., 1986, p. 145). And true to his inheritance from Schelling, Jung says that symbols express themselves in analogies, and that, as an inheritor of a Romantic perspective, the symbolic process is an experience in images and of images.

All symbols are symbols of transformation: they transform in themselves, inside us, between us (e.g. transferentially, erotically or martially), and even, possibly, outside us as meta-personal or spiritual phenomena.

At a personal level, symbols express and reveal a new significance, give and make meaning. They disclose and add a supra-rational and supra-material dimension, are a deep aspect of inwardness, and come from and lead back to a conscious understanding of the unconscious. The symbol, for example, in dreams and relatively unconscious fantasies reveal (in sometimes numinous, fascinating, feeling-toned images and forms) what cannot be expressed in language and, therefore, known in our conscious ego-vocabulary. It was vital for Jung that symbols are understood as extraordinarily meaningful images and processes created out of the transcendence of the deepest unconscious (personal and collective) as expressed manifestations of the otherness of the impersonal layers of the psyche.

Jung's sense of the symbol is of a symbolic representation stemming from and connecting back to earlier, repressed or split-off emotional experiences. Symbols stem from and are coloured by an archetypal and impersonal level of the creative unconscious; that is, archetypal 'levels' form and colour the personal. For example, the 'witch mother' might be a pre-personal image which is then projected onto, if not into, the actual mother, who is perceived subjectively 'as if' she was a witch.

Language and the symbolic

Language is at the core of self-representation and self-re-creation. It is the vehicle for that aspect of psychic reality which makes us affectively symbolising and communicating beings. In the naked revelations of the symbolic and psychosomatically present intercourse of the analytic exchange, it is also where our frustrations and failures can be expressed. That which we either do not or cannot say, or may not consciously know, is the 'between-the-lines' anti-matter for analytic reading and interpretation. We also shape our identity through that which we edit out, do not say or leave silent.

In so far as language is our most potent means through which to communicate in strategic ways, and in so far as language is also used to hide our thoughts, our use of language is a vehicle of symbolising as a way of designing and ever re-designing our way through the contingencies of our inherently delimited, nervous, personal and other-peopled world.

Written words and language are the symbolic vehicles that I am using now. Spoken language, as well as body-language, vitality affects, tone and pitch of voice and artistic expression, aims to represent symbolic relations (analytic experience and thought), their affective psychic weighting and to describe certain common symbolic failures, for example, somatising, literalising and equating. Thus this is where there is a failure of healthy symbolising, memory and imagination that is developed out of the work of true mourning, including the unsymbolised and un-mourned reality of the analyst and the analytic relationship. Yet paradoxically, it is often through failures of symbolising that true symbolic realisation becomes possible. For example, a failure of symbolising function may manifest as psychoid and projective expressions of bodymind equation, this very failure revealing to the analyst vital sources of apprehension and comprehension.

Pseudo-symbolism as a defence

Although my main focus is disturbances to symbol formation, it is also important to discern when pseudo-symbolism can be used as a self-deluding and other-deluding defence, a symbol-like decoy, a misguiding form of signing. Psychodynamic privileging of the symbolic can, at times, lead to a tyranny of ethereal blindness to subtle manipulations and abuses of interpersonal and political power. In other words, we can interpret inappropriately, ideologically, self-servingly. We can be guilty of an abuse of analytic power to interpret away and cleverly symbolise one's own defensive motivations and personal power politics.

Original disappointments and symbolising

What happens *vis a vis* symbolising when, at first contact of infant and parent, the baby is not well met? Matters go very wrong when the psychosomatic family environment is one of emotional incomprehension, panic, oedipal mess, depressive retreat or a hard, robotic, autistic-like non-communication. The unmet infant has to make or find psychosomatic phantasies of order (psychosomatic co-ordination) in whatever way the infant can, as a living being with its buds of consciousness trying to survive in an emotionally malevolent desert. Attempts at self-preservation may remain primitive, be used magically or stay in a realm where body and emotion, image and idea, proto-self and other, subject and object all remain as a pre-separated and pre-organised, inherently confused unit of primary experience.

This is the psychotic core in and behind all neuroses, even our normal nervousness. We healthy symbolic thinkers, linking stuff to the past, who understand and use metaphors as 'as-ifs', who can imagine, play and create, who reflect and do not act out, who never cling superstitiously to the magic of lucky talismans, charms or other fetish idols or ideologies, who never need to or believe in personal gods out there or the beneficence of ancestors as good memories, whose past is never romanticised, who never resort uncritically to the *I Ching* – oh no, *we* never fall or regress into the merest squeak of such infantile panic, such irrational magical thinking fending off fear and angry frustration!

There can be a defensive use of symbolism that can cover over an underlying de-animated depression, an inherent lack of epistemophilic curiosity, perhaps stemming from a fear of the (sometimes sadistic) desire to get to know the insides of mother's mind and body and to get into and between the parents' exciting-frightening-forbidden primal scene and other taboo relations. Where there is no epistemophilic curiosity, there can be no enjoyment in the world and material objects or in intellectual discovery and work. And where there is a lack or loss of primary aesthetic love (i.e. the breast and especially the face of the mother and other senses of her) and of satisfied erotic desire for her body and insides, there can be no real sense of meaningful attachment and thus no emotional reality around symbolising.

Michael Fordham and symbolising

According to Michael Fordham's theory of deintegration and reintegration (Fordham, 1985, pp. 50–63), the primary self deintegrates as it meets and experiences objects and then reintegrates and internalises this experience as images and ideas of the object. This includes psychosomatically satisfying and, therefore, 'good' qualities or disappointing and, therefore, 'bad' qualities, which are either split off from each other or integrated. As this process continues, so, too, do both the managing ego and the self develop.

Fordham's deintegration-reintegration model is, in effect, a Jungian reformulation of both the Winnicottian developmental model and the Kleinian psychogenic dynamic of paranoid-schizoid defences and depressive processes and positions. Fordham's idea of the natural deintegration of the primary self into deintegrates and the symbolised reintegrates describes the origins and development of the psychological capacity for symbolising. The subject-self inherently emerges and develops through meetings and mating as emotional, meaningful and memorable attachments with objects, preferably emotionally and physically good-giving selves. Such relational experience is internalised as personal *imagos* with archetypal qualities.[2]

Warren Colman

In his paper 'Imagination and the Imaginary' (2006), Colman argues that true symbolic imagination depends on being able to distinguish between presence and absence, a capacity which depends in turn on the transcendent function, through which 'the opposites of presence and absence are transcended in the creation of the symbol'. The symbol creates 'a sense of meaning that enables us to bear and even embrace absence and loss, notwithstanding the pain involved' (2006, p. 23). On the other hand, what Colman calls 'the imaginary', is a 'defensive misuse of

2 The *imago* (Jung, *CW* 5) refers to how an internalised image is generated subjectively, according to the internal state of the subject (Samuels et al., 1986, p. 73) (Eds.).

imagination' that attempts to deny those aspects of the world that constitute a check on the omnipotence of fantasy, such as 'absence, loss, difference, otherness etc.' (Colman, 2006, p. 21).

In 'Mourning and the symbolic process' (2010), Colman describes how symbolising emerges out of mourning and is a two-person relational phenomenon (including the analytic relationship). Colman suggests that in developmental trauma, what must be symbolised is an absence. He writes that the 'absence of the object for a child is co-existent with the absence of a mind' available to think and process beta elements. Symbolising loss is not merely the re-creation of the lost object but rather the creative act of bringing a new 'imaginal' reality into being (p. 291). The work of symbolising continues on as new representations of the lost other are formed. It is an active engagement of the tension between love and hate, hope and despair, creation and stasis, life and death. This means that, like symbolising, the work of mourning is ever ongoing.

Symbolising: some observations

It is my observation that it is a healthy development to realise that ideas and imagination are psychic, not material realities. The symbolising function and symbolisation is the *jouissance* uniting and separating desire and law, in the erotic tension between possibility and the forbidden, or wish and fact, poetic imagination and hard neutral nature. Symbolisation arises out of desire and its frustration, out of lack, loss and mourning. It involves surrendering omnipotence, giving up the beloved parent, sibling or analyst as a possible sexual possession and an acquiescent understanding of the desired and/or hated object as a symbol, as an 'as if'.

In primitive emotional states where sensations are unmediated, un-ameliorated and so undeveloped, they thereby become part-object relations, possessive infatuations, fetish dependencies on emotionally over-loaded body bits, desirous and guilty relations to one's own body and its parts, personal and interpersonal zonal and gender confusions. In all such states, there is a failure to symbolise.

The pre-symbolic and the non-symbolic in personality disorders

Only psychotic, schizophrenic, severe borderline, narcissistic and addictive personality disorders, OCD states and autistic handicaps are intrinsically pre-, anti- or non-symbolic. The non-symbolic may be: an incomprehensibly confused non-symbolic state; a primitive and undeveloped pre-symbolic state (somatic, literalising, equational); a destructive/angry anti-symbolic state; or a defensive false symbolic state. In all cases, psychic (as if) reality is confused with material and actual reality.

Psychogenic autism is a defence against massive early depressive anxiety and is usually manifest in the literalism and concrete thinking of those who dare not take anything in, who cannot play or use imagination to construct and create and who dare not play with others. Petrified anxiety and depressive splits from un-mourned and unimaginable loss may lead to an 'autistic' defence against depressive anxiety featuring massive splitting, self-silencing and obliteration of desire. Instead, there is an obsessional and painful attachment to impossible objects (oedipal person or transferential obsession) and no imagination.

Those suffering claustrophobic suffocation of liveliness, a lifeless, airless tunnel with no light at the end, cannot symbolise. Those who blank out, are emotionally petrified, stunned or frozen or who defensively adopt alternative identities with complex psycho-political strategies between their sub-personalities also suffer a lack of symbolising function.

In terms of addictions, not only do the literalism and enactments of additive behaviour militate against symbolising, but certain forms of depression, anxiety, dissociation and addictions sometimes form defences against each other. Many pathologies of symbolising function feature monolithic states of myopic tunnel-vision, lacking imaginal narrative language and so any symbolically enlivening communication. The therapist's imagination may be unmoved, and so cannot 'play back' meaningfully or affectively. Countertransferentially, the therapist feels de-potentiated.

Schizoid personalities who defensively exist in a state of false imagistic/idealistic pseudo-symbolic fascination, a world of magical thinking and superstition, cannot truly symbolise. Paradoxically, this position is the flip side of concrete thinking and the symbolic equation. Superstition is common. Pseudo-symbolisation can amount to a schizoid idealisation and sublimation of fantastic (often imagistic) content, a fascinating 'archetypalising' used as a defence against the shocks of recognition and realisation. We must be clinically aware of schizoid or defensive narcissistic utilisation of fascination with ideas about and/or images of 'symbolism', especially second-hand images, magical ideas or grand words as signs of momentous significance, used to give a deceptive and illusory sense of meaning, perhaps to hold the pain and shame of lack and loss at bay, filling the lacunae with the relief of apparent meaningfulness. These false systems often cover over and defend against an underlying depression or murderous fantasies and impulses, and ultimately against the psychotic core that lies in and behind not only more extreme defensive narcissistic, borderline and other gross disorders but under all our normal neuroses.

Symbolic disfunctions in narcissistic and borderline personality disorders

Let us now consider the internal, relational and analytic problems with symbolisation that are symptomatic of narcissistic and borderline personality disorders. In severe borderline states featuring problems of symbolising there is no distinction between fantasy and reality. Images, ideas, impulses and wishes are taken as concrete and imperative, arising out of an un-mourned lack-loss of a parental figure, an affectively and morally dangerous or ambiguous parent, autistic-like environmental conditions or familial and personal histories of somatising. In place of symbolic thinking, there is a propensity towards impotent outrage, projective identification and infection, lack of impulse control or frustration tolerance. There is no reflective inclination but a defiance of superego. There is an urgent need to communicate impotent frustration and outrage. There is an abject absence of connection, an emotional, erotic lack. Instead of symbolising 'as if' it was real, things are taken 'as real'.

Such symbolic equations may be open to eventual re-conception. Angry, destructive, borderline defences are so literalised and acted out they are paradoxically acutely honest and are so open to true apperception. They can be analytically reflected upon and recycled.

Borderline personalities act through a red haze of murderous hate and destructive impulses, which are often acted out. Such destructive acting-out, literalising and unreflective unconscious splitting is based on relational and emotional lack and frustration as well as confusions between inner and outer, fantasy and reality. In addition, there are oedipal and zonal confusions, behavioural confusion in areas of desire, sexual fantasy and relations. Out of such confusion and frustration, an impulse to attack the most needed good objects erupts, as well as primitive splitting of the hated all-bad and the desperately desired all-good as found in pathological forms of projective identification.

There is a possibility of limited temporary symbolisation. There may be a recognition that the core self is damaged and faulty, that early and subsequent emotional attachments were not enough. Yet the hurt outrage is open to being usefully recycled, harnessed and constructively redirected. To adapt a Spinozan attitude: 'You can love god or nature or the other (parent/analyst), but you cannot expect god or nature or the other to love you back in the same way!'

Borderline destructiveness of the good and strategic narcissistic falseness is the shadow of each other (which is why borderline persons and narcissists tend to hate each other). Both personality disorders arise as a desperate defence against a catastrophic absence (or perversion) of 'primary love' in Balint's sense (1952) and so against a bottomless well of depression. Ultimately, they both defend against a void of absolute lack, a primal absence of any vital bodymind attachment. This means that under the anger and rage, there is a basic core of too-dreadful defeat and depression. However, if this fundamental wound and all-permeating hurt are reached and its abject grief or utter despair is expressed, mourning that engenders real symbolisation may emerge. Addictive- and personality-disordered states tend to be so un-empathic and emotionally manipulative that there can be no symbolic linking, no real imaginal life, no honest critical reflection, no recognition of the subjectivity of projections, no relational alterity and no symbolisation.

The task of analysis involves withdrawing projections with a deep thud of realisation. Projections tend towards exaggeration and literalisation. Mother/father/lover/other is magically, divinely All-Good or is dangerously and disastrously All-Bad. Subjectively, I am, therefore, all good or all bad (as in defeated or angry depression) or all victim (as in narcissistic righteousness or borderline outrage). This is what Klein called the paranoid-schizoid position (Klein, 1935), pre-ambivalent, pre-depressive, without reflection and no affective linking. Nor is there a healthy sense of uncertainty or doubt such as thinking to oneself, 'I don't know for sure'.

Narcissistic personalities are often so brittle, self-righteous and emotionally blackmailing they cannot accept any challenge to their bubble of a system. With their onanistic perspective, they lack empathy and altruistic imagination. Their nervous and recurrent self-deluding defences preclude the development of a relational and social personality. Narcissistic defences are used to avoid underlying depression, anger, borderline outrage and even psychotic impulses. Analytically, there is hope when there is a slow discovery that such underlying murderous hate does not actually kill the therapist (Winnicott, 1949). Such hate-fuelled impulses are actually more relational than the delusions and illusions of narcissistic falseness: they are more meetable, fightable and even playable with and may possibly even lead in the end to a zone of shared irony.

Kernberg (2004) suggests that any less defended expression of underlying borderline outrage is a healthy improvement to false narcissistic self-love. The hiddenness of narcissistic, angry depression covers a basic de-animating, emptiness or meaningless depression, which in turn underlies the fear of shame, humiliation, impotence, ugly desire, openness to punitive rejection or annihilating and painful attack. Narcissism as an effective defence against the destructive rage of borderline impulses hides oedipal fears of both infanticide and castrating parenticide. I would suggest that narcissistic defences are so structurally adamant and so affectively self-deceiving and other-deceiving that they can never really be recycled. Otherwise, there is often regression to pre-symbolic states and/or fragmentation of psychic integrity.

The animating psychoid 'body', the infectious psychosomatic identifications and projections, of beta bits and fragments, as found in the psychotic transference of destructive borderline and angry narcissistic disorders, are the necessarily extreme but affective ways of communicating and relating from an incomprehensible and unsymbolised internal world.

Beta bits are only known when they disturb order; when they are 'out of order'. Like 'matter out of place' (Douglas, 1966), beta disorder only draws attention to itself and only becomes affectively noticeable when it disturbs our psychosomatic co-ordination and our relations. When beta matters are lying latently in the pre-symbolic psychoid materia of normal primal states, even as a pre-ordered unconscious *massa confusa*, they are a neutral and natural 'in-place' aspect of human nature. Just as 'O' becomes evidently manifest through and in its transformations, so too is the beta realm realised and recognised through its disturbances and challenges to conscious alpha functions.

Destructive borderline persons are good at splitting off and projecting their own primitive fear of symbolic realisation, because it is so near to the core, so close and real. That is why, speaking with a touch of irony here, they can make such good analysts – if and when they have eventually learnt to sufficiently contain and control their hate, that is to say, after at least 12 years of at least four times a week well-framed analysis, necessarily through a psychotic transference, which has made the real madness familiar and recycled it into a ruthless passion for moral (and relational) honesty. Jim, the destructive borderline patient whom we met earlier[3] (and will revisit shortly), now works very effectively with disturbed adolescents. He has been asked to head up national think-tanks because he is recognised to be acutely perceptive and a force to be reckoned with – in other words, fiercely recycling his anger and disappointment into radical truths.

Over-sensitive narcissists are very good at interpreting the hidden implications of other people's unconscious symbolic blind-spots (if not their own), helping others realise the meaning of their false-self fantasies and other erroneous significations. That is why they make over-empathic (or nervously falsely sympathetic) psychotherapists, at the cost (to others) of remaining blindly self-righteous, self-pitying, self-excusing and so brittle and defensive in everyday relationships. Christine, as an example of such a narcissistic patient, is now a counsellor-cum-psychotherapist.[4] By her own account, she is 'one of the cleverest and most knowing therapists', even if disliked by her 'mediocre' colleagues and 'most unfairly' unappreciated by her 'selfish' friends and 'disappointing' ex-lovers. In other words, she is still managing her self-conscious loneliness, her underlying empty depression and her primitive fears of destruction and annihilation.

Persons with an affect-less depression, in a state of depressive petrification, are unable to symbolise. There is no reflection, integration or assimilation through normal linking-recognition of loss and absence; instead, there is a clinging to the impossible object, often with split-off and projected obsessional jealousies and irrational objects of hate.

Somatisation is often symptomatic of pre-symbolic, non-symbolic maldevelopment: being stuck in an early body-mind identity, a pre-differentiated psychoid base. This is a regression to a natural base but one with an undeveloped, wounded and defensive internal non-relation. As I understand matters, the psyche is biological, organic in all senses and intrinsically psychoid. Somatising, as well as a symptom of the pre-symbolic, is also a form of proto-symbolising. Psychosomatic pain and/or confusion are simultaneously both a self-defeating defence and a manifest expression of such pain and confusion. For example, harming and cutting of physical parts of oneself may be understood symbolically as a cutting through to the quick and raw pain: an expression and indication of hurt as well as relief. It is an act of affectively somatised proto-symbolisation, a mode of connection and communication. Sexual fantasy is another central zone for the development, mal-development or the atrophying of symbolisation, for active confusion of fantasy and reality, for obsessional restriction, distortion and perversion. It is a psychic realm formed out in the face of taboos, oedipal laws, limitations and often mixed up with zonal confusions, the intolerable frustration of omnipotent gratification, trauma and other private and public fears. It involves sorting out reality

3 See Chapters Six, Seven, Nine and Thirteen (Eds.).

4 See Chapters Nine, Thirteen and Sixteen (Eds.).

and fantasy, desires and repulsions, imagination and empathy and so, of necessary symbolisation. Or it is a realm of non-symbolic, un-reflexive, impulsive acting out. It may represent the potential for psychosomatic recycling of defensive or creative sublimation, of *jouissance*-excess that can be an explosive force of re-creation, where ruthless sadism can return to a more basic and vital motility.

Play, which is based on interpersonal trust in the early familial environment, is always a developmentally vital, symbolic act. Play is about understanding and creating a good and affective (psycho-political) relation to personal and interpersonal powers and their limits, with family relations, with love and hate, lust and disgust, sex and aggression, with impotence, shame and fear.

However, where there is no basic primary trust, potential play loses its symbolic quality, becoming perversely serious, non-unimaginative and literalised: 'as real', rather than 'as if' real. Developmentally, literalised, paranoid-schizoid projections and projective identifications and absolute splits ideally move towards a more complex self-consciousness and so to more reflexive relational behaviour. This requires a good-enough family or analytic container which provides a reflective, reversible, usable and actively responsive psychosomatic bodymind. Sometimes, the development of symbolic reflection and critical self-awareness, of psychological 'as if' thinking and imaginal empathy, of the capacity to play with ideas and play with others, remains limited. This may be for structural reasons or due to the depth of the faults and fears caused by early lacks, confusions, assaults or traumatic shaming and due to the absolute need to maintain and repeat very narrow, evasive or very fierce defences.

'Jim'

To demonstrate the nature of the symbolising function and its emergence and partial development, let us return to the evolving story of borderline Jim and our beta-filled relations after he had attacked the 'church' as my cathedral-body-mind.

I shall first pick two mutative interactions with Jim and try to explain how a psychological understanding (*Anschauungsweise*) and interpretation melted the defences and splits and so moved the relationship in such a way that a degree of symbolic connection and realisation (conception and birth of a third) was formed.

One day, after we had worked for about six years, Jim had to go away for three weeks. He knew he would have to pay for missed sessions. I simply accepted the news and waited. He was frustrated that I was apparently unmoved by this separation and seemed not to care whether he came or went, but above all, he was furious that 'I was leaving him'. In fact, Jim was the one going away, not me. But for Jim, my letting him go away represented an active abandonment of him.

Jim: I hate your stubborn passivity so much that I would just love to stab you.
Me: So I now know that you love me enough to hate me.
Jim: Bloody hell . . . I want to hurt you to the edge of killing you . . . (long pause) . . . Actually, that frightens me, now I say it.

Me: Thinking about stabbing me and nearly killing me.
Jim: When I imagine it, I'd shove it into your belly . . . and I imagine you liking it.
Me: A pleasure.
Jim: Another feeble oh-so-correct word! An orgasm, you fool, an orgasm as you fear that you are going to die!
Me: So, at least you know what you want to shove into me.
Jim: Yes, I know all that. But why does sex have to be so lethal? No, of course, I know why. It's the only way I can get myself and my needs across and into someone. I'd like to stab you with a poison dart, which would give you an unknown deep chronic illness. That'd be fucking great.
Me: So to speak. Anyhow we might say that you've done a fucking good job of that with me over the years.
Jim: Yeah, I suppose I have, haven't I? Fucking great, mate!

About a month later, I told Jim that I was going to emigrate to Australia, so we would have to finish analysis in a year. Although all hell broke loose for that year, so did a process of difficult reflection. He started challenging the boundaries and frames in new ways, particularly over times, not leaving at the end of sessions, ringing between, demanding more, all as a punishment and as a sign of panicky dread. Jim's eventual parting gesture was a new and loaded hit of hurt and angry symbolism. As a leaving present, he gave me a torn-in-half book with a cover picture of a three-spired cathedral. I wondered whether this was a message (symbolic act) or 'how it actually is' . . . He said that it is how it feels.

Jim: Anyhow, for fuck's sake, it's an image, not a bloody church this time. Of course, it's meant to hurt because it's about ruining something beautiful, which I know matters to you, you fairy, and it can't be fucking mended; so there, fuck it. Fuck you . . . . I'll miss you, you sod. And I hope you feel fucking guilty. Forever!
Me: I won't forget you!
Jim: You'd better bloody not.

Not only was Jim a living demonstration of a 'dual-aspect psychosomatic reality', but also, in deeming the cathedral or cathedral image (our cathedral) to be worthy of attack and destruction, he was demonstrating that the beautiful is the good and thus that aesthetics is ethics. This I take to be a relatively mature and sophisticated level of symbolising.

'Adie'

In contrast to Jim, Adie was a person determinedly stuck in non-symbolising, fixed in a state of non-play and non-imagination as a way of avoiding mourning intolerable loss and emotional impossibilities. Instead, she was driven by unbridgeable splits, obsessional jealous (oedipal) fantasies and a hatred of the visible desires of others.

Adie was obsessed with a married so-called 'lover', Don, who paid her virtually no attention, except minimally to keep her quiet and hanging on indefinitely. This presenting state of non-affairs at least made her sad and desperate, but without daring to actually be angry, let alone express it. Adie could never realise that father or lover or I were all unavailable. She had no good memories (or good objects) and had a very limited imagination, let alone capacity for play. She stayed fixedly within her Jewish parents' world, with the fantasy of an unavailable, unreal lover-man, and with me as the magic man who would make the impossible dreams of coming into life and love an actual reality. Adie could only feel obsessional hate for any signs of other people's love life and was totally unable to connect or relate this back to her jealousy of her married non-lover, to her father for loving her mother, to exciting primal scene horrors, to her terrifying forbidden love for her father's carpenter's hands and what they could do and to her mother's and all women's hateful and disgusting small, short women's bodies.

Through her obsession with making pink lampshades (which in itself was linked to her psychic inheritance of intergenerational trauma) and an urgent and imperative/tyrannical task of keeping the family safe by never travelling too far away, I was able to see an intergenerational denial of unimaginably traumatic loss. *Inter alia*, from dream information, I knew that back in her disavowed and untouchable family history, 'lampshades' belonged to the most horrific but unconscious and unrecognised story of unmanageable traumatic loss. Adie could not at all 'get' this not-to-be-sighted and not-to-be-sensed symbolic load. Her world was adamantly small, neat and safe.

One day, Jim passed Adie as he was coming (invasively early) to see me. As he passed her, he mumbled, 'sour-faced cunt'. As he relayed this information to me, I knew that this was a typical Jim-style attack on me, but in a new and troublesome form. In Jim's field of seamless equations, she (Adie) was me (who was always a 'feeble cunt'), was part of my world, which was his world, which was our world, which was his/our disordered 'bodymind' . . . which was simultaneously both forcefully demanding and enviously resenting order.

As always, Jim succeeded in both infuriating and alarming me, but also made me feel protective of Adie; this would surely hurt and frighten her. However, I also thought that he was sort of right! I was dreading her next session; surely she would express volumes of hurt outrage. Imagine my surprise, then, when she apparently took the episode in her stride, only saying, 'What a rude man!' And then later went on and added, 'Perhaps he's right; I wish I could relax and look happier'. She took Jim's remark at non-symbolic 'face value'.

Adie: Do you like me in pink?
Me: You mean, like your father does? Perhaps you wear pink to appear to be Daddy's pretty girl.
Adie: Well, do you?
Me: It depends. I sometimes think it is a mere covering.

Adie: That man was right!
Me: He was a mirror.
Adie: Yes!
Me: I am your mirror.
Adie: Yes!

So somehow arising out of this non-crisis, she had critically 'got it' . . . at least at that moment, she got a homeopathic bit of metaphor and reflection, and even perhaps a bit of serious play. For a long time, that was about as far as Adie could go; otherwise, she remained split, literalising and compulsively phobic about horribly exciting, in-your-face disgusting public 'sex scenes' (as she called them), which were still determinedly never anything to do with her good, clean, bland self.

Or so it seemed. Until, very unpredictably and suddenly, her paternal uncle, her father's younger brother, died of a heart attack. At the funeral, she was overcome by the spectacle of the grief of one of her uncle's two sons. This cousin had a girlfriend with him, whose public display of comforting gestures Adie loathed. A week later, she visited him 'to console her poor cousin'. The girlfriend was not there; he became 'very emotional'. And she said, 'Please sleep with me . . . just for relief'. And they sort of did.

A crisis of guilt, shame and excited desire followed. This cousin was father, was me, was all forbidden incestuous men, was the defeat of the other woman, in fact of all women. Initially, these interpretations were received with her usual impassivity and silence, but slowly, her stillness began to look stunned and became increasingly expressive of a gradual and shocking dawning of connection and symbolic understanding. However, the manic, blind and false-fantastic 'relationship' with the cousin continued, now replacing the hopeless fantasy about Don.

In a session one day, Adie suddenly said, 'For me, Joe's fingers and his penis are the same thing, they really are . . . and of course they are different'. I was stunned. This latter part ('and of course they are different') was hugely significant as the emergence of symbolic thinking. Later, I was able to analyse her very mixed or rather confused and pre-ambivalent ideas about these penis-fingers, as exciting hands, rapacious hands, masturbating hands, dangerous hands, loving father's hands. As to whether these were symbolic equations or symbolic understandings remained unclear . . . due to her fears around these topics and/or to her related general emotional blandness.

When the obsessional 'incestuous' fantasy relationship with this cousin started to go very sour, Adie 'tightened up' again and returned to her old splits and defences. However, she could never forget the reality of this recent upheaving phase of her history and would always now live with certain disturbing memories, sadness, doubts and dreams. She once referred to the whole erotic episode as a 'flurry'. She had to fight not to fall back into her fantasies and melancholic yearnings for her married lover. Otherwise, she felt that her sexual life was now over. Her lampshade-making became a mindless monotonous ritual, fending off the acute pain of her loneliness and sense of loss.

My ongoing countertransferential oscillation of irritation and sadness informed me that Adie was still painfully failing to be able to mourn and manage separation whilst maintaining her desire to keep and not to lose (particularly the good father). Symbolic realisation would bring too much awareness of loss: her own and that of her internalised ancestors. Adie lived out of an internalised family world of a buried 'terrible knowing, too terrible to speak', and if that which cannot be said is too utterly disavowed, split off or absolute, then it cannot be properly symbolised.

The development of symbolising function

What eventually enables the development of the symbolising function and changes of relations to it to emerge? Well, the answer is, I think, in an ambivalent integration of the tension between:

- The laws of nature (actuality) and the psychic reality of personal freedom;
- Laws of the fathers[5] (or frames) and desire;
- Power and impossibility;
- Love and loss;
- Memory and mourning;
- Fantasy and limits;
- Imagination and reason.

These tense dilemmas lead us to having to symbolise as the only possibility for realistic conscious understanding and functioning. What do we do analytically to enable such a development? How does one bring about something mutative? What actually happens symbolically? I suggest three necessary elements are: a real self-position; a process; and a frame.

Analytic position

Regarding a position, I feel and know that I am firstly emotionally healthy and strong enough; secondly conceptually and thoughtfully clear enough; and thirdly both un-defensively imaginative and truly realistic enough to move myself and hence sometimes the other person out of this state of mutual identification and psychosomatic confusion.

5 The term 'Law of the Father' was first coined by Freud in 1897 and taken up by Lacan in regard to the function of the Laws of the Father as mediating desire and order, the limits on the enactment of desire that brings in symbolisation (Eds.).

Analytic process

In regard to process, I suggest that the course of our analytic action is: receptive reverie > contemplation > active reverie > reflection > reason and critical thought > scepticism > responsible interpretation . . . from within our analytic frame.

Analytic frame

The analytic frame symbolically addresses the core of our endeavour and its effectiveness. It invokes our special ritual use of particular laws of the fathers, our psychological and relational taboos, limits and lacks, the inevitable losses, breaks and separations and so the ethical call for mourning. The analytic container and its frames do the work, make the work and *are* the work. The containing frame with its rules and vital rituals may disappoint as much as they may demand. It is these 'irritating facts' that analytically challenge the motor of symbolising and its failures. The frame is the safe, strong scaffolding which allows for and evokes dangerous lacks and the necessary madness of necessary defences. This is Talmudic law, the Mithraic contract, the monastic rule, training requirements, frequency, regularity and boundaries. Therapeutically, the only effective and non-didactic way of engendering the emergence, development and healing of an atrophied symbolising function is through that most frustrating symbolic ritual, the safe analytic frame with its strong ethical laws.

The symbolic is there in the odd and particular analytic relationship. The analyst is a transferential symbol; the analysis and its frame are a symbolic container and dynamic of psychic change and development; the analytic relationship evokes love and hate, desire and fear, lust and disgust, satisfaction and disappointment, hope and inevitable loss and a life of hope, fulfilment, failure and mourning. The analytic frame is an active symbol of all other rules, limits and frustrations, demanding comprehension and constructive and creative adaptation. The analytic container and its limits (taboos, impossibilities, framed exclusions, etc.) re-activates developmental, relational lacks and their normal/abnormal defensive madness. Out of the integration of necessary frustration, true symbolisation or re-symbolisation may begin to develop.

The containing frame provokes, evokes and re-constellates the frustration of all oedipal laws and limits and simultaneously makes it safe for emotional conflict and disorder, for the management, or the disordered mismanagement and destructive outrage (furious psychosomatic infection) to occur within it. The container is also the analyst's reliable, healthy and good-enough 'bodymind'. This is an emotionally attuned, sensitive and thoughtful but also critical analytic mind that meets with understanding (observation, interpretation, discovery, difference and necessary limitations) the needs of the emotional mind of the other but also challenges their defences and realises that the limits make for the work of symbolisation out of the sense of frustration. Part of this mental containing is found in or through ironic differences and limitations of each other.

The frame can also be seen to work like the Euclidian method applied to emotional disorder: not to suppress the pain but rather to point up and so to apprehend, describe and comprehend it. This method requires Socratic doubt, analytic unknowing and interpretation. Through revealing that which is false, an essence of truth and of a truer self may also be revealed, emerge and develop. This is also a method which defines the best possible procedures, ordering and understanding of our place in the world, of our being part of nature, an intuitive knowledge of the connections, links and relations that are our internal and external world. Thus, this disciplined application of a law of the fathers grinds and polishes a lens which further sharpens the analytic focus so we see, know and realise ourselves and other selves, strange warts and all.

Finally, there is the very important matter of the taboo, that alarming, dangerous and so very powerfully affective 'enigmatic realm' which lies between and so outside the clearly defined and demarked. This is the liminal boundary zone, the indefinable, moving or changing frame, where language breaks down or reaches its limits, as does behaviour. We integrate difficult disruptions, slippages, mistakes and conflicts in this taboo-laden zone, with buried (unconscious) land-mines waiting for us to stumble into. Experiences of painful disillusionment, angry or erotic tension can be integrated if the boundaries are found to be basically good and strong enough to survive such shocking experiences. Depressive realisations and symbolic understanding are also challenged by moments of therapy that reveal faults in the frame. An unconscious breaking of the frame by the analyst may represent an unconscious destructive force in the analytic relationship and, therefore, the internalised parental relationship, for example, an unrecognised pattern of passive aggression.

It is here, too, in the analytic cracks, that we are urgently challenged to symbolise as constructively as possible or fail to do so. It is worth remembering that ultimately, as analysts, we can only 'actively observe'; we cannot make meaning for another. Our 'active observation', which is emotionally, thoughtfully and interpretively related, may well be the fertile ground upon which a human and humane symbolisation emerges and develops.

Twenty-one thoughts summarising the theme of symbolising, somatising and not-symbolising

1 The possibility for and degree or depth of transformation of structural, developmental and environmental faults and failures to the symbolising function may be limited.
2 Psychotic, schizophrenic, borderline, narcissistic and addictive personality disorders, OCD states and autistic handicaps are often intrinsically pre-, anti- or non-symbolic.
3 The not-symbolic may be symptomatic of a) a primitive and undeveloped pre-symbolic state (somatic, literalising, equational), b) a zonally/oedipally confused state, c) a defensively false-symbolic state (schizoid, narcissistic), d)

a destructive/angry anti-symbolic state (borderline) and e) other constrictive tunnel-like states.

4 Lack of symbolising implies lack of imagination and atrophy of empathy. Empathic imagination enables one to comprehend relational reality and behave accordingly, so a lack of empathy makes one not understand relational realities.

5 In so far as we are working analytically in a realm in which there are no facts, only interpretations, all analytic work is explicitly and entirely symbolic. For persons with limited symbolising capacities, this relation cannot be fully made use of until such time as an incipient symbolising capacity develops.

6 The experience of true symbols, symbolisation and the processes of symbolising is always a reconstructive disturbance, a catastrophic crisis of conception and re-conception, of de-connection and re-connection.

7 Each and every new symbol disturbs certainty and unsettles meaning. Symbolising, because it is elusive and open to infinite interpretations, can be as deviant, self-deceiving and other-deceiving as words and language.

8 A symbol becomes a mere sign once it is defined by a given meaning and so has to be allowed to die and change disturbingly again and again: all meanings are provisional and temporary.

9 Dreams and fantasies need an amplificatory, associative, linking and interpretive symbolic imagination in order to create an 'objective correlative'[6] where there is none apparent!

10 Since amplifications and interpretations, etc., are symbolic as-ifs, those who cannot symbolise cannot hear their possible symbolic meanings and such symbolic analytic communications have neither effect nor affect.

11 The symbolising function emerges and develops out of the safe containment and transformation of limits to omnipotence, to the realities of contingencies and contingent realities of others, to loss and grief. Such limits, realities and losses force and form imagination, which may become the imaginal, and so, symbolisation.

12 Symbolisation is about the incorporation or non-incorporation of various degrees of normal frustration, which may lead to an acquiescence to the depressive limitations of one's omnipotence, to a realisation of the ambivalence of all relations, to an understanding of the subjectivity of fantasy in the face of adamant contingencies. In other words, this is about the developmentally difficult but necessary, 'normal' and healthy integration of the limits of hallucinatory omnipotence, the limits of power, possession and permanence and the movement from loss, limitation and frustration to grief and mourning. Or if this fails, to dissociation, denial, depression, to the defences of narcissistic false superiority or to a defiant but impotent murderous outrage.

6 The term 'objective correlative' is often attributed to T.S. Eliot, who used it in his essay 'Hamlet and His Problems' (1919), but was first coined by the American painter and poet Washington Allston (1779–1843) (Eds.).

13 In primitive emotional states where sensations are unmediated, un-ameliorated and so undeveloped, sensations and their impulses become over-urgent, gripping part-object relations: compulsive infatuations and possessiveness; fetish dependencies on emotionally over-loaded body bits; desirous/guilty relations to one's own body and its parts; personal and interpersonal zonal and gender confusions, etc. In all such states, there is a failure to symbolise or a narrowing of the symbolising function.

14 If, as analysts, we intuit the symbolic meaning implicit in the patient's unsymbolised material, we cannot symbolise 'for' the patient, only, through shared interpretive analytic activity, symbolise 'with' the patient, such that it ultimately becomes the patient's own symbolic activity. As psychotherapists, we can only a) be open (listen) and be used and b) observe and explore. We cannot make meaning for another. Indeed, where the other has no symbolic capacity, to try do so is vain, an act of selfish violence . . . and is anyhow self-defeating and useless.

15 Symbolising is an emergent solution to variously difficult (and sometimes shocking) opposites, especially the tension between the *jouissance* of life and love and the terrors of loss and death . . . including these in very early infant states.

16 Primary (early) symbolising develops in order to relate and make emotional and ideational sense of two different objects, especially a lusty appetite for life and an existential dread of death. Symbolising is, therefore, a finding and making of significance out of and between: life, love, loss (of loved object) and death.

17 Because we live in a world of presences, absences and losses, we have a past, present and future that is a psychic realm of attachments, hopes and fears and the reality of prospective losses and deaths, including our own.

18 Without our human idea and sense of subjective time and space (and difference), there could be no symbolising.

19 The potential offered by psychoanalysis is a reflectively honest two-person relationship that may help towards the emergence and development of a realistic symbolising function, the symbolisation of previously pre-symbolic, un-symbolised, confused and confusing (literalised) matters.

20 My own formulation is that symbolising arises out of the tension of complex relations between six ontological 'realms of being': a) basic natural biological impulses and unconscious psychic desires and fears (the biological, the neurobiological and the psychic are consubstantial at the psychoid level), b) right brain imaging and left brain thinking, c) unconscious fantasy and unconscious memory (including dreams), d) more conscious fantasy and imagination, e) strategic reasoning (based on a realization of the implications of living in time and space) and f) an ego-consciousness that is much permeated by the moral dilemmas created by the superego. Symbolising (i.e. affective and rational associative linking, a potential for empathy and creativity) emerges and develops out of and through the relations between these six psychosomatic and ontological realms. When any of these elements goes wrong, the relations between them goes wrong or is developmentally disturbed and harmed, then symbolisation goes wrong and is disturbed and harmed.

21 Analytically, it is out of a mix of dream, reverie, imagination, play, association and/or linking, critical empathy, thinking and strategic reasoning that a self-aware and realistic irony may grow, a knowing that we do not know, an understanding that a statement or communication means something other than what is overtly asserted. Such a capacity for healthy irony and scepticism is, I suggest, ultimately the only affective symbolic agency in the face of concrete thinking, un-reflected impulse and 'not-symbolising'.

Concluding thoughts on symbolising and not symbolising

In summary, the task of psychoanalysis is the establishing, maintaining and moving through a critical analytic relationship of frustration, desire, limits, loss, mourning and possible meaning. This sometimes uncovers and enables an epistemophilic and mutative observation of our psychosomatic, emotional and thoughtful mentation rather than aiming to establish a relatively 'stable ego'.

Symbolising is a deintegrative-reintegrative process. But even proto-symbols that are clung to as part objects, talismans, idols (let alone ideals), can be necessary defensive objects which do a normally neurotic job. Here, I am giving respectful place to the needs of our fearful, meaning-seeking human nature. A 'dual aspect' perspective helps me to understand and move self and other in and out of such a world of symbolic equation, unsymbolised acting out or projected psychoid disorder and confusion.

The analyst symbolises the somatised, un-symbolised matter of the patient. This symbolising 'of' should not become a symbolising 'for'. My symbolising of their matters can become (through interpretation) 'our' symbolising . . . and thence the other person's own symbolising. Somatising, as well as a pathology, is a necessary proto-symbolising. For example, harming and cutting (of physical parts of self) is a cutting through to the quick and the raw pain, and is an affectively somatised proto-symbolising, a mode of connection and communication.

Symbolising is, therefore, a finding and making of significance out of and between: life, love, loss (of loved objects) and death. Without our human idea and sense of time (and space and, therefore, difference), there could be no symbolising. Because we live in a world of losses and absences (of presences and gains), we have (conscious and unconscious) memories of the past, we have a present that is also made up of presence and absence, and a future that is an imagination of hopes and fears, as well as the reality of prospective losses and deaths, including one's own. Managing this is the symbolising function of our human nature.

References

Balint, M. (1952). *Primary Love, and Psycho-Analytic Technique*. London: Hogarth.
Bion, W. (1962). *Learning from Experience*. London: William Heinemann.

Bion, W. (1965). *Transformations*. London: Karnac.
Britton, R. (1998). *Belief and Imagination: Explorations in Psychoanalysis*. London: Routledge.
Colman, W. (2006). 'Imagination and the Imaginary'. *Journal of Analytical Psychology*, 51(1): 21–41.
Colman, W. (2010). 'Mourning and the Symbolic Process'. *Journal of Analytical Psychology*, 55(2): 275–297.
de Mijolla, A., ed. (2005). *International Dictionary of Psychoanalysis*. Detroit, MI: Macmillan Reference USA.
Douglas, M. (1966). *Purity and Danger: An Analysis of Concepts of Pollution and Taboo*. London: Routledge & Kegan Paul.
Fordham, M. (1985). *Explorations into the Self*. London and New York: Routledge & Kegan Paul.
Jones, E. (1961). *Papers on Psycho-Analysis*. Boston: Beacon Press.
Jung, C. (1967). 'On the Relation of Analytical Psychology to Poetry'. In *Spirit in Man, Art, and Literature*. Vol. 15 of *The Collected Works of C.G. Jung*. R. Hull, trans. London: Routledge & Kegan Paul.
Kernberg, O. (2004). *Aggressivity, Narcissism and Self-Destructiveness in the Psychotherapeutic Relationship*. New Haven: Yale University Press.
Klein, M. (1935). 'A Contribution to the Psychogenesis of Manic-Depressive States'. *International Journal of Psychoanalysis*, 16: 145–174.
Rycroft, C. (1972). *A Critical Dictionary of Psychoanalysis*. Harmondsworth: Penguin.
Samuels, A., Shorter, B. & Plaut, F. (1986). *A Critical Dictionary of Jungian Analysis*. London: Routledge & Kegan Paul.
Segal, H. (1950). 'Some Aspects of the Analysis of a Schizophrenic'. *International Journal of Psycho-Analysis*, 31: 268–278.
Segal, H. (1952). 'A Psycho-Analytic Contribution to Aesthetics'. *International Journal of Psycho-Analysis*, 33: 196–207.
Segal, H. (1957). 'Notes on Symbol Formation'. *International Journal of Psycho-Analysis*, 38: 391–397.
Segal, H. (1991). *Dream, Phantasy, and Art*. London: Routledge.
Winnicott, D. (1949). 'Hate in the Counter-Transference'. *International Journal of Psychoanalysis*, 30: 69–74.

Chapter 11

Romantic catastrophes and other vital realities

Unpublished, 2009[1]

I will begin with three quotes that inspire my reflections on love:

> The most ideal human passion is love, which is also the most absolute and animal and one of the most ephemeral.
>
> (George Santayana, *Reason in Religion;* Santayana, 1922, p. 196)

> Without love, no happiness.
>
> (Milton, *Paradise Lost: Book VII*)

> Essentially, one might say, the cure is effected by love.
>
> (Letter from Freud to Jung, 6 Dec 1906; McGuire, 1974, pp. 12–13)

In the following, the matter of love is discussed through two areas of interest. Firstly, we consider the influence of the radical subjectivity of German Romanticism, Idealism and the early psychology of Schelling, which is very much a psychology of the unconscious. Secondly, there is a clinical concern with psychosomatic mind-body relations as manifested in the transference-countertransference, a particular interest being destructive borderline and severe narcissistic disorders and their erotic-martial defences against the losses and fears of primary love and intimacy. The two topics are inter-related: firstly, because various aspects of German philosophy and poetry can act analytically as a mental or ideational lens to clarify and amplify clinical thinking; and secondly, the theme of problematic, painfully thwarted primary and subsequent love is a common denominator for both Romantic and psychodynamic attention. A third area concerns the psychoanalytic

1 This chapter amalgamates three unpublished papers concerning love. 'Romantic Catastrophes and Other Vital Realities' (2009) was presented at the ANZAP Saturday Morning Seminar Series: 'A Symposium on Love', in Sydney in March 2009. 'From Pain to Pleasure and Back Again: *Jouissance* and a best possible life' (2009) was given to the C.G. Jung Society of Western Australia on May 15, 2009. 'Difficult Passions' (2009) was given to the Canberra Jung Society in October 2009. Clark also made minor changes to some of these papers, the last being in 2013. We have used his latest versions for this amalgamation (Eds.).

DOI: 10.4324/9781003255826-12

application of Spinoza's writings on love. Let me begin with a brief description of the analytic relevance of the Romantics.

The Romantics

The Romantics both expressed and sometimes lived out their love psychoses to a radical degree, perhaps because they were unable or unwilling to contain their rather infantile, idealistic and sometimes incestuous fantasies and projections. However, although apt to act out destructively, they also defied the cultural superego of the Enlightenment and its passion-killing over-use of Reason. They challenged such a system imaginatively and creatively, re-evaluating irrational passions and associations, the unsystematic and the organic, 'the night-side', the life force and therefore love, its madness and its pains, for its own true sake.

I think especially of Goethe's novel *Sorrows of Young Werther*, written in 1774 and revised in 1787, of Friedrich Schlegel's 1799 novel *Lucinde*, of Kleist and the romantically-inspired *Liebestod* of his double suicide with Henriette Vogel and of the blue flower that first appeared in a dream in a novel by Novalis and became a key Romantic symbol. I think of the wonderful poetic epistolary novel *Hyperion* that Hölderlin wrote before the psychosis-inducing loss of his beloved Diotima in 1800. I recall the sheer brilliant beauty and imaginative creativity of that addicted *puer* Coleridge and of wild Shelley and above all, the painfully playful irony of Heinrich Heine whilst living for years in a 'coffin bed' of physical agony.

I think as well of the empathic cultural pluralism of Herder, of the identity theory and theory of the unconscious within Schelling's *Naturphilosophie*, of the psychodynamic perspicacity of Hegel's master-slave analysis, of Schopenhauer's hilarious and life-enhancing depressive pessimism, his understanding of blind sexual appetites and his angry misogyny. I consider the many German dream theorists and psychologists from von Schubert and Carus, up to the influential swan-song of Fechner's psychological pantheism.

I am intrigued too by the jealous and tragic brother-sister loves of Romantics such as Wordsworth and his sister Dorothy in relation to his wife Mary, Hegel and his sister Christiane, his *Antigone* in relation to Christiane and his wife Marie, Byron and his half-sister Augusta Leigh and even Nietzsche and Elizabeth in relation to Lou Andreas-Salomé.

This subject is a passionate love-zone of my own, but like all good and real loves, it is actually a relation of love-hate. In spite of recognising the possible gains of inwardness, individual feeling and expression of the relationship between love and madness and of personal moral responsibility, I am struck by the narcissistic shadow here. There is irritating sentimentality hiding sadism, an exhibitionism which can be masturbatory, and an excess of feeling that sometimes becomes interpersonally and socially dangerous through a careless loss of good reason.

Tied up with this shadow down-side of Romanticism are schizoid, impersonal and, therefore, depersonalizing, over-generalised imagistic ideas of sexual relations, of the other within and their projection, of a contra-sexual *anima* and *animus*, ideals of oneness, indulgence in death wishes as a suicidal preservation of the ideal good self, which is a denial of time, change, of true disappointment and depressive ambivalence. This is surely more of a fantastic and pathological world of schizoid and narcissistic ideation, sometimes actually precluding both critical reason and the imaginal. A tyranny of the irrational, nationalism and sentimentality that leads to ethnic cleansing can be its horrific products. To translate this to a personal and interpersonal perspective, there is a false and sentimental love that is both a defence against difficult differences and a pink mist that hides sadism.

Before turning to my own shape-shifting reflections on love, let me also bring in another area of interest, that is, Spinoza on love.

Spinoza on love

I have collated and paraphrased the following Spinozan dicta on love, drawn from Harry Frankfurt's short analysis of Spinoza on love and truth in his little book *On Truth* (2006):

1 'Love is nothing but Joy with the accompanying idea of an external cause' (Spinoza, *Ethics*, part III, prop. 13, scholium, in Frankfurt, 2006, p. 39).
2 Joy is a passion by which a person passes to a greater perfection (adapted from Spinoza, *Ethics*, part III, prop. 11, scholium, in Frankfurt, 2006, pp. 39–40).
3 A person's perfection is their *conatus* to be more actively their vital and real self, and the feeling of such increase is joy.
4 A person loves the cause of the joy of such an increase of one's *conatus*-power.
5 'One who loves necessarily strives to present and preserve the things one loves' (*Ethics*, part III, prop. II, scholium, in Frankfurt, 2006, p. 45).
6 Therefore, one loves the truth because it is indispensable in enabling one to stay alive and to live more in accord with one's own nature: one's most powerfully vital and real self (Frankfurt, 2006, pp. 39–46).

The highest aim of this developmentally hard ethical system is to realise, as Borges put it, that 'the mightiest love is that which does not expect to be loved in return' (Borges, 1976, p. 7). Here, I am citing a principle espoused by Spinoza, Goethe and Borges. This is an intellectual love, as of an impersonal 'god-or-nature', but it also applies personally. For Spinoza, Goethe and Borges, it is a philosophical (Stoic and Spinozan) 'going beyond' the psychological need and right to primary love to having one's love fully met and returned from infancy and ever-onwards.

But what is the relation between these two positions? On the one hand, our inherently psychosomatic and affective needs and necessities, and on the other, the toughest realisations and integrations, if not creations, arising out of conscious and unconscious experience of contingencies and limitations. Or, in other words, love as basic need and love as work. But I suggest that a Spinozan ratio-centric, impersonal and one-way idea of love is an astringent corrective to our post-Kantian, individualistic inwardness. It is an older Stoical or Epicurean rational and naturalistic virtue ethic.

Let us dare suggest that ideas precede (or even create) matter and that body is a fantastic 'psychic reality', an imaginative and creative transformation of the actuality that ideas are either dependent upon or are consubstantial with brain, body and biology.

Furthermore, as well as love between loving persons, who love each other, Spinoza emphasises loves that are not returned in kind. With objects of beauty, of music, of nature, the love of ideas, let alone the epistemophilic impulse, emotionally requited love can only be a subjective idea or fantasy, although there may be an intellectual, aesthetic or affective satisfaction and the reward of a sense of increase.

The love of another person is often unrequited, unnoticed or rejected from the earliest relations onward. This may be managed either defensively, creatively or by being sublimated into an idea of a 'higher love'. For example, there is the schizoid-creative love of Spinozan non-durational 'eternity', of Nietzschean 'joy' and of Santayana's 'essences'.

According to Spinoza, we love that person, relation, idea, object of desire or beauty, etc., which we experience as or know to be causing us the joy of increasing our power to maintain our self and our psychosomatic life, the joy of increasing of our power to enhance our essential nature.

Spinoza's ideas about love are highly pertinent to the emergence of the modern ideal of inwardness, of the idea of the unconscious and the irrational, fantasy, emotive memory and association, as well as the vital developmental and cultural role of symbolisation.

Towards a personal definition of love

Let me now attempt some definitions of love of my own. Love, at least erotic love, is the wonderfully creative or sometimes destructive meaning that our passionate and relational 'bodyminds' make of our biology, of our pheromone-fuelled, testosterone-driven and dopamine-connecting natural animal drives and attachments. But for us normally neurotic humans, there is no such thing as absolutely secure attachment. Thus, attachments may be used perversely, desperately and defensively, in so far as we use love unconsciously to fend off our fear of original core existential lacks and loneliness; in other words, to manage our psychotic core. We may use various forms of feigned, false narcissistic pseudo-love to ward off frighteningly dangerous intimacy that would expose an awful and shameful structural flaw, a developmental deficit. There are many unconscious reasons (healthy and unhealthy) why we might resist being identified as being loved, loving or being 'in love'.

Love is nominal and particular, not a floating entity like a winged cupid, although that may be an attractive poetic construct. In other words, there is no such thing as love without lovers loving, even if the lover is a solitary contemplative who is still a lover of something. Love does not exist outside conscious or unconscious human persons. This is my own belief; however, I do appreciate that some people believe such a meta-human, meta-animal, free entity 'Love' exists 'out there'. This is a view common to some religious faiths and to Absolute Idealism and so has a very potent spiritual and intellectual ancestry, a meaningful position and an active attitude which is still very much alive. I understand such a meaning as a psychic reality, but I am sceptical of its substantial actuality.

Making love is an act of physical and emotional trust, of trusting my passionate but vulnerable body and mind with your body and mind, and vice-versa. However, co-existing with such a trusting intimacy is the fact that sexual greed or need can also be essentially impersonal, anti-relational, not striving for oneness, but either blindly demanding and devouring, or centrifugal, fragmentary, polymorphous and amorphous, and thus destructive of loving unions.

Love in its various forms, with its various objects of a variety of genders or determinedly of no gender, is perhaps our most exciting and valuable creation (and recreation). It is an emotional zone that inspires poetry, music and other imaginal and wonderful creations. As noted previously, it can also 'inspire' sentimental kitsch and, in its train, sentimentality's ever-attendant shadow, namely intolerance, cruelty and dangerous fundamentalisms (such as a fanatical Puritanism). Such dangerous shadows lurk, too, in the personal and interpersonal undercurrents of sentimental love. To the extent that intimate relationships or 'marriages' are motivated by either the devouring narcissistic need and greed of mother/other/lover or by socio-economic needs or by the powers of sexual politics, that is not true love.

Lastly, a 'True Love' may be defined as a love that 'goes on being' beyond initial attraction, beyond projections, beyond early disappointment and disillusionment.

Love themes

Most infants literally fall in love and attach to mother, to the breast, her active face, body-bits, sound, smell, to her 'bodymind' and also need and want to be similarly and satisfactorily loved in return. This 'goes wrong' in that the primal need for 'primary love' (Balint, 1949, 1952) is bound to be, to some degree, unreliable. Although our basic need for primary love is inherent and permanent, such love never runs smoothly. We are inevitably thwarted, disappointed, rejected and wounded, and so defences against traumatic losses and disillusionments are necessarily set up.

The issue is, can we love properly, healthily, generously and not over-demandingly, if we have not received primal love or had our love sufficiently reciprocated? I suggest that our subsequent hurt, frustration or depressed defeat is the generator of such solutions as a) false narcissistic charm (hiding hurt, fear and righteous grandiosity), b) destructive outrage, envious hatred and cruelty, c) the finding or creating of a defensive belief in an all-loving personal God, or an absolute ideology or d) an impetus to suicide which is often moved by a fantasy of preservation of and reunion with the good self by killing the bad self?

Lack of love leaves one with an incomprehensible psychosomatic void, a sense of inner emptiness, of there being an inherent fault or handicap, the belief that one is intrinsically unlovable. Thwarted love brings with it a shock of irreplaceable loss, grief and despair. I suggest that the loss or absence of love is our primary anxiety and our greatest psychic pain. It is also our perennial psychic mover and source of true symbolisation and the making of meaning.

Attendant upon such erotic wounds is the apparent inherence of a universal psychic sense of 'right' to receive primary love and to find reliably constant 'good objects'. The failure or betrayal of this natural expectation is experienced as absolutely unjust. I am referring to basic psychosomatic, emotional and relational needs and desires and their intolerable frustration. It is through the various difficult managements or mismanagement of these psychosomatic and emotional pains and struggles that symbolic and affective thinking is made and developed. Out of our most passionate and problematic loves, desire and attachment, their disappointment and defeat, through loss and melancholia, grief and mourning, there may emerge a depressive understanding, a process of creative symbolising, a thinking and linking and the possibility of either 'anxious optimism' or 'cheerful pessimism'.

The primary need for love, its frustration and the urgent attempt to get it 'solved' is the central impetus behind all transferences, including the extremes of narcissistic emptying out of relations and borderline attacks. This is the matter of psychoid and psychosomatic infections and projective contagions, destructive borderline attacks as both offensive defences and as necessary communication. It is also the psychic matter of both the various degrees and levels of the 'basic fault' (Balint, 1968) and the various degrees and intensities of the 'psychotic core' and of their defence systems and behaviours. To some extent, we all have such neurotic and proto-psychotic pockets, conditioning the nurtured nature of our idiosyncratic appetites and defences, both affecting and spoiling our loves and hates and the way we do them!

Love and its hopes are inherently fragile, incorporating inevitable breakages, losses, damages and distortions; love is a close and often sore example of the 'fragility of goodness'.[2] Loves and thwarted loves are complex, incorporating a tense web of conflicting emotions. We learn through the perennial problems and pains of love, love's shocking losses or even sheer lack of love, as from the harmonies of good love or love's goods (good objects).

As Fairbairn (1943) suggests, internalised bad object experience is differently affective and more demanding of hard re-constructive thought and, therefore, perhaps more informative than good object relational experience. To put this another way, our emotional incomprehension and intolerable frustration in the face of loss and lack force us to think and link. As we have seen,[3] our early absences generate the emergence of the symbolising function or fail to do so if the damage-of-absence to primary narcissism is too great. The formation of individual consciousness emerges not only through experiences of good and harmonious relational mix-ups,

2 The phrase 'fragility of goodness' here is possibly taken from the title of Martha Nussbaum's book on Aristotle (1986) (Eds.).

3 See Chapter Ten (Eds.).

but is also motivated through learning from experiences of emotional perplexity, bewilderment and incomprehension of our outer and inner worlds. So, too, all philosophies, metaphysics, ethics and the need for reason and logic are moved by similar discomforts.

As mentioned earlier,[4] as Winnicott doesn't *quite* say in 'The Philosophy of "Real"' in *Human Nature* (1988), philosophers and psychologists are babies whose initial contacts with care-givers were 'slightly less' than good enough, leading to a 'sense of threat of loss of capacity for relationships'. The fear of there being no direct contact with reality 'hangs over them all the time'. It is 'a matter of life and death, of feeding or starvation, of love or isolation' (Winnicott, 1988, pp. 114–115). In other words, psychotherapists often become therapists because they have to do something about their personal problems with love, *ab origine* back then, thereafter and still now.

From pain to pleasure and back again: *jouissance* and a best possible life

Approaching love through its natural intrinsic pains and problems, even as a natural source of 'normal madness', perhaps you might like to ask yourself: 'Am I an anxious optimist or a cheerful pessimist?' If neither of these, then I suggest that you are either an angry depressive, you are in manic denial, pleasantly deluded, you are a higher being or you are psychically dead!

I am working from the idea that human consciousness (the self and the ego) is basically exercised by managing matters that disturb our pain-free peace, which means that consciousness, symbolising, thought and our internal, interpersonal and worldly actions and interactions all arise from 'trying to ease and please' our psychosomatic struggles and pains. It is this painful consciousness that allows us our loves and creativity, our understandings and our imaginative and creative (as well as fantastic, illusory or delusory) ideas of a future, which are also based upon conscious and unconscious past experience. A mature and realistic consciousness has to accommodate the necessity of emotional pains as part of our inherent psychosomatic limitations, inevitable losses, frustrations, disillusionments and disappointments, especially in the area of loving relations.

A basic psychic force makes us juggle and be juggled by our inherent impetus to preserve our vital, good and true self. But this very 'self', our core psychological identity, is made by our creative and/or destructive manoeuvres by which we seek to manage our strong passions, potencies and impotencies and seek to increase our power to preserve our love and the hope that my desired and loved one desires and loves me in return. This reciprocal relation is the essence of my valuable goods and good values.

We are born into an intra- and inter-psychic relational world. We have an inherent need to have overwhelming psychosomatic needs, our incomprehension of

4 See Chapter Seven (Eds.).

unnamed sensations, feelings, images and unformed thinking (our proto-ideas) recognised, taken in hand and in mind and so assuaged or managed. In other words, we need to feel understood and thus helped in understanding our internal and external world and the difference between inner and outer. We all start in the erotic politics of mother and baby, in the erotic politics of the family and in our relational experience viewed through the lenses of oedipal fantasy. Thence derives our strategic manoeuvres to get enough primary love, a degree of oedipal victory, which may mean learning to divide and rule, and simultaneously to not divide, to not harm but rather to establish and maintain the security of love.

We are determined by various levels and degrees of 'repetition compulsions', that is, the compulsion to repeat painful actions, behaviours and relations in order to seek their resolution and to gain understanding and a sense of power over (and of pleasure in) painful defeats of our omnipotent fantasies and desires. Thus, we gain or regain a sense of agency. Indeed, surely our love relations are often compulsive repetitions themselves!

When our need for primary love is thwarted or frustrated, then three defensive and mal-developmental options may occur: dissociation or fragmentation; impotent outrage; and/or a private self-creating and self-managing internal world. In other words, depression, borderline destruction or narcissistic specialness (or becoming a Jungian!) may ensue.

At the same time, we need to keep our valuable core secret and private; we do not want to be too deeply known and understood, as Winnicott observed (1984). The tense relationship between the need to be known and understood and the need to remain hidden and self-protective is variable and can sometimes become a source of great stress and distress.

A psychotherapeutic issue concerns understanding, integrating and changing the internal and relational defensive consequences of early lacks and losses, grief and sadness or depressing defeat, and the possibility of these affects being moved towards meaning, mourning and futurity. Our (mis-)management of failures, disappointments and grievous losses of love, torn attachments and frustrated desire are remade in both the intra-psychic and transferential relations of analysis. A reliable analytic frustration, based on the *agapē* of constancy and frame, facilitates the transformation of limits, disillusionments and disappointments into love even in a time of *cólera*[5] (García Márquez, 1985), depressive ambivalence, understanding and wholeness. A developmental growth of consciousness (self-conscious reality) arises out of analytic frames and boundaries just as much as it does from an analyst being an ever-giving superhumanly all-good mother or magic father, a source of absolute largesse who must correct and fulfil all deficits.

The transferential disappointment with the analyst/analysis and the ultimate loss and mourning of the analytic relationship may become an affective focus for this

5 *Cólera* in Spanish may refer to the disease of cholera, but may also denotes human passion, rage and ire (Eds.).

process. If there is a deep and real enough shared history of emotional understanding and discovery to value and remember in and through the analytic relationship, one is more able to go on living and loving.

The ultimate concerns of analysis are absence, grief, mourning, meaning making and finding new hope, often hope against hope. Where there is loss, there is melancholia, angry depression or destructive borderline offensive defences. However, where there has been a lack or absolute absence of primary love (as with the total absence of a parent or absence of good-enough, loving-enough parenting), then mourning is not possible, rather only an unrelenting state of emptiness, depression and its symptomatic ramifications.

I believe that we are born into a world of external and internal contingencies and exercise an intrinsic demand to find ways to deal with these environmental and personal circumstances. External causes include physical states of affairs, outside conditions, other bodies and their affective actions, culture and political forces, our own body as object, etc. Internal causes and conditions include our own body as a relation of psychosomatic meanings, other internalised object relations, especially internal parental relations (whether united parents or badly dis-united parents), our 'family fate', which is sometimes a psychically near-fatal family. It is our ever-adjusting and ever-increasing conscious understanding and linking of the history and the feeling-tone of these environmental relations that makes for our symbolising function and our creativity, for our sense of active agency and significance and for our sense of meaningfulness. This sense of purpose and responsibility, of free will, even if such free will is, to an extent, illusory, is a psychic reality necessary to our psychic well-being.

Love brings with it other attendant strong emotions, for example: lust and disgust; desire and frustration; appetite and fear; healthy competition and green jealousy; generosity and selfishness; imaginal empathy and projective distortion; joy and sadness; harmony and irritation; security and loss; power and impotence; hope and anxiety. Anxiety, as a fear of losing love, can become strong enough to be self-fulfilling and, therefore, is perhaps the greatest internal threat to love. Finally, I suggest that an intrinsic aspect of love and desire is often aggression. Sometimes, this is manifest as violence, sometimes as the creative energies of sheer life-force and love-force.

Jouissance[6]

Now, I would like to elaborate upon the theme of the complex and tense dynamic of passionate, affective internal and interpersonal relations by saying more about the 'juice of *jouissance' vis a vis* the field of love. Naturalistic *jouissance* incorporates both the conjunction and the keeping apart of affective poles, a dynamic position which cannot and does not demand resolution or an idea of progress/health.

6 The *Jouissance* Grid and explanations can be found in Chapter Seven, p. 107 and Chapter Fifteen, p. 218 (Eds.).

We can actively observe and try to understand this *jouissance* of affects and passions and their complex of fluid relations, inside and between us. It represents the tense relations of attraction and separation between appetite or desire or disgust and fear, pleasure and pain, joyous elation and sad depression, power and its limits or impotence, all incorporated in the psychosomatic *conatus* of the *jouissance* of 'bodymind'. Love, as the seminal relational place for this '*jouissance* tension', is therefore always the field of our psychosomatic and emotional relations, always both internal and interpersonal, always an activity or passivity of fantastically imaginative relations between meaning-laden bodies and body-bits, the stuff of our psychoid 'bodymind' and its organic forces, including natural forces of disunity/non-union. As well as the natural tense relational *jouissance* of all our passions, affects and emotions, there is a recognition of a natural but paradoxical unity of freedom, necessity and responsibility and perhaps an acceptance of the ultimate necessity, namely one's own mortality.

Fragility and mourning

Here, I am thinking of the Aristotelian assertion of the 'fragility of goodness' as it pertains to love and about impermanence and unreliability that is intrinsic to the necessary risk of love. Perhaps it is this very fragility which makes love such a valuable and beautiful, even psychologically essential, creation. But it is for this reason, too, its value and beauty, that it evokes, attracts and invites envious attack. The unloved baby, the thwarted lover, the borderline person who communicates his or her pre-verbal pains by attacking the good, the good self, good bodies and parts and all other goods out there in the desperately needed but ever-failing environment. If an infant experiences mother as emotionally (or actually) absent, unreliable, unpredictable, anxious or fragmented, then the infant cannot go on trusting the object of primary love. Play and, therefore, the development of the symbolising function is damaged, twisted or lost in the energies of neurotic or psychotic defences, including what Michael Balint (1959, 1968) termed *ocnophilic* clinging and *philobatic* evasion.[7] Instead of a healthy development of symbolising and relational capacities, there are defensive splits. These may include: borderline outrage with hate-filled and violent impulses to make the personal public; narcissistic hiding of the wounded self, so secret that it is hidden from the neurotically self-conscious ego; depressive retreats into pockets of psychogenic autism. All of which avoid the underlying depressive 'black hole in the psyche', the unmet and unborn self. Here is the source of narcissistic false facades covering over an underlying

7 Michael Balint first coined the terms the *ocnophil* (lover of closeness) and the *philobat* (lover of space) in 1953 in a letter to David Eichholz. In *Thrills and Regressions* of 1959, they entered the psychoanalytic lexicon. In *The Basic Fault* (1968), Balint describes how as a neonate meets the world at birth, one reaction, that of the *ocnophil*, is to view objects (mother, father, etc.) as safe and comforting, the spaces between being threatening. The *philobat,* or lover of space, views objects (people) as unsafe, and space as safe (Eds.).

destructiveness. The narcissist's fear of the superego splits off latent outrage which could be, paradoxically, constructive and vitalising. Through the shocking recognition of narcissistic defensive strategies, there may emerge an alarming but potent anger and a truer self with the courage to live more honestly. Narcissistic defences are a cover for underlying borderline rage, which is where the truer and more alive self lies wounded and cowering but latently alarming because it is so savage in its fury and force if released.

Borderline persons suffer from relational incapacities, furious demands for love accompanied by hostile attacks on close ones. Borderline persons fight their lacks ferociously, but at least they are alive in the fury of their hurt and hate and are closer to the real enemy within, namely, savage all-defeating depression. Such angry persons, indeed such borderline parts in all of us, make for hungry and fiercely exciting, if also very dangerous, lovers! Furthermore, and paradoxically, due to their imaginative and sensual passion, even if at times destructive, borderline persons are often actually very alive and thereby acutely aware of their own mortality.

A narcissist and analyst converse[8]

Here, I present a caricatured dramatic monologue expressing the internal and interpersonal world-view of a narcissistic position. This is part of each and all of us, so it is not a matter of 'them but surely not me'. Aspects of such fantasies and impulses are common in all close relationships, as are our 'borderline bits'. Perhaps, one wonders, whether a narcissistic position is closer to our common ways of being, in so far as we are all abodes of fear, living nervously in a peopled world, scanning the world like gazelles at the water-hole, often shy and self-conscious, desperate to be seen and liked and/or to keep much hidden and/or be invisible. A narcissistic personality strategically but inwardly re-works their interpersonal world through secretive, fearful, over-sensitive, self-conscious but also deviously adhesive and parasitic defences something like this:

> Look at me and don't look, at least not too closely, and only look at me when I've prepared and arranged my angle; see me but don't see into me, in case you see nothing, an absence, or notice my weak fear of you and all people or see and sense my disgust and cold dislike of emotionally alive persons, but also my desperate need for recognition, for recognition and admiration for my special and great qualities; envy me without resenting me.
>
> I shall get into your wonderful separate life and into your confident, capable, emotional and separate mind, your values, your emotional private riches, and I shall take possession and co-ownership of them.

8 Originally, this paper included both 'A borderline and analyst converse', as well as 'A narcissist and analyst converse' to illustrate how borderline and narcissistic personalities suffer difficulties in their love relations. The Borderline-analyst conversation has been omitted here to avoid undue repetition. See Chapter Nine and Chapter Twelve (Eds.)

> I will do so by making you not notice my intrusion, for my crafty strategies are invisible and secret. I will move you, influence you and your life almost without you noticing by making my extractive leach-bite painless, even pleasurable. Look but don't look, see but don't see, that I'm so loving that you can't help but love me, this best-of-all, most beautiful and interesting me.
>
> You are noticing me, aren't you? You do realise how lucky you are to know me, don't you? I have laid my eggs under your skin. You are my unwitting host. You are my unknowing lover and partner. You can never leave me. I will never leave you. But I keep my powers private and secret and really known only to myself.
>
> I'm not an empty non-person, am I? I'm not dull and boring, am I? I'm not invisible, am I? Do you remember me? Have you gone to sleep on me?
>
> I shall make myself visible and effective through my most subtle manoeuvres, my most secret strategic calculations. I'll get you in the end; in fact, I think I've got you already . . . although you may not realise it yet, you may never realise it . . . but I'll be there; I'm in you forever, living on your insides.

And thus, self-defeating, erotically and socially unattractive defences are most desperately wrought by the narcissist. Under such conditions, it is difficult but vital for a therapist to remember that this person is in a self-conscious grip of primal anxiety and abject loneliness. It is by pointing this out at the right moment and in a way that does not repeat the person's original experience of humiliation, shame and defensive retreats that I become an acceptable and trustable 'emotional reality principle'.

I may thereby disturb such a defensive and falsifying narcissistic system, but in a way that is for the better, namely a stronger emotional reality and relational nerve or courage. But, as I say, this is often such an intolerably depressing recognition or such a precarious change into an unknown world that it is no wonder it is readily and rapidly retreated from, back into the safe old, tried, tested and strategically refined positions.

The analytic task is to address the primitive anxiety, interpersonal terrors and shames. This may lead to a recognition, even a shock of recognition, that their object of fear is a maternal-parental world in which the self is unrecognised, unloved and its healthy exhibitionistic energies crippled.

Both personality disorders originate in being oedipally orphaned; both are also driven by the sore wounds of absolute lacks, abject losses and the repeated sense of there not being enough love, recognition, validation, etc. Envy and resentment are overtly expressed in either the impulsive acts of borderline murderousness or hidden behind a polite feigning in the case of narcissism. The borderline has a possible erotic life lurking within the angry hate, whereas the narcissist may be too fearful to ever dare come out of hiding and live openly, honestly and fully. Primary losses, lacks and consequent disturbances to the symbolising function mean that the developing person cannot integrate, that is, symbolise normal disillusionments and disappointments, and so cannot mourn and move on. This means that other than lust and clinging, there can be no real capacity for the creative play of love, a failure of imagination and the imaginal, which is, to an extent, what emerges out of the management of inevitable absences.

Let us not overlook the possibility that a real love can be pre-symbolic yet still be love and be developmental and redemptive, actually healing of self-defeating but necessary defences against intolerable early loss. For example, the 2007 film *Lars and the Real Girl* features symbolic equivalence (Segal, 1957). Yet it is also a story of an emotionally wounded man able to love and mourn through a relationship with a sex doll (in a non-sexual way). Through this, he not only changes his fear of intimate touch but also redeems his brother's life of denial and, indeed, the various personal defences of the members of the village where he lives. The perceptive and therapeutically able doctor totally understands the essential reparative processes moving Lars' 'symbolically equivalent' love of his doll as a real girl (Gillespie et al., 2007).

Strong and passionate love is a relation that sooner or later makes lovers think through immediate emotional storms, difficult differences, power relations, disillusionment, irritation and anxious fears of loss whilst simultaneously going on loving. And this is what critical transferential psychotherapy recycles and transforms through its processes of symbolising, as a particular framed form of emotional remembering, linking and reflective thinking.

Love necessarily includes difference, change and impermanence, the challenges of betrayal and guilt, loss, separation and mortality, and thus a call through mourning to gratitude and non-melancholic remembrance, an acquiescent letting go and going on, having surely loved and been loved enough . . . or not. As David Malan said, 'The aim of therapy is not to make up to patients for the love that they have missed, but to help them work through their feelings about not having it' (Malan, 1979, p. 141).

All analytic relations, through the dynamics of transference and countertransference, incorporate the mourning of the limitations and failures of the analysis and the immanent presence of our final separation. It is our task to understand why, how and in what way a particular patient cannot live and love well enough, who experiences love as either devouring (whether their own greedy hunger or that of the other), or as too dangerously intimate, too bound to hurt, too exposing and shameful, too much, too dangerous, too distant, never enough, etc. How do I let myself, as a therapist, be used usefully when this is re-constellated transferentially and countertransferentially? Do we respond with sympathy, empathy, interpretation? How much do I challenge a defensive system, how much simply function as a stark mirror of hard home truths, let alone when and how to say something?

Symbolising and love

Love relations and symbolising go hand in hand. The symbolising function emerges through our most passionate and problematic loves, their frustrations, losses, absences as well as their lusts and longings, joys and disappointments, grief and mourning. We also forge our vital thinking, imagination and creativity through our passionate relations.

Psychoanalysis involves moving through a critical relationship our desires, limits, mourning and possible meanings. This uncovers and enables an epistemophilic and mutative understanding of our psychosomatic, emotional and thoughtful motivations. A good therapeutic relationship aids the development of realistic symbolising, out of previously pre-symbolic, un-symbolised, literalised, acted out, confused and confusing matters. Through mourning that which is tragically lost and sadly mourned, through symbolising and finding 'as if' connections, through playing with metaphorical meanings concerning matters of the body and issues of the mind, fantasy and reality, we may find a sense of new hope, a sense of purpose and joyful meaning.

Five penultimate observations on love

Firstly, due to the vicissitudes of primary and subsequent love experiences, there seem to be four possible modes of being, running from the deeply depressed, through the variously mad and neurotic, to the creative and ethical. These are: yearning for a lost ideal; desperately wanting the good; forever searching for something/someone better; and endeavouring to make life (and make love) as well as possible. Love, as healthily and normally experienced, described and defined, is not transferential (that is only an interpretation within a particular context), although, of course, desired and loved persons may well be the objects of all sorts of unconscious part and whole projections!

Secondly, love involves recognition of difference and the otherness of another. Any new other is often initially fascinating, evoking epistemophilic curiosity, attraction and exciting erotic desire. But this relationship can become a possession, a known zone and so a familiarity. The familiar can be either comforting or may breed contempt. The other becomes predicable, thence a bore, thence an irritation. This may be two-way and ambivalent, a relationship in which we are to each other 'a familiar' who is sometimes enlivening, sometimes comforting, sometimes a painful irritation. Most often in therapy (and especially with schizoid splits and narcissistic disorders), we are dealing transferentially with the healthy threat of intimacy, the primitive and conflicted need-fear of being seen and known, of too much exciting-disgusting, warm and wet or stinging intimacy and of being painfully rejected and humiliated or exposed in our naked shame.

Thirdly, I suggest that the opposite of love is neither hate nor indifference (because they are both corollaries or parts of love). Indeed, the Stoic concept of *ataraxia*, meaning detachment, imperturbability, equanimity or tranquillity, is understood as a type of love. I suggest rather that fear, anxiety and depression are love's antitheses because they preclude the ability to love. Depressive anxiety and fear (dread, terror, panic, etc.) prevent love and disturb desire. They de-potentiate and may actually create, perpetuate and exacerbate an even more painful sense of abject loneliness. Anxiety over the possible loss of love (or of the lover) can become self-fulfilling, both because, in extremis, it destroys the necessary trust for love to continue to be and to develop and because it may engender the destructiveness of obsessional jealousy and paranoia. Of course, we wish for love as a balm for loneliness, sadness and worry, but agonisingly, this can be impossible if the precondition is depressive anxiety or cold fear. Furthermore, our next and most self-defeating defences against just such depressive anxiety are schizoid or autistic splits and withdrawals, and these make real or true love even more impossible.

Fourthly, love is also a potency, a condition of 'increase', a realm of self-realisation and other-realisation, a maker of true freedom. This is Spinozan love and also a vital Romantic ideal. I am thinking here of a freedom that is most intensely real because it is felt both amid and because of the coexistence of necessity, contingency and death.

Fifthly, long-term and whole love must include an accumulation of good memories (which were once present good shared moments and plans, desires and fantasies for the future), but simultaneously, a knowledge that these good relational memories shall be lost in death. They are all the more valuable for this natural transience. Although love is transitory, it is also immanently eternal (timeless) and is exquisitely beautiful and most valuable for just this, its inevitable human temporality.

Santayana suggested that normal human madness involves trying to fix in stone that which is moving (Santayana, 1926, p. 41). Translated into love relations, this becomes the intrinsically false idea or ideal of unchanging love ever after.

Final words on love

Love is endlessly represented through tales and depictions of longings, unions, discoveries, jealousies and vengeance: it is celebratory, redemptive, comic and tragic. Love transforms as it is transformed, through its regressions, sublimations and its growth, if and when it accommodates difficulties, difference and otherness. Love is an inspiring, maddening, emotional relational force. It is a relation that we make and remake, an act and interaction of permanent re-creation, or, of course, a relation that un-makes and breaks us. Love lives both creatively and painfully with the psychic reality of ideas of hope and even of eternity, as well as in the face of the hard actuality of mortality.

The development of passionate love into an attachment of satisfying, comforting, reliable companionship and familiarity is a good and natural organic growth, until death us do part. Above all, there is the possibility of going on and increasing our loving through ambivalent relations, a possible virtue in difficult love being possible, including altruistic love and unreturned and unreturnable love. I repeat the principle espoused by Spinoza, Goethe and Borges: 'The mightiest love is that which does not expect to be loved in return', which surely has to be a virtue that is its own reward. That last sentence is, I realise, uttered by a typically schizoid man climbing 'a ladder' up into an impersonal and ethereal love . . . but then, 'all joy wants eternity!' quoting Nietzsche.[9] So, instead of 'And they lived happily ever after', I suggest we more realistically say:

> And they lived fully unpredictably and imperfectly, agreeing to differ on many things, as good normal neurotics, growing ever more true to their own and each other's odd selves, until circumstances (over which they had no control) did them part, in accord with their separate destinies (which was what they made of their respective fates).

I told you I was a cheerful pessimist.

9 '*Denn all Lust will Ewigkeit, will tiefe, tiefe Ewigkeit*' is from Nietzsche's *Zarathustra* (Eds.).

References

Balint, M. (1949). 'Early Developmental States of the Ego. Primary Object Love'. *International Journal of Psycho-Analysis*, 30: 265–273.
Balint, M. (1952). *Primary Love, and Psycho-Analytic Technique*. London: Hogarth.
Balint, M. (1959). *Thrills and Regressions*. London: Maresfield.
Balint, M. (1968). *The Basic Fault: Therapeutic Aspects of Regression*. London: Basic Books.
Borges, J. (1976). 'Baruch Spinoza'. In *Homenaje a Baruch Spinoza*. Buenos Aires: Museo Judío de Buenos Aires.
Fairbairn, W. (1943). 'The Repression and the Return of Bad Objects (With Special Reference to the "War Neuroses")'. *British Journal of Medical Psychology*, 19(3–4): 327–341.
Frankfurt, H. (2006). *On Truth*. New York: Knopf Doubleday.
García Márquez, G. (1985). *El amor en los tiempos del cólera*. Colombia: Oveja Negra.
Gillespie, C., Kimmel, S., Cameron, J., Aubrey, S., Oliver, N., Gosling, R., Mortimer, E., & Schneider, P. (2007). *Lars and the Real Girl* (Feature film). United States: Metro-Goldwyn-Mayer.
Malan, D. (1979). *Individual Psychotherapy and the Science of Psychodynamics*. London: Butterworth-Heinemann.
McGuire, W., ed. (1974). *The Freud/Jung Letters: The Correspondence between Sigmund Freud and C. G. Jung*. Princeton, NJ: Princeton University Press.
Nussbaum, M. (1986). *The Fragility of Goodness: Luck and Ethics in Greek Tragedy and Philosophy*. Cambridge: Cambridge University Press.
Santayana, G. (1922). *The Life of Reason or the Phases of Human Progress. Vol. III: Reason in Religion*. New York, NY: Scribner.
Santayana, G. (1926). 'Normal Madness'. In *Dialogues in Limbo*. New York, NY: Scribner.
Segal, H. (1957). 'Notes on Symbol Formation'. *International Journal of Psycho-Analysis*, 38: 391–397.
Winnicott, D. (1984). 'Communicating and Not Communicating Leading to a Study of Certain Opposites'. In *The Maturational Processes and the Facilitating Environment*. D. Winnicott, ed. London: Karnac (Original work published 1963).
Winnicott, D. (1988). *Human Nature*. London: Free Association Books.

Chapter 12

Embodied countertransference and recycling the mad matter of symbolic equivalence

Routledge, 2010[1]

I wish to emphasise from the outset that this paper is largely theoretical. It has to do with metapsychology and hypothetical models, at times even metaphysics. However, theory here is intended to inter-relate with my analytic positioning and so to my applied reverie, critical clinical reasoning and action, and so can help me see and interpret my way through and out of conditions of destructive psychosomatic attack. I will later attempt to explicate the field I am considering through a brief phenomenological description of the internal and interpersonal worlds of personality disordered persons and their affective relations.

My starting point is to take up Andrew Samuels' (1985) seminal concept of the analytically informative 'embodied countertransference', primarily to suggest that this experiential realm belongs most evidently in analytic relations with states of severe personality disorder, that is, to oversensitive and defensive narcissistic and destructive borderline conditions, to chronically and acutely regressed states, and that it is a highly informative analytic lens into these difficult zones.

In his paper 'Countertransference, the *Mundus Imaginalis* and a Research Project' (1985), Samuels distinguishes embodied countertransference experience from a reflective countertransferential attitude, although vitally, both necessarily share an imaginal condition and capacity. This Samuels amplifies through the work of Henry Corbin on the *mundus imaginalis* (Corbin, 1972), a concept which, Samuels suggests, can link 'soul and corporeality ... intellect and sense impressions' (Samuel 1985, pp. 60– 61). In the analytic context, we could say that the *mundus imaginalis* functions

1 Originally published as Clark, G. (2010). 'The Embodied Counter-Transference and Recycling the Mad Matter of Symbolic Equivalence: a Re-evaluation of Samuels' Idea of the "Embodied Counter-Transference"'. In *Sacral Revolutions: Reflecting on the Work of Andrew Samuels: Cutting Edges in Psychoanalysis and Jungian Analysis*, G. Heuer, ed. London: Routledge, pp. 88–96. This chapter includes some material not in the published version of the paper. This was added by Clark in unpublished revisions before and after this paper was published. We have also omitted material repeated verbatim from earlier chapters (Eds.).

DOI: 10.4324/9781003255826-13

as a linking factor between patient and analyst (Samuels, 1985, p. 60). Regarding embodiment, Samuels explains that

> 'embodied' is intended to suggest a physical, actual, material, sensual, expression in the analyst of something in the patient's inner world, a drawing together and solidification of this, an incarnation by the analyst of a part of the patient's psyche . . . If our psyche tends to personify, as Jung suggests, then 'embodiment' speaks of the way the person/analyst plays his part in that.
>
> (Samuels, 1985, p. 52)

He goes on to suggest that 'it is necessary to see our field of reference in analysis as seamless and continuous' and so to realise that 'the coin is three-sided: to body and image can be added relationship' (p. 68).

One implication of Samuels' hypothesis is a possible re-visioning and extension of the concept of the psychoid into analytic transference and countertransference interaction. My clinical hypothesis is that this psychoid realm is one of psychosomatic mutuality, a pre-verbal relational field that is a conduit for urgent communication, often sickening or seductive, but demanding internal recycling into a more integrated co-ordination and a separation out of identification into differentiation. Thence, what have always been intolerable lacks, losses, limitations and frustrations can be painfully grieved and perhaps mourned, and meaningful causal links can be made, and so there may emerge a more realistic symbolic functionality.

A regression into a psychoid state,[2] often induced or re-constellated by a psychotic transference or split-off primitive beta bits, is necessarily communicated by projective identifications and so experienced in psychosomatically-sensed (as well as imaged) countertransference. This makes for a mutual field that is partially pre-symbolic or a realm of 'symbolic equation' (Segal, 1957) where beta-disordered fragments may yet eventually become ordered into a functional alpha state. The analyst is made and/or psychically informed (and/or temporally deformed) by this process and thence can help the patient grieve and mourn their lacks, losses, limitations and angry frustrations, and so possibly make for the emergence of a truer and more satisfying liveliness.

The analyst is forcefully moved 'down' into a primitive 'psychoid' level or realm from which he/she is made to operate as from a position of psycho-sensing perception; this may bring change from beta body-mind confusion and symbolic equivalence to a more functional order.

I find the idea of the psychoid to be one of Jung's most fertile and clinically useful concepts. However, we also have to be careful not to fall into fantastic thinking in this realm of 'using the psychoid' as a clinical theory and practice. An application

2 The following two paragraphs come from an unpublished version of this chapter and are not in the 2010 publication (Eds.).

of critical reason, healthy scepticism and therapeutic pragmatism are needed. We also need to be clear about the issue of whether to understand the psychoid as an object for scientific investigation or as a symbolic 'as if', a unit of meaning, or as both simultaneously.

Ann Addison (2008, 2009) has most usefully synthesised, developed and extended Jungian and post-Jungian clinical thinking about 'the psychoid'. She traces how Jung conceived the idea of the psychoid based on the teleological and vitalist orientation of Hans Driesch (1867–1941) and the more causal and self-determining approach of Eugen Bleuler (1857–1939), who held that psyche and soma act on similar, parallel principles (psycho-physical parallelism), and called this *Die Psychoide*. Jung had worked with Bleuler at the Burghölzli Hospital. Jung's idea of psychoid processes, first articulated in his Ascona presentation of 1946 (Jung, 1947), was that they are 'quasi-psychic' and 'lie somewhere between vitalistic phenomena and psychic processes' (Addison, 2008, p. 4). In *Mysterium Coniunctionis*, Jung writes that 'deepest down of all is the paradox of the sympathetic and parasympathetic psychoid processes' (Jung, 1970a; *CW* 14, para. 279) and in 'On the Nature of the Psyche' (Jung, 1970b, the final English version of his initial presentation at Ascona) he suggests that

> [s]ince psyche and matter are contained in one and the same world, and moreover are in continuous contact with one another and ultimately rest on irrepresentable, transcendental factors, it is not only possible but fairly probable, even, that psyche and matter are two different aspects of the same thing.
>
> (*CW* 8, para. 418)

Here, Jung is using a dual-aspect theory. If it was not for Jung's use of the word 'transcendent', this sentence is surely close to the substance monism and dual-aspect theory of Spinoza, which I use to argue my ideational system. Addison's own hypothesis is that

> psychosensory phenomena, occurring varyingly along the body-mind axis in the transference/countertransference, may be expected to arise during periods of regression to early states when issues concerning separation and bodily integrity are at the forefront.
>
> (Addison, 2008, p. 10)

Furthermore, she suggests that 'such experiences represent evidence of the emergence of psyche from soma', and so have to do with the 'development of mind' (Addison, 2008, p. 6).

I would say that psychoid processes are not only regressive but are also a potentiality and a potency. They can also be understood as a basically emergent and vital organic force, like a seed with the DNA of its form inherently or conatively determined to make manifest, realise and develop in both a species-typical and an individually idiosyncratic way and thence be re-formed by environmental (conscious and unconscious) experience. To put this into a language appropriate to analytic experience: an emergence through psychoid and psychosomatic identity to symbolisation, the separation and creation of meaning (out) of matter. Transferentially/countertransferentially, the 'dual aspect' of the psychoid realm makes for 'consubstantial' psyche-soma experience at the level of the autonomic nervous system, which emerges out of, between, around us both in analysis, whence it calls out for functional symbolic ordering which can move us to a more relational state.

Analytic work at the psychoid level or through psyche-soma as a 'bodymind' self (Grotstein, 1997) is induced and activated by those pre-symbolic or anti-symbolic regressive behaviours that belong to the pathological nature of destructive borderline relations. This is a realm of fragmented beta disorder which relentlessly compounds its own sense of frustration, of concretised emotions expressed through psychosomatically infectious, defensive, projective, urgently communicative and informative forces and of archaic symbolic equations.

I would further suggest that when such strong affects are experienced countertransferentially with persons with over-sensitive, thin-skinned (and secretively grandiose and righteous) narcissistic defences, then they could be a signal of the split off but underlying angry core that has hitherto been so fearfully avoided by such persons. Furthermore, much embodied countertransferential communication and information that is experienced even with normally neurotic persons (who are not personality disordered) derives from pockets of early beta pre-order or disorder.

I must, however, acknowledge that this sort of openness to analytic work with embodied psychosomatic countertransferential experience, let alone to a related interest in the psychoid and in consubstantial body-mind identity states, can be symptomatic of the analyst's need to co-ordinate, re-order and integrate his/her own psychosomatic and relational disorder. This possibility must come into his/her assessment of the relative informative usefulness or degree of personal subjective neurosis in such an equivocal field of experience.

Mind-body identity[3] and interpersonal identification have a natural base at the psychoid level, but it is a beta chaos and confused realm of symbolic equivalence that makes a 'night in which all cows are black' (as Hegel said of Schelling's philosophy of Absolute Identity) and calls out for functional clarification. This is achieved through the analytic relationship enabling psychosomatic co-ordination and more functional internal and interpersonal relations, an interpretive process that emerges out of 'selected facts', which themselves eventually arise out of protracted reverie and careful thinking through.

It is, therefore, vital that I try to understand whether and how analytically my psychosomatic 'bodymind' is being affectively made by the analysand; thence, I have to decide on a mutually mutative interpretation. This is also about discerning the source and meaning of psychosomatic (infectious) information and defensive projection: whether it is a syntonic and concordant communication or a product of

3 The following two paragraphs are not in the 2010 publication (Eds.).

one's own (analyst's) neurotic vulnerability and identification. I must acknowledge that this sort of analytic openness to, work with and interest in embodied psychosomatic countertransferential experience, let alone a related interest in the psychoid and in consubstantial body-mind identity states, can be symptomatic of the analyst's need to co-ordinate, re-order and integrate his/her psychosomatic and relational disorder. This possibility must come into his/her assessment of the relative informative usefulness or degree of personal subjective neurosis of such affectivity.

To further adapt Samuels' point, I would say that the psychoid is always simultaneously 'sensuous body matters' and 'emotional mental images and ideas'. In other words, we can say that, at the psychoid level, body, image and idea are a unit, an identity experienced or expressed as a dual aspect, as different attributes and modes of 'bodymind' as a 'single substance'.

I have written elsewhere[4] about how a neo-Spinozan substance monism and dual-aspect theory help my psychosomatically responsive analytic position. In brief, I described how the *conatus* (the innate psychic and organic endeavour for self-preservation and the enhancement of powers to maintain the self) is related to the concept that the mind is the idea of the body, corporality and embodiment, of body, body-bits and bodily relations. I then further extended this re-conceptualisation of the *conatus* and mind-as-idea-of-the-body into an ideational and practical model of internal and interpersonal emotional and embodied relations, 'ideas' of bodies and body relations and the natural tensions between these affects, tensions which are essential to the ongoing formation of identity. I call this dynamic grid a *jouissance* of affects and their relations. *Conatus* as *jouissance* is the 'passions of the bodymind' and incorporates all psychosomatic forces, affective states and their relations, and simultaneously both joins and keeps apart, unites and separates, incorporating the tension between desire and repulsion, joy and sadness, power and limitation. It is of both *mind and body, may be represented through either, but must be* conceived as though representing a *dual aspects* of a single substance and understood as *substantially univocal.* It is important, concerning the psychoid, to view these Spinozan theoretical concepts as both practical and 'as if' realities.

This helps me to understand those analytic states that are psycho-sensually close to psychoid processes, where emotional images, mental ideation and body matters are 'as one', where self and other, fantasy and reality are unseparated, where we are pulled back into a pre-symbolic or anti-symbolic world which is often transferentially expressed through psychosomatic contamination and mind-body confusions, through projective identifications, destructive acting out and sexualised pressures that attack our necessary boundaries and frames. This is all regressive, anti-imaginal and maddeningly literalising.

Segal (1957) described how, in a mental state in which 'symbolic equations' proliferate, symbolic thoughts (and original objects) are treated not as thoughts but as literal things. In her later papers, and especially in the book *Dream, Phantasy*

4 See Chapter Seven (Eds.).

and Art (Segal, 1991), Segal, following Bion, viewed pathological forms of projective identification as responsible for disturbances in symbol formation. She made connections between her work on symbol formation and Bion's alpha and beta elements: concrete symbolic equations can be understood as beta-elements, which have the possibility of becoming alpha functioning. In other words, early concrete equations and pre-symbolised objects belong to a state latent with potential symbolic development. I would say that symbolic equations are 're-conceivable' or recyclable into the imagination, thought and creation.

Britton (1998) explains that 'symbolic equation' arises from

> an arrested development of the symbolic process at the point of relinquishment of the original object. The object is preserved by a sustained projection of the self into the place vacated by the absent object and which denies its disappearance . . . . In such thinking there is no world outside the mind: existence of self and object world are coterminous.
>
> (Britton, 1998, p. 138)

'Symbolic equation' manifests as a pre-ambivalent or paranoid-schizoid position, a realm of identity confusion and identification, arising out of an attempt to deny the intolerable loss or lack of a needed but also envied and murderously hated loved/loving object. In chronic borderline and acutely regressed states, the psychoid pre-order, psychosomatic disorder and pre-symbolic confusion of body and mind, of body bits and zones of meaning, are desperately evacuated and projected. This is where the psychoid processes feel as if they are the mad matter of symbolic equation. The borderline baby-bomb off-loads and communicates an intolerable toxicity, dissociation and fragmentation through projective identification into the countertransferential psycho-sensing 'body' of the analyst, which is a needed containing, digesting, processing and 'feeding back' (interpretive) object.

The phenomenology of the borderline relational world[5]

To create a phenomenology of the borderline relational world, such a person may think, feel and angrily express their transferential urgency something like this:

> For me, mind and body, fantasy and reality, inner and outer, my mind and your mind, my body and your body, you and me, are and must always be fused as one . . . (but you must and must not simultaneously sort out this confusion).
>
> My desperate (impotent) need is now to somehow make matters such that your mind is my mind, and your body is my body.

5 See also Chapter Nine (Eds.).

> Because I am starved of enough of anything good and have never had the necessary power to get the primary love I should have had . . . you must, therefore, love me now . . . even though I know that you never shall do so enough, and you must love me forever . . . even though I know that you never shall.
>
> My hurt makes me hate, attack and destroy all that is enviably good and loving . . . everyone (such as you) who gets and gives to others the love that I so desperately want.
>
> Because I love you, it is outrageous and intolerable that you do not love me back, and for this, I hate you, and because of this, I will forcibly affect and infect you, or I will seduce you, arouse and move you irresistibly.
>
> I shall get into and possess your separate body-mind by disturbing and infecting you psychosomatically. I shall confuse your thinking, attack your linking, and somatise your symbolising function . . . as mine is.
>
> Realise and understand (as I do not) that making war is my way of making love.
>
> My anger knows no bounds.

In this evacuative and sickening attack on or seduction of what I have called the 'concretely fantasised' analytic breast-body-mind (using concrete images as units of thought), there is what Bion (1959) refers to as a part-object relationship with physiological rather than anatomical functions, 'not with the breast but with feeding, poisoning, loving, hating' (Bion, 1959, p. 312).

From the other side, my analytic mind might operate from an internal position something like this:

> I have received in mind and body your furiously urgent message, namely your absolute, compulsive, angry, hungry, ever-frustrated need and thwarted desire. Your emotionally pained mind has regressed to and become your passionately pained body, craving an impossibly absolute connection. I represent the possibility of a linking and thinking bodymind relation, an analytic relation that here and now represents all loves, limitations and losses, and so a relationship which itself must be mourned.
>
> However, the necessary and ethical law of this human world is: No, you cannot have it all (me, others, parents) as you will; you cannot make me disclose and open my separate private self to your devouring hunger to know and have power over my mind and body, for that would preclude necessarily frustrating fantasies; you cannot make me, by force or seduction, love you the way you wish. There is a limiting frame that others (me now) do and shall embody: a Law of the Fathers, necessary parental and social limits.
>
> Your desires, frustrations and hates are here now for us to understand.
>
> Your hurt makes you hate, attack and destroy the good and the possibility of love that you so desperately need . . . because for you, they are never enough.
>
> Indeed, as you say and show, your anger recognises no bounds . . . no boundaries.

> But my boundaries and the world's necessities are actually your truest gain: a free necessity. I shall reflect before I act. I shall use my separate thinking mind. Out of a mass of emotional information, I shall find selected facts and interpretations.

Thus, borderline persons evacuate and communicate their impotent rage through their affecting/infecting/disturbing the integrity of my embodied analytic self, thereby having their impossible desires and furious passions received. This chronic state of global rage and frustration may then become a slow mourning that taps into the concomitant sadness and depression. However, much remains perennially un-mourned, which means an ongoing sense of impotence, loss and destruction: the hungry core of outrage and defiance of the superego continues to bite and burn.

This all-devouring destructive hunger is exactly the emotional psychic reality that the narcissistic personality defensively and over-sensitively avoids (makes void) both internally and interpersonally. A grandiose false self is a defensive response to the pain of their losses, failures and doubts; to a core reality that is too fearfully and angrily depressed to be consciously acknowledged and expressed.

Here, the perennially split-off anger is a strenuous and tense manoeuvre, and both the disguised, even reversed, anger and the tactical tension can be evoked and constellated in the analyst through subtle 'passive relational activity'.

Although the adhesive identifications of narcissistic need are not so crudely acted out, they can surely be nearly as psychosomatically infectious as the projective identifications of the borderline person because they function as a defence against their own hidden destructive rage. Adhesive identifications and extractive introjections do 'get right under my skin', 'make my flesh creep' and often make me 'sick with disgust'.

The whole strategic system of narcissistic defences can be challenged and melted down by naming the person's secret fear of being an oedipal failure and realizing their fear of their lethal anger and resentment that is hidden in the righteous disdain. I may thus disturb the narcissistic universe in a way that the whole strategic, secretive, defensive system of what Kernberg (2004) calls the 'malignant self-love' is recognised as being self-defeating. As Kernberg points out, to challenge, and so sometimes enable, strong and repetitive narcissistic defences to break down into a realisation and even expression of the underlying fearful (borderline) murderous hate and anger is actually a healthy development towards a more emotionally real and vital self than the false deceptions (i.e. self-deception and a feigning of persona) of narcissistic 'malignant self-love'. A real sense of outrage and a real attack or fight is actually analytically enlivening, and its energetic truth can be integrated.

Both disordered states are basically driven by toxic envy and resentment. They are defensively and desperately re-constellated through transferential inducements in and communications through the body and mind of the analyst's countertransference: their projective poisons get into my auto-immune self-system, but thence a necessary process of self-preservation is activated. With borderline states, there is, by definition, a strong tendency to act out because there is no functional symbolisation, no self-containing reflection, no impulse control, but rather a compulsion to affect the matter and mind of others. However, as well as managing the possibility of actual violence and actual psychosomatic disturbance, the analyst can also find various metaphors for the experience of being in a shared atmosphere of such primitive, destructive, borderline relations.

The 'wounded healer' actually heals through their survival, management and recycling of their own wounds and madness. This contains and processes the maddening wounds of the other.

I am initially countertransferentially open (at a psychoid level) to psychosomatic infection, projective identification and psychotic beta confusion, but thereby my analytic bodymind is psycho-sensually used, informed or necessarily deformed by primitive pre-symbolic and anti-symbolic psychosomatic infections and by forceful projections, by transferentially evacuated pains of intolerable lacks and losses and the furies of thwarted primary love. But thence, out of my countertransferential experience of consubstantiating processes, out of psychosomatic infection and contagion, I have to find healthy separateness, related reverie, creative imagination, reflection, critical reason and the eventual emergence of intuitive knowledge or of 'selected facts', and so to a transformative interpretation.

Thus, due to their very real passion, and when analytically well-contained, borderline persons may be able to grieve and mourn their impotent desires and frustrations and so develop a greater degree of agency, a relatively functional symbolic understanding, and a capacity to live more constructively and creatively.

References

Addison, A. (2008). 'Reframing the Unconscious: A View of Jung's Psychoid Unconscious Then and Now.' *Paper Given at Journal of Analytical Psychology Conference*, Orta, Italy. Unpublished.

Addison, A. (2009). 'Jung, Vitalism and "the Psychoid": An Historical Reconstruction'. *Journal of Analytical Psychology*, 54(1): 123–142.

Bion, W. (1959). 'Attacks on Linking'. *International Journal of Psychoanalysis*, 40: 285–300.

Britton, R. (1998). *Belief and Imagination: Explorations in Psychoanalysis*. London, Routledge.

Corbin, H. (1972). *Mundus Imaginalis, or the Imaginary and the Imaginal*. In Spring. Dallas: Spring Publications.

Grotstein, J. (1997). '"Mens Sane in Corpore Sano": The Mind and Body as an "Odd Couple" and an Oddly Coupled Unity'. *Psychoanalytic Inquiry*, 17(2): 204–222.

Jung, C. (1947). 'Der Geist der Psychologie'. In *Geist und Natur*. Vorträge gehalten auf der Tagung in Ascona 26. August bis 3. September 1946. O. Fröbe-Kapteyn, ed. Zürich: Rhein-Verlag (Eranos-Jahrbuch XIV/1946).

Jung, C. (1970a). *Mysterium Coniunctionis: An Inquiry into the Separation and Synthesis of Psychic Opposites in Alchemy*. Vol. 14 of *The Collected Works of C.G. Jung*. Translated by R. Hull. 2nd edn. London: Routledge & Kegan Paul.

Jung, C. (1970b). 'On the Nature of the Psyche'. In *The Structure and Dynamics of the Psyche*. Vol. 8 of *The Collected Works of C.G. Jung*. R. Hull, trans. 2nd edn. London: Routledge & Kegan Paul.

Kernberg, O. (2004). *Aggressivity, Narcissism and Self-Destructiveness in the Psychotherapeutic Relationship*. New Haven: Yale University Press.
Samuels, A. (1985). 'Countertransference, the "Mundus Imaginalis" and a Research Project'. *Journal of Analytical Psychology*, 30(1): 47–71.
Segal, H. (1957). 'Notes on Symbol Formation'. *International Journal of Psycho-Analysis*, 38: 391–397.
Segal, H. (1991). *Dream, Phantasy, and Art*. London: Routledge.

Chapter 13

Unconscious structures and defences

Unpublished, 2010[1]

> For two personalities to meet is like mixing two different chemical substances: if there is any combination at all, both are transformed. In any effective psychological treatment the doctor is bound to influence the patient; but this influence can only take place if the patient has a reciprocal influence on the doctor. You can exert no influence if you are not susceptible to influence.
>
> (Jung, 1993, *CW* 16, para. 163)

In analysis, both patient and analyst enter a contained process of emotionally intense and intimate psychic observation and exploration, a shared relational realm of such forceful pain and pleasure, impotence and power that both are mutually infected and informed. Taking place through deeply unconscious psychic and somatic as well as conscious communications, this encounter may be life-changing – perhaps more for one party than the other, but to some degree for both. Out of this mix, the transcendent function may emerge.

When two people decide to meet regularly within the containing frame of analysis in order to explore the effects of psychological forces (through fantasies, dreams and the re-experiencing of emotional relations), then there may be an affective psychic and psychosomatic meeting at many levels. This, I suggest, represents a radical re-visioning of my place in the force-field of my intra-psychic and inter-psychic nature and nurture. It catalyses a Spinozan 'intuitive knowledge' that emerges out of deeply processed transferential and countertransferential informational matter (that is, passionately embodied matter). Thereby both of us may be profoundly moved and changed in our 'emotional minds' and in our 'sensitive bodies' too. This is 'psychosomatic'. I am not referring to psychogenic physical illness, but

1 This chapter is based on an ANZSJA Professional Development Seminar given in Christchurch, New Zealand on March 19, 2010. The original seminar included two full clinical vignettes concerning 'Jim', included in Chapter Seven, and 'Christine', found in Chapter Nine and also included in Chapter Sixteen. We have taken out the verbatim repeats and so refer the reader to the presentations concerning Jim in Chapters Six, Seven, Nine and Ten. For Christine, we refer the reader to Chapters Nine and Sixteen (Eds.).

DOI: 10.4324/9781003255826-14

using this term in the sense of the psyche-soma unit, that is, as a representation of (Spinozan) dual-aspect theory, where mind and body are different aspects of a single 'substance'.

In 'Problems of Practical Psychotherapy' (Jung, 1993), Jung, with certain prescience, recognises a mutually shared, inter-subjective psychic field as a third agent of the analytic relationship, in and through which both persons are changed, the transcendent third. Perhaps Jung didn't say quite enough about what changes actually happen to the person he calls 'the doctor' in this analytic alchemical bath, in the black rain, the contagious atmosphere, the psyche-soma union, the *participation mystique*, the erotic oceanic bliss, the emotional battlefields of analysis. Nor does he elaborate on what 'the doctor' can do with these sometimes radical movements, how to interpret them (as distinct from amplify them), when and how to feed them back to the analysand or not (and if not, then why not) and how this profound relational transformation really works.

It is a *sine qua non* that the problems and personality of the patient-as-other are paramount and are the locus and driver of our concern. The therapist embodies an attentive, receptive, reflective and interpretive mind, a mind that is there to be therapeutically 'used' consciously and unconsciously.

In my own writings, I have continued to elaborate on the clinical hypothesis of an infectious consubstantiating animating psychoid body which is affective through *participation mystique* and through transferential and countertransferential weather. I am referring in particular to the storms of desire, love, disappointment, loss, grief, angry depression or even through the affects and effects of an absence of primary love, of frustration and impotent rage, and so through projective identification as a forceful defence and communication. There are the doldrums of loneliness, defeat, self-loathing and passive suicidality.

In the emotional storms and doldrums of deep psychotherapy, we find ourselves asking: What is this relationship and process that we are in together? What is happening to or between us? What are we doing to each other and to ourselves? How much can we really know? We may entertain a necessary illusion of the possibility of change, understanding, choice and agency within an actually unfree, pre-determined material 'necessity', certainly a neurobiological and contingent nature within and without. Our genes, our biology, the extent and depth of our unconsciousness, political and cultural forces and contingent events all make relative our so-called 'free will'. Two psychologically necessary illusions which are valuable subjective 'psychic realities', might be teleology (or purpose and meaning) and free will. As Schopenhauer said, 'A man can only do what he wills to do, but he cannot determine what he wills'.[2]

Personally, I find that a realistic acquiescence to the contingent limits of my freedom of will, choice, agency and knowledge is psychically liberating. As Calvino wrote of Diderot's novel *Jacques le Fataliste*,

> Diderot had worked out that actually the most rigidly deterministic conceptions of the world are the ones that generate in the individual will an urge to move

2 '*Der Mensch thut allezeit nur was er will, und thut es doch notwendig*' (Schopenhauer, 1860, p. 98).

forward, as though will and free choice can only be effective if they carve out their openings against the hard rock of necessity.

(Calvino, 1999, p. 110)

However, this acquiescence to 'the pre-determined' and hard contingent facts coexists with an ego-developing Hegelian defiance. In other words, belief in the lack of actual freedom simultaneously sits beside an animal faith in and a phantasy of the psychic reality of free will and agency.

Perhaps, as Jung emphasises, analytic interpretations, linking connections, amplification and new understanding can lead to an increase in true symbolising. A realising of 'as if' symbolic connections and causes in one's life, behind our impulses and feelings, may enable a stronger sense of agency and understanding of the 'choices' we have made, as well as taking responsibility for such choices.

As said previously, a severely undeveloped, faulty symbolising function means that a person lives in and lives out a primitive literalness and is passively pushed around without reflexive understanding by unconscious impulses.[3] There are impulses to split off and spit out impotent rage through projective identifications. Such psychic-somatic confusion is infectious, at times engendering mutual panic or transferential love, which, if a 'love psychosis' is like a fairground ride, exciting and frightening at the same time. And we are both on this ride.

Analysis is a bit like being on a long walking trip taken together, sometimes slow and hard, sometimes a monotonous slog, but when we come to the top of a hill and cross the brow, we see the unexpected glory of the Himalayas before us, or a landscape of desolation and destruction or a depressing desert. This emotionally-loaded spectacle, this shock of symbolic recognition, moves us both deeply.

The psychoid revisited

I cannot deal with these issues, with this subjective and inter-subjective realm, without revisiting Jung's concept of 'the psychoid', the shared emotional psychic and somatic alchemical bath, which can be experienced, interpreted and so described as either an erotic *participation mystique* or as being together in an infectious or contagious atmosphere, in a dangerously toxic violent realm.

The psychoid concerns a substrate level at which the psychic and the organic are consubstantial, are as one where they meet; the psyche is intrinsically psychoid. In the context of borderline and other disordered personality relations, the psychoid substance is particularly evident in the transferential infectious projections and in the countertransferential information received through the urgent communicative forces operative at this primitive psyche-soma level. As Addison[4] suggests, this arises particularly in periods of regression to very early stages involving 'the

3 For a fuller account of undeveloped and faulty symbolising function, see Chapter Ten (Eds.).

4 See Chapter Twelve for a fuller account of Addison's hypothesis and Clark's own theorising on the dual identity of the psychoid realm (Eds.).

emergence of psyche from soma' and has a 'teleological function in the development of mind' (Addison, 2008, p. 10).

Psychoid processes are also emergent forces, the innate psyche-soma ground from which 'archetypes-as-such' emerge. This is what Jean Knox (2003) calls 'image schemas', unconscious patterns, without content in themselves, that emerge from very early and repeated interactions with significant others in the environment. Mind (or meaning) emerges from body (*via* neurobiology) and from bodily relations, which become meaning-endowed relations. Both patient and analyst may experience an emergence through psychoid and psychosomatic identity to new forms of symbolisation, the separation and creation of meaning out of matter.

When such strong affects are experienced countertransferentially with persons with over-sensitive, thin-skinned narcissistic defences (which are secretively grandiose and self-righteous), then they can be a signal of a split-off underlying angry core that has hitherto been fearfully avoided. Much embodied countertransferential communication experienced even with 'normally neurotic' persons derives from pockets of early beta pre-order or disorder.

At the psychoid level, bodily matter, mental image and idea are but different modes of the one substance. Mind arises out of bodily relations. Being an emergent and dynamic force, the psychoid is also a potentiality and a potency. This connects to Hanna Segal's (1957) idea that symbolic equations are potentially symbolic and Bion's that beta elements can develop into alpha functioning. For matter or body to be given meaning, such matter, body and bodies must exist in the first place. This could imply epiphenomenalism, the idea that mind and consciousness emerge out of matter. The only other two alternatives are either that 'body matter' is a product, expression or representation of mind, which is an extreme form of Idealism or that matter (or physical body) and mind (or idea) are substantially identified: two differently identifiable aspects of a common 'substance'. This is the attitude that I prefer.

Perhaps this 'panpsychic perception and position' can be said to derive from the psychoid substrate of the *conatus*; implying that the psyche is intrinsically psychoid. Transferentially/countertransferentially, this dual aspect of the psychoid realm, of 'bodymind', makes for 'consubstantial' experience and for its possible transformation. It emerges out of, between, around and, therefore, to both of us in analysis, whence it can move or be moved from somatic sensation or somatisation to symbolic reverie and to thought. And thence, it may be given back to the patient in so far as he or she is receptive.

Such constructive 'in-formation' is always at a certain level psychosomatic, of the 'bodymind'. Therefore, as we shall soon see, paradoxically acted-out destructiveness is often a most affective active form of communication (as well as of defence). Mutual change or transformation can be a psychic (and psychosomatic) infection and contagion. The task is, therefore, a process of separation out of such fusion, of individuation and real personal symbolisation.

It is through this affective psychic immersion that we remember, re-construct and re-live our idiosyncratic feeling-toned internalised images of past relations, not only good and loving relations but also unresolved and difficult primary family relations. We realise how intolerable lacks and losses, frustrating, failed and fearful relations have been so internalised that they have unconscious but powerful effects on ourselves, our relations to others and to the world. Related to this, there is the issue of the development of the symbolising function, particularly when it is a matter of failures of symbolisation and how, through the interpretive action of the analytic relationship, such malfunctions can be potentially rectified.

Analytic therapy is a particular relational (or anti-relational) and psychically alive (or deathly, if not deadly) world of communicated emotional experience, of the therapist being with and working for another in an environment that is often alive with the slings and arrows of projective identifications, as well as the arrows of *Eros*. I am speaking about being an affected but still thinking mind, even when caught up in emotionally disturbing latent and actual explosions, which may also be moments of creation: dreaming, imagining, reflecting, thinking, interpreting and talking through emotional storms, earthquakes and battles, difficult loves and passions.

We come into psychotherapy seeking to be loved and understood and to solve problems relating to our frustrating and depressing hurts of love and understanding. When primary love does not go well, we feel psychically defeated and frightened. Indeed, lacks are experienced as attacks and sometimes there are real abuses and acts of violence. And so, in different ways and to different degrees, our various defences are necessarily set up. These may be normally neurotic defences or more psychotically disordered states. I am thinking here of schizoid splits, fearful narcissistic decoys, destructive borderline outrage, dissociation and psychogenic autistic pockets.

Defensive systems are either unconscious, hidden from others and oneself, or distorted and lost under complex layers or are angry and destructive. All defences are based on an impetus or *conatus* for self-preservation. They can be fierce, angry or fearful, assertive or evasive. However, they all reveal the needs of the underlying lost truth (true self) through dreams, fantasies, unconscious projections, transferential desires, hates, disappointments and even through the recognition of narcissistic fears of non-existence, absences of real emotional connection or sense of being a real self.

Analytic reverie, thinking and interpretive action fly in the face of transferential psychoid storms and deathly calms, which are also the dangerously vital (sometimes near deadly) volcanic stuff at the unconscious core of all of us. Our relative sanity is normal neurotic madness put to good use, but at the fundament of our emotional mind is our maddening primal 'beta' chaos and disorder (the *prima materia*).

Let us remember that Jung, unlike Freud, formulated his models and ideas of the psyche through his experience (including his own psychotic pockets) and work with near-psychotic and psychotic patients, initially at the Burghölzli Hospital. This is why his psychology so helps us work with difficult personality disorders and their primitive pre-symbolic and anti-symbolic realms. The 'furious storm' is exactly what the narcissist spends his or her strategic false-life trying to avoid, displaying instead a false calm. It is this violence through which the borderline spends his or her psychotically destructive life trying to reach a real love and meaningful order, although any love and order is always simultaneously envied, resented and murderously attacked. In destructive borderline relations, there is at least the real intimacy of fight, whereas with the fearful narcissist, there is a more strategically hidden 'sucking hollow' of lonely hurt and anger. I refer the reader to the clinical vignette of 'Jim'[5] for the former and 'Christine'[6] for the latter.

Christine, again

This is a story of how Christine moved from righteous but fragile and fearful narcissistic false superiority, through nervous adhesive identification, to disappointment and disillusionment, to angry depression, to borderline invasion and to an eventual scepticism and the irony of 'cheerful pessimism'. It is the story of how she took me with her to places I did not know I would or could experience.

Christine, you may recall, described herself as 'a brilliant artist' but felt unappreciated. She came to see me to complain about how her 'ever so helpful suggestions', based on the 'wisdom of my vast experience', seemed to fall on deaf ears. Despite being so 'altruistic, loving and spiritually wise', she couldn't understand why 'people drop me and continuously let me down. Perhaps I am just too kind and giving for this competitive and greedy modern world'.

Finding her sentimentality, grandiosity and lack of self-awareness annoying, I had to remind myself that her hollow superiority covered over a lonely sense of inferiority and insignificance, and this, in turn, covered up disappointed outrage. This angry core might be real and alive, but it was dangerous as she feared it would make her even more alienated from the peopled world.

A seminal dream depicting her core 'basic fault' in Balint's sense was of her stomach and vagina being full of writhing maggots with featureless faces except for hungry 'nasty little mouths'. This we interpreted as representing not being able to let anything good in nor bad out.

A major shocking shift occurred when she suddenly and out of the blue asked me if I found her disgusting (like these worms). However, having been put to sleep by her endless droning monotones, out of my stupor, I made a careless response, 'No, but at last, I am really interested'. This unleashed a tirade of outrage: I was heartless, unprofessional, insensitive . . . just like everyone else. Furthermore, she now blamed me for filling her with the proverbial hungry maggots.

5 This paper originally included a detailed account of the clinical case of Jim but this has been removed here to avoid repetitions. It can be found in Chapters Six, Seven, Nine and Ten. Some additional material on Jim occurs further on (Eds.).

6 This paper originally featured a fuller clinical vignette concerning Christine. We have removed verbatim repeats from earlier chapters, but this paper includes new material which has been retained here. See Chapters Nine and Sixteen for other versions of the case of Christine (Eds.).

One night, after a session with Christine in which she had been expressing a very angry disappointment with her unappreciative male colleagues (i.e. with me), I dreamt that I was dressed in wolf-skin and my task, against my impulse, was to not kill Christine, however angry (hungry?) I was. With no obvious connection, I happened the next day to give a seminar in which I used Housman's well-known poem from *A Shropshire Lad*, with its reference to an 'air that kills' coming from the 'land of lost content' with its 'blue remembered hills' (Housman, 1906, p. 57).

Two days later, Christine came with this dream:

> Walking along a country road, I came over the brow of a hill and saw the wall of the high Himalayas before me, a range of rolling blue hills beneath. So startling and awesome that I nearly fainted. I was overcome with grief and turned to my boyfriend (who was suddenly with me) and said, 'We have to make love, right now'.
>
> I was about to do so when I saw that he was covered with red scales; he was malevolent and dangerous. His skin was poisonous to the touch.
>
> He showed his teeth in a canine snarl; was he rabid?
>
> I was too late; I hadn't either run away in time or shot him. So I knew I'd had it and was now going to be savaged to an agonisingly slow death; I would be eaten alive.
>
> Would sex by seduction save me?
>
> No, I knew that seduction and sex with an evil reptilian or rabid wolf-man was a non-starter . . . because he had no human empathy at all. And anyhow, I was too frightened to even try sex.
>
> Or prayer?
>
> I realised that the answer to prayer would be that I must acquiesce and die as resignedly as possible.
>
> Perhaps he was a dark aspect of God . . . or was this just wishful thinking?
>
> I got ready to die, remembering the vast Himalayas and the sad blue hills.
>
> I woke up.

The Himalayas and the blue hills could be interpreted as the strong and good parents, an internal union to resignedly and peacefully die (back) into. For Christine, the alarmingly and monstrously transformed boyfriend (analyst) represented the lethal danger of desire. For Christine, the needed and desired love objects always go bad and become deadly.

In spite of our imagining, feeling and thinking into this dream, some days later, I became ill and was off work for a whole week, for the first time in my analytic life. When we recommended a week later, I continued to think and interpret our way through the unconscious poisonous atmosphere. However, Christine repeatedly retreated back into her familiar and 'safe' position of hiding her dangerously potent real self.

The analytic task in such situations is to address the primitive anxiety, interpersonal terrors and shames. This may lead to a shock of recognition that the analysand's object of fear is a maternal-parental world in which the self is unrecognised and unloved and its healthy exhibitionistic energies crippled. Thus clever, strategic and secretive, but very counter-productive, self-defeating defences are desperately wrought.

As described in Chapter Nine, Christine had originally secretly hoped that therapy would enable her to 'stop being a frightened gazelle and become a leopard'. In the end, she realised that 'sometimes I enjoy being a gazelle'.

Was that a 'good enough' ending, I wonder?

Kernberg (2004) has described how narcissism, which is essentially a fearful defence, a hiding and a falseness, a secret adhesiveness, a private righteous superiority precariously covering failure and loneliness, attempts to strategically defend against a very frightening anger. Therefore, when a narcissist moves out of their secretive and false self-world into a realisation and expression of outrage, their underlying impulse to angrily attack the lacks, then they are truer and more alive.

Jim, again

Jim, you will recall,[7] dreamed that he was screwing the spiky, hard, sharp transepts of a Gothic cathedral, and as he does so, it becomes soft, wet and disgusting, a foul, wet cunt. It disappears beneath him, leaving him exploding into empty space. I interpreted this to represent a destruction of myself, the transcendent function between us and any attainment of a depressive position. After a further four years of love and hate, of closeness and attacks from close range, I had to let Jim know that I was going to emigrate in a year's time. A month before the end of our analytic relationship, he had the following dream:

> I am in a First World War trench. There is another soldier next to me with a bandaged or scarfed face and wearing a tin-helmet, so his face was doubly invisible. Was he a dead enemy soldier or my mate?

I reflected, 'Your beloved enemy . . . or your hidden companion', Jim sobbed.

As we saw earlier, ours was initially a trading in primal primitive body meanings, in body fears and desires, powers and impotencies, where our bodies are indeed our minds and are our uses of our bodies. For Jim, there was initially no differentiation between subject and object: a primitive mind-body identity, a psychoid psychosomatic unit of experience where beta emotions move both body and idea because they are experienced as 'the same thing'. There was also no differentiation between fantasy and reality, inside and outside, self and other. Jim enacted a double identity position in relation to self and other. In addition, a good object for him was one that was worthy of attack and destruction. In so far as he realised all this, he achieved a relatively mature and sophisticated level of symbolisation.[8]

7 See Chapter Seven (Eds.).

8 This paper originally featured a long segment titled 'Phenomenology of borderline relations' but this has been omitted as it occurs in two earlier chapters. See Chapters Nine and Twelve (Eds.).

The analytic battlefield of extreme transferential and countertransferential relations

In the analytic battlefield of a 'psychotic transference' in which poisonous feelings are split off and evacuated into the psyche-soma of the other/others, the analyst is sometimes made to have or become the body and neurological energy for and of the other and thence to feel, think, feel, link, observe, explore, interpret and recreate our way through and out of these passions and pains.

As said before, as wounded healers, we heal through our wounds, through recycling our madness. It is our personal areas of idiosyncratic emotional and physical vulnerability that are open to being disturbed and moved. Countertransferential information is received through our psychosomatically 'weakest' areas; it is through our 'strongly' reactive 'Achilles' areas from which we are made to work.

Projective poisons can and do get into my emotionally receptive 'bodymind', even at times into my auto-immune self-system, but hopefully also into my analytic mind. I necessarily need to think non-reactively and clearly through and out of this infection or contagion to focus my reverie (intuitive knowledge of other, me, us) and eventually, with applied understanding, to speak and interpret in a way that is mutative. As one such patient once sang to me, quoting the Quaker poet John Greenleaf Whittier, 'Speak through the earthquake, wind, and fire, O still, small voice of calm!'[9]

There seem to be several metaphors for the experience of being in a shared atmosphere of such primitive, destructive, borderline matters and relations. They include: earthquake and volcanic eruption; invisible, psychic projectiles; infections and contagions; being poisoned; a numbing or paralysing nerve gas which stops ongoing functions, above all thinking and speaking; invasion and possession by alien forces; being overpowered; being bombed; being attacked by a suicidal terrorist; being ambushed by a dangerous animal or reptile; being coerced; being inveigled and seduced by nearly irresistible inducements and enchantments; excessive sexual pressures, pulls, intrusions and suctions; an excessive tension of *jouissance*; a global anti-mind of chaotic beta bits whose confusing fragments are maddening. Sometimes, these are the only form (or deform) for urgently needed and effective communication, the making and sharing of intolerable disorder which has somehow to be understood and 'sorted out' by the analyst's clarifying mind and by the internalisation of a good-enough analytic relationship.

Conclusion

Work with borderline personality disorders demonstrates a primal psychosomatic unity through states of zonal identification and confusion, personally and interpersonally and even between mind and the world. Such disorder is not so much a

9 This line is taken from the hymn 'Dear Lord and Father of Mankind', adapted from a section of Whittier's 1872 'The Brewing of Soma' (Eds.).

matter of cause and effect but is only perceived thus. It is a matter of identification, not connection. The substance of such psychic activity is psychoid and, because of its somatisation of the symbolic, symbolically equivalent or sometimes psychotic. At a very basic and often invisible level, these primal pre-separated and pre-verbal psychoid realms, where subject and object, inside and outside, fantasy and reality, mind and matter, can be a force-field that draws us into its disturbing *unus mundus* state, are either or both a place of mystical unity or of psychosis, our psychotic core. This is the level at which it is demonstrated that 'mind and body are two different perceptions of one activity',

As an analyst, in the countertransference I am at times made to feel as if I want to blow up the narcissist's false security and to order the borderline's forces of disorder; thus, I, too, am affected. But ultimately, from between these two positions, there may emerge a healthy sense of lively psychic energy and of sceptical irony; this vital sense is mutual, though also personal and different, because, after all, we are each our separate selves.

Such personality disorders necessarily induce in their therapist a primitive embodied countertransference (which is sometimes hate-filled, the stuff of Winnicott's 1949 'Hate in the Countertransference') and, therefore, (also necessarily) a reflexive thought-demanding 'complementary' transferential relationship.

Both borderline and narcissistic states are basically driven by venomous envy and resentment: overtly expressed in impulsive acts of borderline murderousness; denied and hidden behind polite invisibility and the art of feigning in the case of narcissism.

Narcissism is a defence against loneliness, anxiety and anger; borderline outrage is an aggressive defence against depressive defeat and autistic non-connections. Both are trying to manage a basic fault: a foundational lack of primary love. The narcissist assuages the superego and tries to hold self, others and the world safely together, as in an idealised or false mandala (centripetal forces). The borderline defies the superego and tries to blow self, others and the world apart, but where such destruction of the idealised good makes for an intensely real aliveness (centrifugal forces).

This primal or primitive and sometimes savage stuff is also common to and typical of the forces at the origins, depths and core of all of us. Although we may not all be oedipal orphans, we are all oedipally sensitive. In all deeply shared realms in psychotherapy, in normally neurotic relations as well as in more primitive near-psychotic zones, the life of our internal and interpersonal dramas are dreamt, reflected upon and reflected back, remembered, grieved, thought through, linked up and so seen symbolically. We come to better understand why and how we feel and do as we do, and so are less blind and more aware – which is not necessarily comfortable. Suffering with your eyes more widely open! At the same time, we know just how much we do not know. This is surely an achievement of a mature ironic scepticism.

In spite of successful splits and defences against our difficult, frightening and passionate selves, our crafty self-delusions and blank voids of dissociation, if we survive the intensity of this particular intimate meeting, how can any of us undergo such elemental and emotionally-loaded journeys into our darkest and most dazzling churn of unconscious forces without being seismically moved, vitally affected and deeply transformed?

Sometimes this can be about being moved to an abode of psychic stillness and calm; however, even such an apparently peaceful state may turn out to be the still centre of a cyclone, a calm before another storm, another whirlwind.

References

Addison, A. (2008). 'Reframing the Unconscious: A View of Jung's Psychoid Unconscious Then and Now'. *Paper Given at Journal of Analytical Psychology Conference*, Orta, Italy. Unpublished.

Calvino, I. (1999). *Why Read the Classics?* New York: Pantheon.

Housman, A. (1906). *A Shropshire Lad*. New York: John Lane (Bodley Head).

Jung, C. (1993). 'Problems of Modern Psychotherapy'. In *The Practice of Psychotherapy*. Vol. 16 of *The Collected Works of C.G. Jung*. R. Hull, trans. London: Routledge & Kegan Paul.

Kernberg, O. (2004). *Aggressivity, Narcissism and Self-Destructiveness in the Psychotherapeutic Relationship*. New Haven: Yale University Press.

Knox, J. (2003). *Archetype, Attachment, Analysis: Jungian Psychology and the Emergent Mind*. Hove and New York: Brunner-Routledge.

Schopenhauer, A. (1860). 'Über die Freiheit des menschlichen Willens'. In *Die beiden Grundprobleme der Ethik*. Leipzig: Brockhaus.

Segal, H. (1957). 'Notes on Symbol Formation'. *International Journal of Psychoanalysis*, 38: 391–397.

Whittier, J. (1872). 'The Brewing of the Soma'. In *The Pennsylvania Pilgrim and Other Poems*. Boston: James R. Osgood.

Winnicott, D. (1949). 'Hate in the Counter-Transference'. *International Journal of Psychoanalysis*, 30: 69–74.

Chapter 14

On psychosis

Unpublished, 2010[1]

I take it as a *sine qua non* that there can sometimes be endogenous, neurological (biological or chemical) causes of psychosis. Schizophrenic disorders of thought and speech, the emotional states of extreme bipolar and depressive psychoses, etc., are partly caused by organic conditions. When dealing with psychosis, some analytic issues are: to what extent are manifestations of psychotic states open to symbolic interpretation, to finding or making meaning and to the possibility of (relational) change? As well as endogenous schizophrenic, bipolar, depressive and anxiety psychoses, there are also psychotic-like aspects to addictive, OCD and borderline states, in states of regression and cases featuring failures of symbolisation. All such partly psychotic states are not uncommon in analytic relations.

Two related classical Jungian hypotheses about psychosis are the theory of the dissociability (splitting) of the psyche and the idea that the ego may be swamped, possessed or disordered by split-off, irrational and affectively laden archetypal unconscious content. We may also fear that we might 'crack up' or 'break down' through too much consciousness, for example, by too much emotional tension or moral conflict (with no possible resolution or no transcendent function, etc.), by too many bad memories or excessive worry about the future, fears of impending losses, let alone fear of death itself. However, these conscious worries, anxieties and dreads are normally neurotic and are not usually psychotic. We get to know our own psychotic parts in other ways: through nightmares, possessive fears and unconscious phantasies, obsessions, bad drug experiences, delirious states (sometimes caused by fever or pain), from 'love psychoses' (where we are overcome by infatuation, jealousy and loss), states of extreme anxiety and panic and experience of irrationally destructive parental and family interactions. We may also temporarily 'lose our mind' through other 'psychotic' relations, including analytic relations when we experience a loss of control of our emotional, thinking and ordered/ordering mind.

If our conscious and unconscious behaviour is to a varying degree motivated by neurotically normal, necessary defences of the self, for example, by strategic and tactical defences such as schizoid retreats, narcissistic hiding and falseness, angry

1 Originally given as an ANZSJA training seminar in 2010.

DOI: 10.4324/9781003255826-15

borderline outrage and destructiveness, splitting or melancholia, then psychosis represents a state of defeat of such neurotic defences or a state where the defences have become literally self-defeating of psychosomatic order. Above all, psychosis here is a state without effective defences against non-ego or anti-ego forces that are therefore seen as overly 'other' or 'alien'.

Defences against psychosis can be psychotic themselves when driven and conditioned by fearful psychotic objects. Psychotic persons create a psychotic rationale to make idiosyncratically 'comprehensible' their world-view and self-view, which is pre-symbolic and anti-symbolic, perhaps a perverse defence. From a developmental perspective, this may originate as a defence against the intolerable lack of or perversion of needed and expected primary love. This lack is experienced as an attack and so is defended against through fight, flight or panic, depressive, paranoid states, dissociation or psychogenic psychosis. However, the psychotic rationale is not only a relationally generated defence; it may be a defence against (and thereby unconsciously reveal) an original structural fault with an inherent pathological over-sensitivity. Or it may be an expression of an inherent distortion of psychosomatic receptors or of other structural faults of perception and apperception.

Normal human madness involves wanting to change the fixed or unchangeable, and wanting to fix and keep the changing, the going and forever gone. As Santayana put it, 'every living body is mad in so far as it is inwardly disposed to permanence when things about it are unstable, or is inwardly disposed to change when, the circumstances being stable, there is no occasion for changing' (Santayana, 1926, p. 41). *Nequid Pereat* ('Let nothing perish') is either a madly foolish or a heroically defiant ideal. We want the good objects to survive, the good parents to be immortal, but the good is fragile, unreliable and impermanent; it 'goes bad', or may become part of a depressive ambivalence. Often, the good becomes but an idealised melancholic memory. There is also the omnipotent wish for that which cannot be changed to change (e.g. the laws of the father and the necessities of nature). All such 'normal human madness' is re-constellated in the transference and so becomes the passionate analytic work. However, the question is, how can this ever become the work in cases of psychosis?

The essence of psychotic experience is that of a person pushed around by a monstrous internalised, split off and projected 'alien force' which evokes 'incomprehensible emotions', as one psychotic person put it. These maddening forces may manifest in the form of hallucinations, dissociation, out-of-body experience, overwhelming ideas or emotions, intolerably conflicted passions and an impossible moral tension that is beyond reflection, understanding and control.

This deeply disturbing 'alien force' may manifest through a disturbance to the coherence of thinking, which I discuss more fully further on. In turn, this makes word-finding and the flow of words difficult, disjointed and incoherent. This may reflect a symptomatic relational projection of internalised family disjointedness, lack of family psychological coherence and mixed moral messages. Or it may be symptomatic of sexual and oedipal confusion, of an intolerable internal moral tension and internalised lack of coherent identity, which becomes expressed through disordered communications (including in the flow of interpersonal conversation).

So what is going on here? The psychotic other is being driven, as by alien forces (not 'as if'), through a myopic tunnel, a perception and apperception through which they see, experience and know a particularly peopled world-view (and its world-law and its world-history), and so act accordingly.

Borderline psychosis

The anger and destructive outrage of borderline states can also become so extreme that it, too, is experienced as an alien force possessing the person. It, too, can become a seemingly autonomous, uncontrollable and terrifyingly violent force. Such borderline destructiveness is determinedly offensive-defensive, evacuative, projective, infectious, informative and urgently communicative. The psychotic aspect of borderline impulses occurs when the self-destructive and murderous impulses become compulsively acted out. Primitive borderline body-mind and self-other confusion are latently psychotic; what Jung referred to as 'borderline schizophrenic'. Thus, we can see it is hard at times to differentiate where borderline stops and the psychotic begins: perhaps it is a matter of degree.

Psychogenic borderline states derive from a relation of particular parental failures, primary self characteristics and the nature of the defences against the frustrations of these lacks and limitations. This may include lack of original psychosomatic containment and safe, good primary love, a lack of order and sanity leading to the experience of a disordered or distressed maternal 'bodymind'. It may refer to the absence of any necessary law of a strong and clear father or an environment of confused-confusing moral messages. Lack may be due to a sadistic, perverse or autistic absent parent or destructively confusing parental relations such as a parental non-union or oedipal confusions.

I have spoken of narcissism as a defence against fearful borderline destructiveness and taken up Kernberg's understanding that for narcissistic personalities to begin to manifest borderline traits is a sign of relative health. This is because it is an expression of the split-off emotional reality or 'truth'. However, we also need to unearth the never-to-be-touched narcissistic wound embedded in borderline proto-psychotic states.

The *jouissance* grid and psychosis

My *Jouissance* Grid[2] is also relevant to the topic of psychotic extremes. As we saw earlier, the *Jouissance* Grid is about the psychosomatic subject as object and so helps me with my psychosomatic knowing, containing and thinking. It also incorporates the possibility of psychosis: a destructive (rather than vital) excess of '*jouissance* tension' (that separates and joins affects) may become psychotic. The *jouissance* that joins and separates the emotions can become a psychotic zone if the

2 For the *Jouissance* grid, see Chapter Seven, p. 107 and Chapter Fifteen, p. 218 (Eds.).

tension becomes destructively (rather than vitally) excessive and conflictual or if there is a defensive/repressive split and one affect becomes over-dominant and the other becomes unconscious.

Psychogenic psychosis can be engendered by an excessive tension between conflicting emotions and/or the intensity of an affect that is unmitigated and unmediated by a contrary affect (e.g. unfiltered desire, pleasure or power). Similar excessive tensions or one-sided intensities may be caused or exacerbated by endogenous psychosis. But, remaining within a psychogenic perspective, we can understand how such tensions and unbalanced intensities could leave an infant, child or adult struggling with desperate responses, such as psychotic rationales, fantastically perverse or distorted interpretations of self, others and world, as well as defensive rather than developmental 'actions for self-preservation'. Such people may try in vain to make sense of and manage their psychosomatically incomprehensible internal and external world. Distinctions between internal and external are lost in the terrible and chaotic confusions of zones, of subject and object (self and family), of good and bad, etc.

There is often a fantastically elaborated or distorted memory of parental disorder and lack. Elaborate phantasies and psychotic rationales preclude the possibility of a healthy internalisation of well-united (safe and morally clear) parents and preclude the process of symbolisation. This is the world of the uncontained, betrayed and hurt child who can only know bewildering confusion, desperation, hopeless need and global hate. The person resorts defensively into dissociation, depression or narcissistic retreat. There is, above all, a lonely and defenceless self with an absolute fear and intolerance of absence and of the limits of the power to get and possess one's desired objects, an oedipal defeat and loss, which precludes any possibility for imaginal oedipal victory.

These internalised confusions are often the cause of overwhelming and incomprehensible emotions. These may manifest symptomatically in disorganised, reversed or incoherent thoughts. This is an agitated thinking which, when pushed by a pressure of words, stutters the flow of language and thereby also affects the analyst's thinking-linking and word-finding abilities and ability to form a clear clarifying sentence with any interpretive or even any real communicative effectiveness.

In the face of intolerable frustration with internal and external realities, magical phantasies may be constructed about the impossibly desired/thwarted objects, phantasies of power over objects or phantasies of being persecuted by the terrifying powers of those objects, or both. These terrible objects commonly include a psychic experience of the annihilation of life or of the greatest good, or annihilation by the unmediated original and absolute All-Good object. There is the phantasy of some sort of salvation, rebirth or eternity. Beyond or beneath such compensatory phantasy, there is an internalised and thence repeatedly acted-out attack on thinking, linking and common sense, a total disorder of reason and of well-decided action and inter-action. This is an attack by an explosive, exploded and fragmented mind on the parental mindlessness which caused this very lack.

The mutual transferential-countertransferential realm becomes a field of psychoid contagion, involving communication by angry and agitated identification, attempts to share a state of familial incomprehension. There is both a desperate call to think and simultaneously a projection of forces that prevent the ability to think. The goals of the destructive projective identifications are a combination of fusion and fissure. The psychotic content is frightening, bizarre and sado-sexual. Or it may be fanatically religious, numinous, tremendous or fascinating (*à la* Otto). It is apparently supra-personal and archetypalised.

Psychogenically, this may be generated from living with an oedipally-sexually, morally mixed-up, unclear and confused or absent parental mind. There may be such a degree of parental dissociation (emotional and relational absence) that it is psychogenic of infantile (and subsequent) psychosis. Or it may be generated from living under the terrors of an over-strong or tyrannous law of the father, the internalised all-seeing and knowing superego who judges and punishes the guilt and shame of transgressive oedipal thoughts and intentions. However, to various degrees, the now-psychotic subject may have been a schizogenic child who evoked or exacerbated a disorder in family relations and behaviour. This evocative behaviour may be due to an inherent organic condition such as autism, etc.

This creates a therapeutic field determined by a severely confused mind with crazed ideas about body, bodies and body relations, including my analytical 'bodymind' and relations between our 'bodyminds'. Psychotic defences against reality and persecutory ideas, images and phantasies are un-symbolised. Interpretations are often experienced as a dangerous attack on the concrete un-changeability of psychotic relations and are met by angry irritation or depressive defeat. Previous discussions on the psychoid are relevant here, since in the psychotic transference-countertransference dynamics, mind and body are often equated rather than differentiated as two aspects of the one substance.

A major analytic issue is how to think and act (interpret) analytically through a welter of un-symbolised concrete equations, emotional storms of divine or demonic superego persecutions, paranoid splitting and contagious psychosomatic projective attacks, seductive inveiglements, bizarre incomprehensibilities. How can we, as analysts, withstand a barrage of repetitiveness that induces boredom, weariness and eventually a self-preservatory dissociation? The problem in psychotic relations is whether any interpretive thinking, linking and understanding can be received effectively at all or whether such thinking is actively attacked with such absoluteness that it is utterly therapeutically impotent. How can clear thinking and reasoning emerge when my analytic thoughts are experienced as dangerously bad because they challenge the absolutist codes of the psychotic mind? How can the analyst's symbolising function and alpha functioning facilitate an ameliorating position of reflection about persistently psychotic non-symbolisation or destructive borderline acting out?

Firstly, it is through knowing that I am seen in the transference to be sane and well and, therefore, able to bring about sanity and wellness in my peopled world. Secondly, it is through the emergence of a sense of trusted alliance. Thirdly, it is through my healthy imaginative psychic world, my symbolic 'as ifs' and interpretations. Fourthly, it is through my healthily united internal parents, through my stamina and my on-going constancy, reliability and safety, through thoughts and/or interpretations based upon my understanding that repetitive, bizarre, perverse, self-defeating manoeuvres and contorted behaviours are yet driven by the conative striving for psychic and psychosomatic self-preservation. This analytic mix of theoretical thought, empathic imagination and the strong containing law of the frame is the sort of sanity and robustness that a person comes into analysis hoping to meet. It is this very health that is both needed and enviously resented, so blinkered out by psychotic delusions or near-psychotic self-deceptions.

Psychosis has the same meaning or lack of meaning as a nightmare. We can try to find or give meaning (interpretive links) to bizarre psychotic content and action. However, such a given meaning may or may not be effective, perhaps depending upon the degree of narcissistic retreat, actively destructive compulsion or petrifying vision.

The monstrosity of this out-of-control psychic experience expresses itself through nightmarishly bizarre archetypal fantasy, imagery and hallucination. This psychotic matter (and its relations) may be not only nightmarishly 'bad' but also, as Rhode (1994) suggests, be a primal monstrosity of the dangerously unfiltered Good (what I see as an overabundance of *jouissance*), an excess of the Good, or the Good become monstrous. The force of incomprehensibility makes eternal and psychic realities strange and over-strong, 'an excess of reality', an object-experience that is so idiosyncratic and irrational as to be delusional. As my case example that follows will show, this monstrous force becomes a projected or depressively introjected relation. The analytic task is to psychosomatically know, contain and thoughtfully understand and so interpret this overwhelming disorder and its incomprehensible emotions, in spite of attacks on and preclusions of thinking and linking.

In the 'wild weather' conditions of psychosis, the analyst cannot easily do what Bion, Winnicott, Fordham and others have said is the task of the analysis. I am referring to the state of mind, referred to by Bion (1962) as reverie, where one is utterly receptive to what is true and seeks to convey that truth. Fordham described an analyst's task as one that 'is primarily concerned to define, in the simplest terms possible, the patient's state of mind in relation to himself' (Fordham, 1991, p. 186). Similarly, Lear suggests that the analyst may become '(subjectively) a scientific observer to the extent to which he is able (subjectively) to observe the patient and himself in interaction' (Lear, 2003, p. 43). It is just these sorts of analytic reflections and understandings (symbolic connections), in the form of mutually clear and comprehensible interpretations communicated to the patient's unconscious mind, that are forcefully blocked by literalising, concrete and impulsive psychotic non-symbolising and non-reflective tunnel blinkers and sometimes by a psychotic incapacity to hear and respond appropriately to a coherent string of worded ideas because the psychotic's own ideation and thinking is so incoherent and chaotically crazed and disordered.

Psychotic patients express their disorder and incoherence, needing my thinking mind and my control of it. They need to make me identify with the frustrations of their destructive familial disturbance. Simultaneously, they also need me to sort, order and clarify their chaos, to think and link and to be sane enough to do so. However, such potencies and abilities are also envied, resented and repeatedly destroyed. Fordham says that in a psychotic transference, the analyst must go on interpreting. I don't know if I agree that that is the immediate task. I think it is to listen, to be sensed as reliably going on imagining and thinking about the patient's disjoined and disturbed 'bodymind' and to be able to survive its attacks on joined relations and coherence. However, the analytic task is still to search to psychosomatically know, contain, thoughtfully understand and so to interpret the otherwise overwhelming disorder and its incomprehensible emotions.

'Kim'

This case concerns a man obsessed and driven by compulsive sexual and other 'bad' thoughts, torn by incestuous or oedipal conflicts, zonal confusion, punitive moral guilt, having almost hallucinatory conversations with God and a recurrent nightmare of a 'genital spider'. Some of our work incorporated odd and eccentric rituals. Kim's psychological trajectory included: incest equated to sex with God; knowledge of the sin of transgression against the greatest of taboos connected to unforgivable guilt; OCD as a ritual punishment where obsessive ideas and their objects were themselves psychotic. The engine of Kim's psychosis derives from the terrible connection between the guilt and the OCD impulses. Although diagnostically, this is an obsessional neurosis, in so far as unsymbolised obsessive thoughts become delusional and paranoid, motivating certain destructive actions, they are also psychotic. Although Kim could see that some of his intrusive thoughts and contorted rituals were irrational, the God who spoke to him was 'the real and actual God himself' and was 'known' beyond any doubt and in no way an 'as if'. In other words, there was no healthy scepticism at all.

Kim came from a family of sexual repression, confusion, acting out and incestuous acts. His family was Armenian, and there was also a disavowed inheritance of intergenerational genocide. He lived with an internal family of incomprehensible contradictions under a reign of terror conducted by a super-moral, superego God. At the beginning of therapy, Kim was apparently calm, relatively coherent and strikingly articulate. Then, there were two disturbing developments: the emergence of conspiracy theories, followed gradually by persecutory ideas and obsessive thoughts. Symptomatically connected to this obsessional ideation was a combination of verbal gush, like a verbal dysentery, and abrupt and awkward verbal constipation in which his flow of speech and verbal communication tripped up or stopped in its tracks:

> Just like wanking, I can't get there, it won't cum because it's all too interfered with and the attempts to get back on flow are so convoluted that I can't breathe.

Not being able to breathe was the somatic manifestation of not being able to think. In so far as speaking is an embodying and breathing out of thoughts, he became unable to speak flowingly. As he revealed his history, Kim became increasingly disjointed and disturbed by invasive ideas and images that were, for him, affectively real. Attendant upon these thoughts, he developed relentless repetition compulsions, mainly in the form of shockingly shameful thoughts, often expressed through a tangle of shattered word-salad non-talk, with variously long or short pauses between words, but always ending with a sense of him 'buggering God':

> A cock, spunk, sister's thighs, dad's hands, fingers, sucking God, buggering God.

Then he'd instruct me:

> Just don't say anything; shut up; keep right there, shut up, you.

And, indeed, he did shut me up because, at the time, I could not find the right analytic words or, indeed, any form of appropriate response. It felt to me as if the whole room, our space, was filled with his out-of-control penis and its messy beta products.

For Kim, analytic interpretations were an attack on God and on his duty to God. That is, the God who had to suffer years of Kim's unforgivable sexual transgressions and 'putrid soiling', his compulsive sexual thoughts and impulses which were to him actual. Disgusting and unforgivable crimes were repeatedly inflicted on parents, siblings, me and, above all, on God's body. According to Kim, God said things like:

> You need to be forgiven. You must confess to everyone affected, and they must know and understand fully and must be able to forgive you. Only then will you be free. However, what you have done is so bad and foul that I, God, cannot and never shall forgive you.

This was not a hallucinated auditory voice but a received idea of 'the words of the one and only real God'. This could obviously be seen as, and indeed is, a symptom of a familial oedipal mess: incestuous, patricidal, homosexual. It is laden with murderous guilt, shame and a punitive superego, relentless, obsessive and compulsive; bad thoughts and words as compulsive repetitions.

Repetition compulsions do a lot of work. The fantasy is that one comes to understand more and enough through the repetitions; to get the incomprehensible pain solved and salved; and to get understood and loved in spite of, even masochistically, because of the problematic self.

Kim once said:

> I have a messy body with shit on the inside and sexual organs, sperm and their dangerous animal impulses all determining my behaviour out into the world of others.

He had a recurrent dream image which originated as a childhood nightmare concerning a menacing giant curly-haired spider, a frightening creature with a soft body, wiry hair and a poisonous barb hidden somewhere in its body. This image was surely a representation of his genital (zonal), gender and parental confusion. I cannot say it was a symbol because, for him, it was something literally demonic within, which made him 'a mistake', an aberration to God and, therefore, inherently unforgivable.

Eventually, Kim's relentless, obsessive-compulsive ideas became mind-numbing in their repetitiveness. Was I punch-drunk on his verbal and ideational pummelling? Was there any symbolic mind, play and creation for him to integrate? I discovered that I simply had to let him off-load the 'shit', not into me but around me. I found that I could listen, attend and respond only from a state of reverie. This related to the therapeutic need to clarify his mis-minded mind-body by daydreaming and thinking through our conscious and unconscious psychoid relations.

Analytic tasks in psychotic situations

Analytic work involves being and working in a transferential/countertransferential field. This involves a thoughtful re-ordering of our effected and affected mind, of our mutual mental and emotional confusion and thereby reflecting upon, clarifying and symbolising the other's psychosomatic disorder. The task of analysis involves thinking and linking symbolically and interpretively, reflecting together through emotional storms and so observing, experiencing and understanding unconscious structural defences and their dynamics and consequences. It is also about the internalising of this analytic relationship and possibly thereby realising a structural transformation. In cases of psychotic relations, the issue becomes: How can a transferential process of symbolising and an internalising of analytic relations occur in this realm of psychotic states and conditions?

The seminal activity of my position and work as an analyst arises out of the more passive matter of my mind being made by its ideas of other minds or other bodyminds. My reasoning, thinking, linking and thence interpreting of this psychically, mentally and somatically received information is often a process of trying to order anti-verbal beta disorder, of the development of psychosomatic co-ordination and re-formation. This depends on my ability to use my ambivalent, depressive position through its being in a dynamic relation to my paranoid schizoid forces to split. This is what I mean by a cheerful or even optimistic pessimism. It is based on both enough good object relations (joined parents) and good objects in themselves whose foundations are pre-conception. They belong to a timeless or eternal realm, pre-meeting with and mating with one's own body and maternal body. However, this original internal All-Good object, this Absolute, must be both latent with its intrinsic (not yet inherent) and necessary psychosomatic impulse to meet and mate with other material objects and with an intrinsic need to be mediated (by deintegration and reintegration). Otherwise, it is overwhelming and maddening, lethal to thinking, reason and sanity, a too-vast and therefore uncontained, supra-human (impersonal), abstract but also too-powerful pure idea. In Spinozan terms, an idea must have a body, brains and other bodies as objects to have ideas of or ideas about.

If we say from a psychological position and perspective that the body is a unit of meaning (and so can be called psychosomatic) then meaning must have a body to find or make meaning.

Analytic thinking is slow because it is a hard grind of mental work, a thinking through and into emotional storm and surge. It is a day-dreaming that avoids escape and is informed by the dream of the person at hand. Thus, for me, psychoanalytic stamina implies a symbolic and interpretive thinking that cuts a deep ethical groove, a radical change of direction, an incremental dawning of clarity that is paradoxically also a shock of recognition.

In psychotic transferential relations, I need to think clearly through and out of psychosomatically disturbing infection or contagion. I often imagine letting the contagious disorder and disease, the fragmented beta-bits, 'fall all around me', which lessens my identification with the aggressive, invasive and infectious projections and other psychotically crazed forces flying about in our psychosomatic field. However, it is still my difficult task to focus my reverie and regain 'intuitive knowledge' (of other, me, us), and so eventually find the right words and interpret affectively, which I think must imply a mourning of failure and of irreversible traumatic losses and lacks – and an understanding of the apparently counter-intuitive psychotic defences against these losses and lack.

Kim, again

One day, after Kim had told me yet again of his repeated nightmare of the pubic-haired spider, I found myself dozing off into a state of identificatory near-sleep in which I had a fleeting dream of an elephant shackled with chains. It was dangerously in musk, and I heard it shake and rattle its chains. To my shocked surprise, I heard myself saying out loud, 'Ultimately, this is about going on with the damage attached forever; how can it be otherwise?'

Then, out of self-protection, I quickly added: 'I think that's what you may be saying'. Perhaps Kim had, in fact, been saying something along the same lines while I had dozed off because, to my surprise, he answered, 'A seed of hope! Time to start clearing the mine-field'. He became considerably calmer. However, over the continuing years of analysis, quite a few land-mines continued to be stepped upon, explosively and destructively.

Because of my daydream, I realised that my analytic mind plods slowly and with carefully chosen footing, but at times also forcefully, like an elephant negotiating an unstable and thin-skinned volcanic landscape. Agitated, outraged, explosive or implosive patients can sometimes imbibe my plodding but careful elephantine mind, my slow Spinozan bodymind, as it is informed by and attends to their unstable world. This is my imaginal elephant's countertransferential dreaming, let alone the reverie of my proto-mammalian, psychoid bodymind (or perhaps even of our mixed and mutual unconscious-unconscious psychoid bodymind). Thence, through a sudden and very unconsciously produced 'intuitive knowledge', which yet arises out of long, slow and careful thinking, linking and reasoning, I eventually comprehend Kim's living nightmare world and so be part of the process of recycling it, in so far as possible.

If this sounds a little over-metaphorical and a bit vague, it is actually poetically precise, focused vagueness with carefully and critically chosen analogies. And it makes the incomprehensible more comprehensible and less of an alien force. In the case of Kim, we didn't get the family genitals into their right places. That was and is impossible, but we could better see where they were, what damage they had done and how to 'go on being' as best one can with the spider's webs of psychotic entanglements still attached.

References

Bion, W. (1962). *Learning from Experience*. Northvale, NJ: Jason Aronson.
Fordham, M. (1991). 'The Supposed Limits of Interpretation'. In *Analyst-Patient Interaction: Collected Papers on Technique*. London: Routledge, 2003.
Lear, J. (2003). *Therapeutic Action: An Earnest Plea for Irony*. London: Karnac Books.
Rhode, E. (1994). *Psychotic Metaphysics*. London: Karnac Books.
Santayana, G. (1926). 'Normal Madness'. In *Dialogues in Limbo*. New York: Scribner.

Chapter 15

Herder's force

Pluralism, expressivism, mind-body relations and empathy

Montreal, 2010, 2012[1]

The works and teachings of Johann Gottfried Herder (1744–1803) have helped shape virtually every discipline within the humanities and the social sciences. Herder's work was of radically constructive significance in many ways, as well as more ambivalent in others. Among the constructive elements were his relativistic challenge to Kant's conceptual and moral hierarchies; his original studies of the philosophy of mind and the emotions; his original studies of anthropology and of world history, which made him the originator of historicism as a distinct discipline; his philosophy of language; his stressing of the importance of critical textual studies, making him a precursor of philology; and his position as the first proponent of critical hermeneutics. He was a major influence on the *Sturm und Drang* movement and on German Romanticism.

Herder also developed a novel notion of the tense relations between plurality and commonality, of multiplicity in a common humanity and so of the revelatory possibilities of a hard heteropathic empathy across and into difference. His strong argument for a radical pluralism and promotion of political and cultural cosmopolitanism coupled with his idea of 'critical heteropathic empathy' or *Einfühlung*, helped shape a central component of the modern world-view.

More pertinently for this chapter, his assertion of the value of individual 'inwardness', of 'limitless internal depths', imagination, dreams and their revelatory meanings, made him a seminal figure in the emergence of the idea of the unconscious (30 years before Schelling's *Naturphilosophie* and Schopenhauer's 'Will'). He was also a key figure in bringing about a revival of interest in the work of Spinoza, introducing Goethe,[2] among others, to Spinoza's 'personally indifferent pantheism'. He helped to initiate the rethinking of Spinoza's work within and beyond German-speaking lands in relation to the new social and cultural context of

1 This chapter was originally given in 2010 to the XVIII Congress of the International Association for Analytical Psychology. Published in P. Bennett, ed. (2012). *Montreal 2010. Facing Multiplicity: Psyche, Nature, Culture: Proceedings of the XVIIIth Congress of the International Association for Analytical Psychology*. Einsiedeln: Daimon Verlag. Minor editing has been applied to this version (Eds.).

2 Goethe is said to have partly based the character of his Faust on the extraordinary epistemophilic appetite of Herder.

DOI: 10.4324/9781003255826-16

the late 18th and early 19th century (this included his mutative addition of aesthetics into the rational and 'geometric' metaphysics of Spinoza).

Like Spinoza, Herder saw humans 'objectively' as being 'a mere part of nature', as having a 'mediocre' (*mittelmässig*) place in the scheme of things. This position of hard naturalism sits in creative tension alongside his strong evaluation of personal subjective feelings and their expression. Anticipating 'Romantic irony', he saw a tension between our understanding that although we are a part of nature (we are thus also united with each other), we also think and act as though separate from nature (and from each other). He furthered the Spinozan idea that we have very limited free will, even that it is a necessary fantasy. Similarly, our sense of personal and/or social teleology needs to be subsumed under a recognition of the fateful realities of infinitely greater natural processes. Unlike Hegel after him, he did not proclaim a belief in 'the progress of history towards an ideal perfection' but rather saw history as being a ceaseless and fluid 'changing' of different civilisations, cultures and values (Herder, 1997).

There is much more that one could note about Herder, including his revolutionary ideas on the comparative significance of popular culture, folk music and songs and fairy tales (which he thought were culturally differentiated expressions and re-formations of the deeply unconscious world and contents of dreams); his theories of sculpture and painting; his revaluation of Gothic architecture (part of his pluralistic challenge to the accepted ideals of French classicism and its cultural hegemony); and finally, his more disturbing ideas of *das Volk* and of the virtues of irrational (or anti-rational) inwardness and 'expressivism'. For Herder, these were healthy cultural and psychological concepts, but as it turned out, they helped engender dangerous nationalistic political forces and a sometimes narcissistically inward-looking (intra-psychic) and socially blind psychology.

In the following exposition, I will only take up seven interrelated concepts from Herder's work. These are:

1 How Spinoza's monistic dual-aspect 'substance' became an organic 'Force of all Forces' (*die Urkraft aller Kräfte*);
2 How Spinoza's *conatus* (the endeavour for self-preservation, self-enhancement and self-expression) became *conatus*-as-culture and so an idea of cultural expressivism and of cultural pluralism;
3 How this is an expressivism of conscious and unconscious inner depths and forceful impulses, of dreams, imagination and creativity and so of the primacy of the subject self;
4 How Spinoza's dual-aspect theory of mind-body relations became 'irritation' (*Reiz* or *Reizbarkeit*) . . . and so a concept that was perhaps proto-psychoid;
5 Which, in turn, implies a biological determinism and so an ethic of 'free necessity';
6 Herder's advocation of a hard heteropathic 'empathy' (*Einfühlung*) into different others;
7 My own Herder-inspired neo-Spinozan idea of *conatus*-as-*jouissance* as a dynamic model, which I use analytically as an interpretive grid.

I read Herder (and other neo-Spinozan philosophers) as objectively and as empathically as possible (for Herder, the two are the same), but I also grind and polish an ideational lens through which I critically view psychodynamic theory, colour my clinical reverie and structure my interpretations.

Herder's neo-Spinozism substance as force

It was Herder's engagement with the so-called 'Pantheism Controversy' that made him the first intellectually important neo-Spinozan. This controversy arose out of Jacobi's and Mendelssohn's argument over Lessing's atheistic, deterministic and rationalistic Spinozism. Frederick Beiser's *The Fate of Reason* (1987) is the best analysis of this topic, and his work permeates much of the following discussion of Herder's significance.

The two most relevant Spinozan perceptions are, firstly, that extended matter and thinking mind are substantially identified, or, specifically, that body-and-brain and emotional-thinking mind are differently perceived aspects of a single 'substance'. Secondly, the *conatus* is an intrinsic energetic striving for self-preservation and for self-expression. Herder vitalised this 'one substance' as an organic *Urkraft aller Kräfte*,[3] and saw the *conatus* as also being operative in cultures, in their diverse expressions and in the tense relations between them.

Herder, in *God, Some Conversations* (1940), re-interprets and inflects Spinoza's philosophy whilst still sustaining its monism and naturalism. As Beiser describes:

> Rather than seeing Spinoza's God as a substance with two heterogeneous attributes (thought and extension), we should regard it as a power with an infinity of manifestations. Spinoza's dead substance then becomes an active, living force, and his God becomes the monad of monads, the *Urkraft aller Kräfte*. This notion of power not only replaces extension as the essence of matter, but it also mediates between mind and body, so that they are no longer distinct attributes, but different degrees of one and the same primal force. This . . . pantheistic vitalism or vitalistic pantheism . . . [injects] life into Spinoza's static universe.
> (Beiser, 1987, p. 163)

In *Sources of the Self* (1989), Charles Taylor says that Herder's idea that this inner organic force strives to express itself externally through cultures and through different persons implies that:

> Nature is now within . . . This is closely tied to the idea of a self, a subject. It is no longer some impersonal 'Form' or 'nature' which comes to actuality, but a being capable of self-articulation . . .
>
> Expressivism was the basis for a new and fuller individuation. This is the idea which grows in the late eighteenth century that each individual is different

3 Literally, the original power or motive force, the power underlying all powers (Eds.)

> and original, and that this originality determines how he or she ought to live . . . [our differences from each other] entail that each one of us has an original path which we ought to tread; they lay the obligation on each of us to live up to our originality. Herder formulated this idea in a telling image: 'Each human being has his own measure, as it were an accord peculiar to him of all his feelings to each other'. . . . Here we have the notion that the good life for you is not the same as the good life for me; each of us has our own calling, and we shouldn't exchange them. Following you may be betraying my own calling, even though you are being faithful to yours . . . We are all called to live up to our originality.
>
> (Taylor, 1989, pp. 375–376)

Herder's pluralism

Herder argued for a non-hierarchical historical, anthropological and cultural pluralism, incorporating a drive to expression whilst understanding inherent tensions and conflicts. Importantly, this tense issue of cultural pluralism and commonality applies also to persons or selves. Herder,

> in tension though not contradiction with his principle of sociality, holds that (even within a single period and culture) human minds are as a rule deeply individual and different from each other – so that in addition to a generalizing psychology we also need a psychology oriented to individuality.
>
> (Forster, 2010, p. 30)

We can see this as relevant to Jung's concept of individuation and also how each patient requires of the analyst a different theory.

Herder's radical combination of immanence, inwardness and expressionism was of seminal significance to the emergence of Romanticism and secular modernity and also to the idea that subjective feelings, imaginings and dreams are personally and culturally valuable and vital (by vital, I mean both necessary for health and energetically loaded). However, the shadow of this subjectivity and inwardness is that it harbours an idealised, elitist and privileged narcissism, let alone a blindness to social injustices and political realities.

Spinoza's concept of the *conatus*

Before going on to describe Herder's notion of the cultural *conatus,* I remind the reader of how the *conatus* was conceived by Spinoza.[4] The *conatus* is the individuating impulse or endeavour for self-preservation of life and of an idea of my (good) self and my products, and is, therefore, basically a healthy defence (though such defence can be offensive). It is also the individuating endeavour or impulse to increase my powers for self-preservation and the individuating urge to express myself, whether creatively or defensively or destructively. However, this *conatus*

4 See Chapter Seven (Eds.).

for self-preservation can manifest as an impetus to destroy others (each with their own *conatus*) and may itself be a victim of the destructive *conatus* of others. It can be paradoxical or counter-intuitive, for example, in acting upon the idea of preserving or restoring the good self by destroying the bad self through suicide. It can become pathologically paranoid or perverse because its defensiveness is affected by unconscious (and conscious) emotional tensions and manoeuvres. This is the stuff of the forces, tensions and conflicts of the *conatus*-as-*jouissance,* as seen in my *Jouissance* Grid (see Figure 15.1).

Herder on culture and the *conatus*

Herder applied the concept of the *conatus* to culture, arguing that all these personal forces and qualities also apply to the *conatus* of different cultures, for example, self-preservation as defence or offence, the use or the abuse of power, the assertion of idiosyncratic values and virtues, distinctive artistic expression, various religious beliefs and ethics, the politics of commonality, difference and negotiation, as well as aggression, war and paranoid terror. As with the internal and interpersonally-related individual (with a range of difficult relations of tense or conflicted affective forces), similarly, a cultural or political entity struggles over its moral and power dilemmas, such as cultural or religious tolerance.

In *Spinoza and the Specters of Modernity: The Hidden Enlightenment of Diversity from Spinoza to Freud* (2010), Michael Mack says that

> we may justifiably describe Herder as the inventor of the concept 'culture' . . . Herder's notion of culture is a creative development of Spinoza's conatus. Spinoza's conatus describes the ways in which the particular participates in the universal: by preserving oneself one contributes to the preservation of the entire universe of which we are all an infinitesimal part.
>
> (Mack, 2010, p. 8)

This concept also implies 'the twin issues of self-preservation and self-destruction' (Mack, 2010, p. 30). For Herder, 'In true Spinozist fashion each entity has the right and duty to preserve itself in its distinctiveness', but Herder then crucially adds that 'the self is only sustainable in its distinctiveness if it cooperates with what is different from itself' (Mack, 2010, p. 53). Mack also writes that

> according to Herder, humanity can only survive if it reflects upon and thus learns from the past. In Spinozist terms one could describe his notion of reflection as the conatus that is specific to humanity. Indeed Herder mentions self-preservation [and therefore reflection and the related impetus for expression] as the raison d'être of existence . . . By interpreting mental work as part of humanity's material or existential condition, Herder enmeshes the mind into the sphere of nature and the environment at large.
>
> (Mack, 2010, p. 63)

According to Herder, each culture is distinctive according to its time in history and its place in the world, and each culture forcefully strives to both express and differentiate itself linguistically, through religion and beliefs, in ethics, values and rites and artistically.

Herder also added aesthetics into Spinoza's geometrically rational metaphysics. He accomplished this by extending the concept of the *conatus* as also being the force behind the diversity of cultures through history and through their different languages, customs, expressive folk arts, etc., and thence to demonstrating the value of empathic studies thereof. For Herder, all cultures differ due to their historical time and place and forcefully strive to both express and differentiate themselves linguistically, through religion and beliefs, in ethics, values and rites and artistically. Groups and their forceful expressions are both differentiating (or individuating) and universal.

Mind, irritation and the psychoid

Beiser further develops his theme of how Herder's neo-Spinozan concept of *Kraft* unites our notions of mind and body in that they are not different in kind but only in degree:

> Herder's theory postulates a single principle, a single concept to unite our notions of mind and body; the concept of power (*Kraft*). The essence of power is defined as self-generating, self-organising activity . . . The difference between mind and body is not a difference in kind, then, but only one in degree: the body is amorphous power, the mind organised power. It also follows from this theory that we can treat both mind and body in either mental or physical terms: the mind is a higher degree of organisation of the body, or the body is a lower degree of organisation of the mind, depending on our perspective.
>
> (Beiser, 1987, pp. 146–147)

For Herder, this 'avoids the pitfalls of dualism and reductivism. The theory is clearly not dualistic since it defines the mind by its purpose, the control and organisation of the various functions of the body'. Nor is it 'reductivistic' since 'mind is the unity of the various functions of the body, and such a unity is seen as a whole that is not reducible to the mere sum of its parts'. The body 'is a living organism'. Mind and body 'are not heterogeneous substances and are instead only different aspects of a single living force' (Beiser, 1987, p. 147). Herder declares: 'In my humble opinion, no psychology is possible that is not physiology at every step' (Herder, in Beiser, 1987, p. 148).

Herder also drew on the phenomenon of 'irritability' (*Reizbarkeit*), which he took from Albrecht von Haller, as inferring 'that there is one and the same living force in the mental and the physical'. Herder saw this irritability 'as the missing link between the material and the mental' (Beiser, 1987, p. 148). Michael Forster (2010) also describes how Herder tries to explain the mind in terms of the phenomenon of 'irritation' (*Reiz*): 'a phenomenon which, while basically physiological, also seems to exhibit a transition to mental characteristics' (Forster, 2010, p. 28). Irritation and irritability were idiosyncratically interpreted by Herder as related to vital force, the energetic quantity and quality which is the life of 'bodymind', the sensation and sensibility common to both body and emotion, a generative (sexual) friction and a creative frustration and even a painful deprivation or threatening attack which can destroy the matter of life.

I suggest that Herder's hypothesis of *Reiz/Reizbarkeit* as the primal psycho-physical force may be understood as an early precursor of the concept of the 'psychoid'.

The psychoid

Throughout my writings, I use the term 'psychosomatic' to refer to the psyche-soma unit as a representation of (Spinozan) dual-aspect theory, mind and body being seen as differently identified aspects of a single 'substance', and where 'the mind is the idea of the body'. This I have related to Jung's passages about 'the paradox of the sympathetic and parasympathetic psychoid processes' (Jung, 1970a, *CW* 14, para. 279) where 'psyche and matter are two different aspects of the same thing' (Jung, 1970b, *CW* 8, para. 418). The Jungian concept of the 'psychoid' is about a substrate level where the psychic and the organic (mind and body) meet, at which they are consubstantial. Psyche being intrinsically psychoid, so, too, are our affective relations.

The psychoid is simultaneously the source and expression of sensuous body matters and of emotional, mental images and ideas of such matters. This primitive unity is most evident in regressed, pre-symbolic (and pre-verbal) states, in borderline disorders and relations, in the 'psychotic transference', which is a field of projective identifications and urgent communication. The psychoid is also a latent, emergent and dynamic psychophysical force inherently determined to make manifest, realise and develop in both an individually idiosyncratic and species-typical way. Therefore, the psychoid is not only primitive or regressive, but also a potentiality and a potency. I would add that the psychoid may be experienced transferentially as an interpersonal, communicative, consubstantiating or infectious force.

The 'dual aspect' of the psychoid 'bodymind' unit makes for consubstantial (contagious or relational) psychosomatic experience and for its possible transformation. It forms out of, between and, therefore, to both of us in analysis, whence it can move or be moved from the autonomic level and from somatic sensation or somatisation to symbolic reverie and to thought. And so thence be given (back) through interpretation to the patient – but of course only in so far as he or she is receptive.

This constructive primitive psychosomatic 'in-formation' is always operative at an autonomic level, an affective form of defence and communication of the self as an auto-immune system, indeed of the 'psychoid self' as a social, interpersonal and relational auto-immune system. We might say that through the 'irritations' of our psychoid substrate, we take the psychosomatic into both the creative-expressive and into the passions of the interpersonal, including into our limitations, frustrations and separateness, and so to the issue of how we learn to live as well as possible with these realities and contingencies. This is surely a core task of analysis.

Perhaps Spinoza's and Herder's form of (forceful) pan-psychism where matter and mind are substantially identified as two differently identifiable aspects of the single substance, can be understood as a source of my idea of the psychoid substrate of the '*conatus*-as-*jouissance*'.

Determinism and 'free necessity'

Such neurobiological 'natural materialism' implies a considerable degree of 'necessitarianism', a recognition that even our apparent freedom of will and choice is basically pre-determined, let alone that our ideas of personal, social and historical teleology must be seriously qualified by a recognition of the reality of infinitely greater natural processes that can have no intention or goal.

It is both Spinozan and Herderian to see or make a virtue of free necessity (see Lloyd, 2008, p. 234). This a paradoxical sense of psychic freedom deriving from an acceptance that we are essentially determined by our neurobiology, by the unconscious neural priming of 'freely' chosen voluntary actions, by genetic inheritance, gender, the biology of our bodily conditions, our basic forms of attachment, our largely unconscious and tense forces of desire and self-preservation, by internalised unconscious object relations, family values and tyrannies, social and political powers and by all other internal and external contingencies.

Yet, we have to consciously and unconsciously manage these contingencies. Our apparent freedom of agency is, to a great degree, a 'normal illusion', necessary for our psychic health. This *Anschauungsweise* or attitude is the radical virtue ethic of 'free necessity'.

Herder's *Einfühlung* or empathy

Forster says that as a crucial and practical culmination of his cultural and psychological pluralism, Herder proposes 'that the way to bridge radical difference when interpreting is through *Einfühlung*, "feeling one's way in"' (Forster, 2010, p. 19). Thus, Herder initiated critical empathic studies of different cultures, their values and beliefs and a comparative ethnography of popular artistic expression. For Herder, the application of such cross-cultural or interpersonal empathy is heteropathic, empathy across difference, not on the basis of similarities, a product of not only feeling but also informed imagination and, above all, hard intellectual work and reasoning across difference.

Forster summarises Herder's idea of empathy through six components, which are remarkable both as ideas that were seminal to comparative cultural studies and anthropology and also when considered in the light of our ideal analytic positions and practices. Firstly, the interpreter faces radical difference between his own mentality and that of the interpreted subject, making interpretation a difficult task. Secondly, such 'critical empathy' should 'include thorough research, not only into a text's use of language, but also into its historical, geographical and social context' (Forster, 2010, p. 19). Thirdly, 'in order to understand an interpreted subject's language the interpreter must achieve an imaginative reproduction of his (perceptual and affective) sensations'. Fourthly, 'hostility in an interpreter towards the people he interprets will generally distort his interpretation and must therefore be avoided'. Fifthly, 'the interpreter should strive to develop his grasp of linguistic usage, contextual facts and relevant sensations to the point where it achieves something like the same automatic immediacy that it had for a text's original author and audience' (Forster, 2010, p. 19). Lastly, the interpreter's own 'difference' must be reflectively used as an aspect of such 'critical empathy'.

Moving Herder's neo-Spinozism into the clinical: '*conatus-as-jouissance*'

To conclude, I refer the reader back to earlier writings about my own somewhat Herderian, neo-Spinozan concept, the '*conatus*-as-*jouissance*'. My *Jouissance* Grid,[5] as a diagram, represents the natural dynamic of psychoid and psychosomatic affects and their personal and interpersonal relations. These are tense relations of unconsciously and consciously attractive and repulsive emotive forces, between desire/love and fear/hate, pleasure and pain, joyous elation and sad depression, power and its limits (or impotence) . . . all incorporated in the *conatus* of the bodymind's *jouissance.*

Conatus-jouissance grid

I have written about how I use this grid to think through informative transferential and embodied countertransferential communications and through the psychosomatic confusions, emotional storms, uncertainties and blind-spots in the clinical encounter with a 'radical other'. Thence, from my reverie and critical empathic thinking, there may appear a comprehensive 'selected fact' or, in Spinozan terms, 'intuitive knowledge'. The '*jouissance* grid' forms a conceptual structure to interpret analytic relations with destructive borderline and defensive narcissistic disorders in a field of projective identifications, extractive processes and sticky narcissistic adhesiveness. However, it can also be used in a critical analysis of the phenomenology of various forms of depression and to understand the dynamics of severe disorders of the self, for example, where repetitive compulsive acts and/or extreme dissociative (or psychogenic autistic-like) states are operating as defences against massive depressive anxiety. I suggest that in these cases, it is through our empathic (imaginative, emotional and thoughtful) analytic understanding and its communication that we might find or engender life in apparently lifeless states: a relational vitality and its symbolisation may thus emerge from the pre-order of our common psychoid ground.

5 See Chapter Seven for the first use of the *Jouissance* grid, p. 107. An Appendix to Chapter Seven, pp. 107–108, gives Giles' explanatory notes to the grid. We have omitted the explanatory notes here to avoid repetition (Eds.).

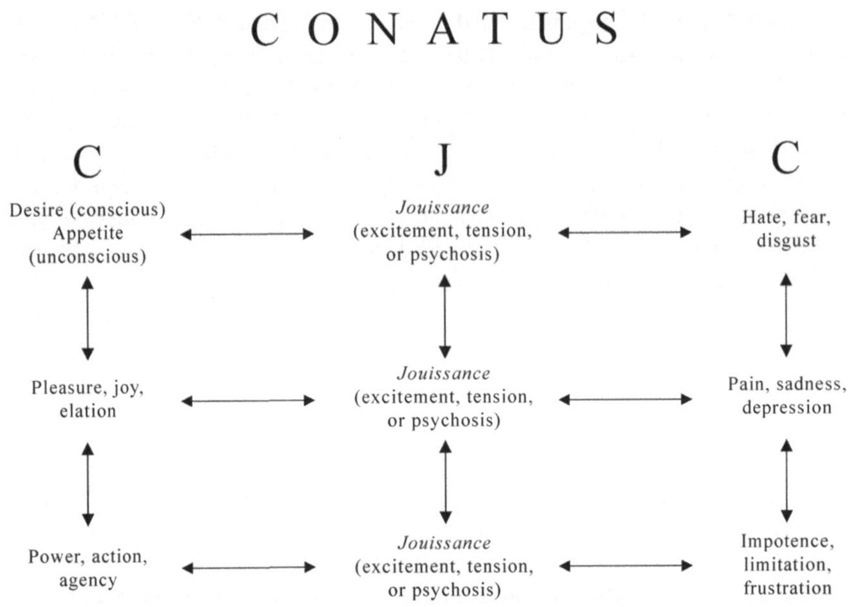

Figure 15.1 *Jouissance* Grid (2010 version)

References

Beiser, F. (1987). *The Fate of Reason: German Philosophy from Kant to Fichte*. Cambridge, MA and London: Harvard University Press.

Forster, M. (2010). *After Herder: Philosophy of Language in the German Tradition*. Oxford: Oxford University Press.

Herder, J. (1940). *God, Some Conversations*. Translated and introduction by F. Burkhardt. New York: Hafner (Original German, 1787).

Herder, J. (1997). *On World History*. Edited by H. Adler & E. Menze. London: M. E. Sharpe.

Jung, C. (1970a). *Mysterium Coniunctionis: An Inquiry Into the Separation and Synthesis of Psychic Opposites in Alchemy*. Vol. 14 of *the Collected Works of C.G. Jung*. Translated by R. Hull. 2nd edn. London: Routledge & Kegan Paul.

Jung, C. (1970b). 'On the Nature of the Psyche'. In *The Structure and Dynamics of the Psyche*. Vol. 8 of *The Collected Works of C.G. Jung*. R. Hull, trans. 2nd edn. London: Routledge & Kegan Paul.

Lloyd, G. (2008). *Providence Lost*. Cambridge, MA: Harvard University Press.

Mack, M. (2010). *Spinoza and the Specters of Modernity, The Hidden Enlightenment of Diversity from Spinoza to Freud*. New York and London: Continuum.

Taylor, C. (1989). *Sources of the Self*. Cambridge: Cambridge University Press.

Chapter 16

Psychoid relations in the transferential/countertransferential field of personality disorders

IAAP, Copenhagen, 2013, 2015[1]

Jung's concept of psychoid processes is both prescient and increasingly of practical clinical significance. It is pertinent to our understanding of the embodied countertransference, relational inter-subjectivity, analytic field theory and the psychotherapeutic implications of recent neurobiological research. The work of Addison (2008, 2009) has particularly established this re-evaluation, and I have written elsewhere about my own theoretical and analytic use of psychoid processes (Clark, 2010).[2]

My hypothesis is that all intra-psychic and interpersonal psychic relations are psychoid relations. Therefore, psychoid processes are always part of the clinical situation, especially in regard to countertransference. At the psychoid level, body and mind are a basic psyche-soma unit, an identity experienced and expressed through dual aspects, different modes of 'bodymind', which is also a single psychoid substance. As quoted before, Jung writes that 'deepest down of all is the paradox of the sympathetic and parasympathetic psychoid processes' (Jung, 1970a, *CW* 14, para. 279) and that 'psyche and matter' are 'two different aspects of the same thing' (Jung, 1970b, *CW* 8, para. 418). I understand 'the psychoid realm' and 'psychoid processes' as being simultaneously both an object for scientific investigation and phenomenologically as a symbolic 'as if', a unit of meaning: as both organic function and as intuited idea or symbol of instantiated phenomena.

Santayana and Spinoza

A philosophical hypothesis that supports my clinical theme is Santayana's concept of 'the organic psyche', or that 'the psyche is an organism' (cf. Santayana,

1 This was originally presented to the IAAP congress in Copenhagen in 2013 and published in 1915 in E. Kiehl (Ed.), Copenhagen 2013: *100 Years On: Origins, Innovations and Controversies*. Proceedings of the 19th Congress of the International Association for Analytical Psychology. Damon Verlag, Einsiedeln, 2015, pp. 850–859. We have incorporated material from a longer version of the paper that Giles continued to work on, his last edits being made on December 4, 2017. We have also removed several verbatim repetitions from earlier chapters (Eds.).

2 See Chapter Twelve.

DOI: 10.4324/9781003255826-17

1930). For Santayana, 'the psyche' is the life of the human body with all its functions and actions, including consciousness; it is our inherent physical or organic biology (including neurobiology) and its inherent functionalities and processes of self-regulation and self-preservation (until death or other natural contingencies supervene). So, we could see 'psyche' as involving the emergence, development and ongoing flux of psychoid processes.

According to Michael Brodrick (2013), Santayana's concept of the psyche could be described as 'amphibious', by which Brodrick meant that it had elements of both body and psyche. He quotes Santayana who, in *The Realm of Spirit* (1940), says that from the outside, psyche is 'the self-maintaining and reproducing pattern or structure of an organism, conceived as a power' (Santayana, 1940, p. 15, in Brodrick, 2013, p. 247). However, the 'inner nature of psyche . . . is that of a "moral unity" that consists of impulses, feelings, perceptions, memories, and in some cases concepts' (Brodrick, 2013, p. 247). In other words, Santayana's 'amphibious' concept of the psyche is an understanding of the body and its processes as primary but inherently incorporating other emergent epiphenomena such as consciousness, subjectivity, ideation, feeling and attachment. The 'theory of mind-body relations relying on the concept of psyche as amphibious avoids the traditional mind-body problem, rendering epiphenomenalism and other classic theories of mind-body relations obsolete' (Brodrick, 2013, p. 248). And as John Lachs describes it, psyche is the 'essence of natural biological life', including physical structure and drives (Lachs, 2006, p. 47). This is a representation of Santayana's critical Spinozism as a theory of mind-body relation based on the concept of psyche as 'amphibious', of matter and mind as different aspects of a unit, that is, a dual aspect theory.

Santayana rendered Spinoza's proposition that 'the mind is the idea of the body' (*Ethics*, 2, P14 – P30, in Curley, 1994, pp. 162–170) into the more elaborate statement that 'the body is an instrument, the mind its function, the witness and reward of its operation' (Santayana, 1910, p. 206). Santayana's concept of the self-maintaining organic psyche is also partly derived from Spinoza's idea of the *conatus*.

Santayana's philosophy is an expression of the dramatic (and creative) tension (and oscillation) between matter and spirit, reason and imagination, dialectics and the poetic, strategy and animal impulse/reaction: between the ideal and normal madness. For Santayana, consciousness or 'spirit' is epiphenomenal (i.e. dependent on material body and brain processes), an aspect of psyche and materially ineffectual. It may sometimes be a pure intuition of non-existent Essences (which are also ineffectual and so preclude a literal essentialism). Thus, Santayana's ontological system found expression in his contemplative (sometimes non-relational) spirituality, a spirituality without any theistic belief or dogma. Santayana understood matter as primary, 'psyche' as basically physical and 'spirit' or consciousness as a natural, sometimes beautiful, sometimes mad, but always impotent epiphenomenon of (physical) 'psychic' (neural and bodily) functioning.

Santayana's 'normal madness' (Santayana, 1926) also includes our taking as actual (and acting upon) our normal, 'mad' (imaginary) illusions, such as the projections and literalisation of the pathetic fallacy, and, for a Spinozan, also illusions such as teleology and free will, which are subjective psychological 'realities', necessary for normal psychic health, but which are not objectively real or actual.

A word of qualification. Santayana can never be, for me, an idealised self-object. His anti-Semitism, fascist sympathies, snobbish aristocratic values and the cold (and sometimes cruel) ruthlessness of his relational detachment (his lack of erotic love) preclude any such idealisation. Yet at the same time, his 'detachment' is also a contemplative solitariness that is both personally (psychically and spiritually) valid and philosophically valuable (when put to good use).

Analytically, especially when working with difficult personality disorders, I filter my reactions, reverie and thinking through both a Spinozan lens (Clark, 1996, 2006)[3] and from a perspective of Santayana's materialist, epiphenomenal ontology. My term 'psychoid *conatus*' is a composite of Spinoza's *conatus* and Santayana's 'organic psyche'. Its interaction with others and with the world is both biologically determined (matter) and a meaning-endowed intuited relation (essence).

Before going any further, I need to emphasise that neither Spinoza's monistic dual aspect philosophy nor Santayana's naturalistic ontology explains clinical experience, but together they help clarify my thinking about problematic clinical relations, particularly thinking through what is happening between us psychosomatically.

Adapting and utilising the argument of Santayana's essay 'The Suppressed Madness of Sane Men' (Smith, 1921, pp. 8–9),[4] I would say that our personal and interpersonal 'psychoid consubstantiality' incorporates both our self-preservation and our self-destructiveness, our reason and our passion, our animal faith (practical common sense) and our delusions, our self-consciousness and its superego saturated conflicts, our anxieties and our mad panics.

This is the 'normal madness' (Santayana, 1926) of an ego-consciousness that distorts and confuses symbolic understanding, which cannot reflect and reason sufficiently, which believes that our subjectivity, our memories and dreams, perceptions and projections make for knowledge of objective reality and so acts (and acts out) accordingly.

Thus, our relations to the psychoid *conatus* become disordered. It is a field of projective identification and primitive psychosomatic communication and information, a relational realm of fierce or fearful styles of attachment, of closeness-distance tension, of the intimate passions of desire, possession, frustration and loss, of psychosomatic infection and contagion. Addison observes that such psychoid matters arise particularly in periods of regression to early states involving the emergence of psyche from soma (Addison, 2008, p. 10).[5]

The psychoid and psychotic transference/countertransference is the most effective vehicle for both the evacuation and communication of primitive

3 See Chapters Five and Seven (Eds.)

4 Marion Milner makes critical use of this essay by Santayana in her book *On Not Being Able to Paint* (Chapter Five, 'The necessity of illusion'), as a stimulus for her personal psychoanalytic reflections (Milner, 1957).

5 Further discussion of Addison's hypothesis can be found in Chapter Twelve (Eds.).

preverbal, unsymbolised, somatised beta matters, in so far as my 'bodymind' is open to the emotional bodymind of the patient. For the analyst to remain psychosomatically unaffected or unmoved in such primitive relations is surely a dissociative defence against acute (depressive) anxiety. An analyst needs to have the necessary openness to his/her own wounds, to recycle their own madness and to have the reflective ability to think through, link up and so interpret the patient's damaged relational and developmental necessities, i.e. the lacks that drive these infectious projections, evacuations, forceful communications and pulls of identification.

Damasio and neurobiology

From the perspective of neurobiology, the *conatus* could be seen as 'the aggregate of dispositions laid down in brain circuitry that, once engaged by internal or environmental conditions, seeks both survival and well-being' (Damasio, 2003, p. 36).[6] So, too, the 'psychoid realm' relates neurobiologically to what Damasio (2003) has termed 'the body-sensing and body-mapping brain regions (which) are the neural location of body-self and other-self ideation' and that '[t]he contents of feelings are the configurations of body state represented in somatosensing maps' (Damasio, 2003, p. 36). As Stuart Hampshire succinctly puts this, 'the brain maps the body, and the mind maps the brain' (2005, p. li).

These regions are the cingulate cortex, the somatosensory cortices, namely the insular and SII, the hypothalamus, the right amygdala and several nuclei in the brain stem tegmentum (Damasio, 2003, pp. 105–106). These brain functions are needed for empathising with the emotional and physical states in others. This has to do with the very early primitive perceptual representational system and the implicit, pre-episodic memory. It also has to do with the autonomic nervous system, which Roderick Peters (1987, p. 4) calls the serpent mind. So, I would add that interpersonal psychosomatic affectivity is also mapped.

It is these regions of the brain, these primitive proto-mammalian and reptilian areas, that are active in the psychoid transferential field that I am describing.

Christine

Let us revisit the case of Christine,[7] who first came to see me because she was 'deeply hurt' that no one appreciated either her artistic talents or her abundance of 'kindness and goodness'. Like many narcissists, rather than develop greater insight and self-awareness, unconsciously she sought to have her defences justified and enhanced. Her internal world had been developmentally atrophied and

6 A fuller neurobiological explanation of the *conatus* according to Damasio can be found in Chapter Eighteen (Eds.).

7 See Chapters Nine and Thirteen (Eds.).

distorted by a demanding mother and a weak but doting father. She was ashamed of her desires, terrified by real sexual relations and so had none. She was bulimic; any appetites and goods were always going bad. Her defence against her insecurity was an indignant self-righteousness and a judgmental grandiosity. She was thin-skinned and prickly, timorous, arrogant and seething with suppressed anger. She was not easily likeable.

My difficulty in liking her was, on one hand, a complementary countertransference, an introjection of her mother's inability to love her. Yet she unwittingly made herself quite disagreeable: as a child towards her mother and now towards me. She said her eating problems were her mother's fault. I said that she used her internalised mother as a buffer against her sense of emptiness and her angry hurt and that this mother was 'good food gone bad'. I was more able to tolerate Christine's narcissism when realising that I was dealing with her internalised maternal narcissism. It later emerged that she also had a desperately shameful and suppressed fear of her incestuous feelings towards her father, who was caught in his own sentimentality but unable to really emotionally meet and safely mediate Christine's oedipal desires. But mostly, Christine complained about her parents without qualification. There was no imaginal empathy for their separateness, their alterity, that they, too, might be persons in their own right. Her inability to reflect, link, acknowledge self-doubt, empathise, symbolise, play (or even laugh) was all-permeating. There were many experiences of her hard but brittle grandiosity and disdain and of her suppressed but seething, seeping anger. Such narcissistic defences were driven by the need to avoid the pain of primal lacks, depressive emptiness and shame.

In her first period of analysis, which lasted around four years, Christine had come three times a week. She was well-defended and her malignant narcissistic self-love remained largely intact. Such brittle thin-skinned narcissism cannot be met head-on. Rather, the analytic task is to address primitive anxiety, interpersonal terrors and shames. I therefore addressed her strategic false-self system with 'big picture' or 'general human condition' interpretations to avoid provoking her narcissistic defences by focusing in on idiosyncratic personal traits.

Other people were 'never up to scratch'. For example, her fellow trainees in a counselling course were not in her league:

Christine: They dither so much and have nothing important to do. Not like me. What's worse is that they get away with being ever so second-rate. For some reason, everybody confirms their supposed success.

Me: And you are frustrated . . .

Christine: Intentionally over-looked, ignored, always put down.

Me: Do you think that they envy you?

Christine: 'Well yes . . . they've got a lot to envy, of course.

Me: And do you envy them?

Christine: No, I simply resent the unfairness of it all.

I found myself relying on theoretical knowledge and clinical thinking to overcome feelings of distaste and reach a degree of heteropathic empathy and an ability to interpret usefully, reminding myself she was basically an oedipal orphan and behind her seeming superiority lay feelings of inferiority, etc.

She brought me a series of her paintings. They were her 'great theme' – textured acrylics of icy surfaces, sometimes with a dry leaf or flower-head lying on the ice. She said that she was partly inspired by the Dutch artist Hendrick Avercamp but above all by her own realisation of the 'eternal beauty of natural ice'. I thought that they were aesthetically attractive and technically well-executed but also noticeably unpeopled. Privately, I thought that while Avercamp's ice scenes are about people, Christine's work was about the surface beauty of ice: impersonal, hard, cold matter, with touches of formally beautiful death but without any human life: a representation perhaps of her schizoid narcissism.

She was entering a competition, and I anticipated that she might well get hurt. The exhibition had its opening evening. She was on a proud high. Then, a catastrophe: she overheard a (very careless) judge say:

> Christine's pictures are basically twee little decorations.

This obviously hurt her but did not ostensibly enrage her. After spending three sessions expressing her hurt, she suddenly asked me:

Christine: You don't find them twee, do you?
Me: That's not the word I'd choose, no.

Why had I answered her question, and not interpreted it? For example, I might have suggested that perhaps she wanted me to be the good judge/father who loved her work/her.

Christine: What do you mean . . . what word would you choose?
Me: Beautiful cold surfaces . . . (and then added) . . . icy parts of nature.

Again, it was an answer rather than an interpretation and, furthermore, not a single word was asked for. I was obviously out of my analytic self-control. My wordy non-interpretive response was a product of countertransferential panic, of being caught out by her narcissistic vulnerability and unconsciously falling into an enactment of hurting her in her most wounded places.

Christine: You don't understand them. This means you don't understand me.

I decided to challenge her, I thought, in a sensitive way:

Me: I wonder how much you want me to really understand (know) you?
Christine: How could you say that?! I am so upset. I must go. Let me go. Please. Thank you.

I simply replied: 'See you next week'. She fled. She did return to her next session and sat sobbing, which she continued to do for three weeks. After several more weeks, I felt it timely to ask:

Me: I sometimes wonder, what lies under the surface?
Christine: What do you mean? The ice is the point. How could it matter what goes on underneath?
Me: I mean under your surfaces.
Christine: O God . . . you've done it again. This is about painting, not me.
Me: I think that it's also about an absence of people, disappointing or frightening people who need to be kept out, kept away, but which also feels very lonely.
Christine: I'm not sure.
Me: I am also talking about keeping me at a distance.
Christine: Oh God! I must go again . . .

And she left again in tears, but again she came back. What should I have said? How could my relentless interpretations become usefully irritating and so get under her skin, thus wearing thin her defensive skin? More generally, how can one challenge such narcissistic fragility based on such a fierce, righteous envy? How to get to the hurt and hate? She could not symbolically realise that the water under the skin was her own emotional insides under her brittle defences. Where were her real angry hate and her disgust of others and of herself? Very much later (in our second phase of analysis), she said in reference to these episodes that I was a heartless, insensitive and cruel so-called analyst, 'my careless cruelty had undermined her universe'. Whilst trying to maintain my capacity for clinical thinking and interpretation, I felt restricted, and increasingly I found myself feeling loathing for her false-self defences. My 'bad' countertransferential reaction (semi-consciously due to irritation and not liking her) was, to an extent, a complementary re-constellation of parental indifference. However, her offended, hurt and fleetingly angry spitting out of her inside feelings was the beginning of an expression of healthy aggression. The healthy aggression, though, was quickly repressed and fled from and crafty narcissistic defences were determinedly set up again. So when therapy ended because she was moving to another area, I thought perhaps we had reached the limits of therapeutic change.

Christine's return

Three years later, Christine attended a lecture that I gave. In the course of this lecture, I quoted a passage from Winnicott and said that it applied to the malignant narcissist's defensive strategy of emptying out of real (analytic) relations. She contacted me and said that she wanted to return for more therapy. Against my normal frame that once an analysis had finished, the limitations of that analysis had to be accepted and the ending of the analysis mourned, I agreed to see her again. Later, I was to interpret her coming to the lecture as a means of re-activating an unfinished analytic process. In retrospect, I realised that the real analysis only began when we could dare to confront the emotional realities of lost love and murderous rage, dare to be infected and affected and then finally be ready to separate and mourn more truly and honestly.

In her second period of analysis, a new crisis occurred. Her father had been found by her mother to have been having a six-month affair. Christine said, 'How could he do that to me?' This revealed both her oedipal anger and the force of narcissistic wounds. More significantly, it also emerged that she was deeply disappointed by and angry with me for having failed to get to the bottom of her illusions and delusions in the first round of analysis. The basic message conveyed was: Did I believe I had done any good for her? No, I had not! Did I ever really care about her? No, I couldn't have done!

Christine: Back then I did not realise that I was yearning hopelessly for what was never there and what will never be. Now, rather than sad, I am increasingly full of resentment.

I knew that this included resentment with our previous therapy, for what she had never gotten from me, that which never came into being in herself and between us. She expressed her disappointment, sometimes with a vengeance:

Christine: It's your fault. You just accepted me as I was. You failed me exactly like my father. Now I want to frighten you out of your self-satisfied smugness. I feel like spitting venom.

And she did. I had been moved from being an object with whom she adhesively identified to a proto-transitional object and now to an object of frustration, envy and murderous hate. However, unlike Jim's borderline 'acting out' and 'acting-into', Christine did not enact such murderous destructiveness. She was still held back by her narcissistic fears and defences. Rather, her projective identifications operated through a more subtle process of adhesive identification and extractive introjection. Sometimes, there were flashes of 'looks that could kill' followed by a very nervous checking and repairing. I often felt 'a bit murdered'.

Outside analysis, Christine started having catastrophic sexual relations, impersonal encounters only made possible by being very drunk. These events were dangerous, shameful and unsatisfying. She realised, though, that they were driven by desperate and intolerable loneliness. Her addictions (bulimia, alcohol) and other somatic matters became increasingly severe. She was psychosomatically hungry, desperate, angry and frightened.

Christine's addictions also incorporated self-harm: she started to cut herself, which I saw as representing a cutting through to the quick of her own deadened self. Her self-harming and offensive-defensive attacks on me were vicious and visceral. They were effective psychoid projectiles into the psychoid 'bodymind' of her too-separate analyst, into her 'selfish mother' and 'weak father'. We found ourselves in a proto-symbolising psychosomatic field, a primitive psychoid realm.

Previously, her self-righteous indignation, lack of reflection and thin-skinned woundedness irritated and bored me. Now, split-off outrage and desire for revenge erupted. I was put on 'self-protective alert' when she brought a dream about 'a giant, long-bodied spider that kept scuttling away and hiding in cracks in her room'. This, she said, was a 'venomous spider that liquefies its prey's insides'. Initially, she said that the spider 'is probably my mother'.

I said, 'Perhaps it's more to do with your own deep impulses'. She replied dismissively but slightly nervously, 'Oh, I just don't know about that'. This nervousness betrayed the emergence of an incipient moral symbolic sensibility.

More interpersonally, I felt that the spider was an affective image of the unsymbolised psychoid projectile she was now launching into me. In order to possess my body and mind, she had to get into my head and under my skin, even into my muscles and blood. I felt that I was fighting for my psychosomatic health. I became ill. My symptoms were worse during and sometimes shortly after Christine's sessions, which felt like somatic reactions to Christine's transferential attacks on the envied good analyst and on my psychosomatic forces for self-preservation, an undermining of my necessary defences, even a disabling of my auto-immune and autonomic nervous systems: in other words, a real threat to the psychoid *conatus* of my own self.

The goods of others (mother, father, me) were a red rag to her envious hate. I had to struggle against both internal flight (sleep) and an impulse to retaliate:

Christine: You are all right. You've got it all. You don't know what it's like to be intentionally overlooked and not recognised and appreciated.

Me: Repeatedly resented, even hated . . .

Christine: Yes. Most people get loved back. Can't people see the amount of love I've got to give?

Me: Perhaps they pick up on your resentment . . .

Christine: But they get me wrong. I am good. They just can't see my goodness. Their injustice is blind. And cruel.

Me: Sometimes you retaliate.

Christine: Of course!

Me: Cruelly, too. As in your attacks on me and the analysis.

Christine: God, sometimes I hate you.

On another occasion, a close family member of mine had died, and I said that I would have to miss the next three sessions for unforeseen reasons.

Christine: Has someone died?

I was surprised and shocked, and felt invaded by the acuity of her 'intuition'.

Christine: Well . . . so, has someone died?

Rattled, exposed, open to disclosure and perhaps even retaliatory. I answered: 'Yes.'

Christine: You should pay more attention to the living than the dead.
Me: You mean . . . to you?
Christine: Yes, of course!
Me: I am still here.

Again, I was left thinking about what I might have better said. I certainly should have said, by way of interpretation, 'This has touched your place of feeling second best' . . . or some such. However, I think that my increasingly frequent moments of 'psychosomatic infection' were a communication, through our shared contagious psychoid field, signalling and informing us of the first inklings of a symbolic life.

As well as feeling attacked and invaded by Christine's somatically sickening angry assaults, at other times, I began to enjoy a sense of her emotional reality, her passion and vivacity, her moments of playfulness. She might still be difficult to like, but she was now more 'real' and so paradoxically more interesting to be with, even likeable. We had finally established a degree of basic trust.

One day, Christine launched a vitriolic and envious attack on my presence and demeanour, on the 'ways of my body' and 'the ways of my mind'. I was somewhat stunned and initially lost my presence of mind. Then, after re-gathering my alpha functioning and with a sense of 'intuitive knowledge' I eventually said:

Me: You are afraid of going mad in your explosive but also fearful loneliness.

After a long pause, she responded:

Christine: But now I think that I may actually be sad and mad enough to survive. . . [Another long pause, then she added] . . . I know that if I don't kill myself, I can make my sadness and madness a sort of strength.

I thought, 'And if you don't kill me'. Then, to my surprise, she said quietly:

Christine: And if I stop wanting to kill you.
Me: Killing me . . . who will not become what you want, and who can never be enough.

I had said this many times before, but now it was affectively as if I was saying it for the first time. Her reaction was:

Christine: You are always just so 'over there' . . . so maddening. Fuck you!

This was communicated with anger but also with a slight sense of humour, a degree of ambivalence that indicated the possible emergence and integration of oedipal limits and relational reality.

Over the next nine months, Christine became more able to contain, harness and re-direct her aggression more constructively. She became more self-aware and aware of her relations with others. She was more self-critical and genuinely empathic. Because of a growing capacity for trust and a sense of irony, she was more able to be, and enjoy being, playful.

She had moved from a pre-ambivalent split state to a more depressive reality, from the melancholic defences of a false self, through angry grief and thence mourning to a more many-sided self-reflexive life. She had begun to recycle her madness. There was an acquiescence to the limits to change. These characteristics are a manifestation of the emergence of a relatively functional and true symbolising function, although what she called 'the poisonous snake coiled at my core' was still alive and would still sometimes strike with venom. Just as there had been a split-off angry borderline substrate underlying her narcissistic defences in the earlier stage of our analytic relations, so now there remained a narcissistic element to her angrily expressive self.

When we eventually ended the second period of analysis, we were able to separate through a process of real mourning: disappointment, sadness, gratitude . . . and relief.

Twelve observations about narcissistic and borderline relations

Firstly, a move from the false (self-deluding) fear-based, sometimes masochistic defences of the narcissist to the overtly destructive behaviour of the borderline personality is a relatively healthy development because at least the latter is more savagely real and relational – torn between love and hate, hurt expressed as hate, lonely need and outrage, splitting and ambivalence. It is a recycling of madness. Here, I am drawing on both Kernberg and Winnicott. Kernberg observed that any expression of the underlying borderline rage is a relatively healthy intra- and inter-psychic development beyond malignant narcissistic self-love. He observes that:

> underneath the pathological grandiose Self is a lack of integration of a normal Self, an identity diffusion. And when you dissolve the pathological grandiose Self the identity's diffusion comes to the surface . . .
>
> So, pathological narcissism is a secondary complication to borderline personality organisation . . . . The ordinary borderline case is more a matter of uncontrollable impulses, and intolerance of frustration and anxiety, yet it is better able to relate to people and to be clingingly dependent, in contrast to the narcissistic personality . . . . [i]n the course of treatment, the borderline pathology emerges in the transference and can then be treated like any borderline pathology.
>
> (Kernberg, 2001, p. 13)

Winnicott warns:

> the patient may even mobilise a psycho-neurotic false self for the purpose of finishing and expressing gratitude. But, in fact, the patient knows that there has

> been no change in the underlying psychotic state and that the analyst and the patient have succeeded in colluding to bring about a failure.
>
> (Winnicott, 1969, p. 712)

Secondly, the over-sensitive, thin-skinned narcissist's strategic adhesive identifications (false intimacies) and the borderline person's destructiveness (of the envied good) are both defences against each other. Developmentally and, therefore, internally, they are closely related. From a Jungian perspective, as personality types and traits, they are the shadow of each other. Projectively, they hate each other (as can be seen in some training groups).

Thirdly, for brittle narcissists, real intimacy is generally and transferentially so fearful and shameful that it is turned into an apparently gentle adhesive-seductive-extractive pull of false intimacy. Furthermore, strategic defences are so necessary that they are quickly rebuilt. These recurrent defensive manoeuvres only compound the shameful loneliness and so backfire. Increasingly desperate sado-masochistic repetitions may develop.

Fourthly, narcissistic defences are fiercely resistant to change, such change being perceived as either deathly shame or an opening to too-dangerously destructive impulses. The best hope for change is either through a shocking accident or the slow discovery that murderous hate does not actually kill the therapist (i.e. the loved and needed other is also he/she who is unfairly not enough and an intolerably separate person). However, such underlying borderline outrage edged with psychotic impulses is actually more real than the delusions and illusions of narcissistic falseness. These underlying borderline impulses do at least have fantasies, and these fantasies are meet-able, fight-able with and even play-able with a relational zone for possible symbolisation.

Borderline relations also defy change *inter alia,* because a change for the better or for the good belongs to the envied other, the analyst. However, a more borderline person, though often concrete to the point of fantasy-reality equivalence, is more able to develop a relatively healthy symbolising function and a reflective self-awareness through a strong and long-term analytic relationship where hurt expressed as hate can also (to an extent) lead to some critical reflection.

Fifthly, narcissistic falseness empties the analytic relationship (and all relationships) of real emotional connectedness, thus making any change arising out of shocks of linking, recognition and realisation virtually impossible. Narcissism renders the analytic relationship affectively void. Psychoid and physical life is thereby rendered tired and dull, if not narcotised. My analytic reverie is therefore solipsistic and countertransferentially unrelated and un-informative. In contrast, because aggressive borderline relations are physically and emotionally urgent, my reverie is countertransferentially loaded with primitive psychoid force and vital information (even if in fantasies of retaliatory and hate-filled fight) or is driven by a defensive flight from or freezing in the face of the barrage of projective identifications, for example by falling asleep.

Sixthly, a narcissist's ambivalent attachment/detachment communicates the message: 'Look at me, understand and know me well . . . Don't look too closely, do not get to know me too deeply'. The use of the couch helps to manage this tension, but it can also be used as a disembodying defence, an aspect of the narcissistic voiding of the relationship. A borderline person often attacks the couch. This is an attack on the analyst's enviably strong/healthy/good 'bodymind', on the containment/constraint of the analytic relationship and on their own needy dependence. Relationally, it is somatically loaded and affective at a psychoid level.

Seventhly, both disorders arise as a desperate defence against a catastrophic absence or perversion of 'primary love', against a pit of anxiety and depressive defeat. There is a too-painful reality of lack, a failure of early relational and erotic attachment, and so an anxious or an angry depression. Only if and/or when this depression becomes an honest (often shameful) process of grief and mourning can there be real structural change and a real symbolic life.

Eighthly, both disorders are based on a common early developmental failure or lack, both are defences against this common fault, and both disorders are a defence against each other. Consequently, there is always a borderline substrate to narcissism (which is sometimes actualised), and there is always a narcissistic defence within borderline states (which is sometimes actualised).

Ninthly, further split off and buried under the defences set up against an early absence of emotional connection, there lies a sense that this primary lack is actually infanticidal: a basic psychosomatic panic in the face of total abandonment, being left to die or being killed. Such annihilation is the terrifying object of the psychotic core, which often generates a paranoid fundamentalism and fanaticism that cannot tolerate and so cannot make use of any analytic interpretation).

Tenthly, the savage urgency of a borderline's preverbal and unsymbolised beta chaos, their zonal and relational confusion, is enacted and communicated through pre-emptive offensive defences. Their paranoid splitting and ruthless sadism make the analyst their needed victim and thereby also aim to provoke a revengeful countertransferential counter-attack. In other words, this is the matter of evacuation and communication through a psychotic transference and an embodied countertransference, through well-aimed projective identifications and extractions, through psychosomatic infection and consubstantial contagion which may affect and disturb the nervous and auto-immune systems. However, this is at least a process of inter-action and dangerous (destructive) relations, unlike the unrelatedness, the un-reality and the (interpersonal and internal) emptiness of the narcissistic false self. Thus it is that more borderline defences may allow for the development of a self-reflexive, self-critical symbolising function; fearful and abject narcissistic defences are so adamant that they can allow for no such developmental possibilities.

Eleventhly, both disorders are anti-symbolic and have not developed a mature symbolising function. This leaves both borderline and narcisstic cases blind to critical reflection and self-awareness and with limited empathy. They are also stuck in states of unconscious somatisation, which are sickening not only to the subject but also to the needed other. However, whereas a borderline personality is impulsively destructive of envied objects, a narcissist's lack of empathic imagination may render their relations more coldly impersonal and unconsciously cruel.

Twelfthly, it is work in this realm of disturbance and psychosomatic disorder that calls upon my analytic thinking and linking (whilst remembering that analytically we can only interpret, never know), on my ability to reflect, contain and symbolise rather than enact countertransferential impulses of retaliation, flight or dissociation. Such containment may, in turn, facilitate some self-reflection, self-containment and functional symbolising in the other. It is such disturbance that moves us between near-death and new life, being wounded and healed through the preservatory work of the psychosomatic self, 'the psychoid *conatus*'.

Conclusion

We can only hope to recycle our madness and put it to better use. We do this through hard reasoning, trying to understand our psychoid complexes, conflicts and tensions, our forceful desires and revulsions, pleasures and pains, powers and impotencies, through the shock of linking and recognising the developmental causes behind our neuroses, defences and destructive impulses. It also involves taking responsibility for our limitations and their consequences, deepening and extending our (always subjective) symbolic understanding (which implies having moved out of primitive concrete thinking, acting-out and absolutist splitting), and through mourning our lacks and losses. Such integration and acquiescence help us to re-make meaning (again and again), forge a relational faith tempered by healthy scepticism (which implies not-knowing and ambivalence), develop a sense of irony and so live well within a contingent nature.

References

Addison, A. (2008). 'Reframing the Unconscious: A View of Jung's Psychoid Unconscious Then and Now'. *Paper Given at Journal of Analytical Psychology Conference*, Orta, Italy. Unpublished.

Addison, A. (2009). 'Jung, Vitalism and "the Psychoid": An Historical Reconstruction'. *Journal of Analytical Psychology*, 54(1): 123–142.

Brodrick, M. (2013). 'Santayana's Amphibious Concepts'. *Transactions of the Charles S. Peirce Society*, 49(2): 238–249.

Clark, G. (1996). 'The Animating Body: Psychoid Substance as a Mutual Experience of Psychosomatic Disorder'. *Journal of Analytical Psychology*, 41(3): 353–368 (Chapter Five, this book).

Clark, G. (2006). 'A Spinozan Lens onto the Confusions of Borderline Relations'. *Journal of Analytical Psychology*, 51(1): 67–86 (Chapter Seven, this book).

Clark, G. (2010). 'The Embodied Counter-Transference and Recycling the Mad Matter of Symbolic Equivalence: A Re-evaluation of Samuels' Idea of the "Embodied Counter-Transference"'. In *Sacral Revolutions: Reflecting on the Work of Andrew Samuels: Cutting Edges in Psychoanalysis and Jungian Analysis*. G. Heuer, ed. London: Routledge (Chapter Twelve, this book).

Curley, E., ed. and trans. (1994). *A Spinoza Reader: The Ethics and Other Works*. Princeton, NJ: Princeton University Press.

Damasio, A. (2003). *Looking for Spinoza: Joy, Sorrow, and the Feeling Brain*. Orlando: Harcourt.

Hampshire, S. (2005). *Spinoza and Spinozism*. Oxford: Clarendon Press.

Jung, C. (1970a). *Mysterium Coniunctionis: An Inquiry Into the Separation and Synthesis of Psychic Opposites in Alchemy*. Vol. 14 of *the Collected Works of C.G. Jung*. Translated by R. Hull. 2nd edn. London: Routledge & Kegan Paul.

Jung, C. (1970b). 'On the Nature of the Psyche'. In *The Structure and Dynamics of the Psyche*. Vol. 8 of *The Collected Works of C.G. Jung*. Translated by R. Hull. 2nd edn. London: Routledge & Kegan Paul.

Kernberg, O. (2001). 'Narcissism: The American Contribution – A Conversation of Raffaele Siniscalco with Otto Kernberg'. *Journal of European Psychoanalysis*: 12–13.

Lachs, J. (2006). *On Santayana*. Belmont, CA: Wadsworth.

Milner, M. (1957). *On Not Being Able to Paint*. London: Heinemann.

Peters, R. (1987). 'The Eagle and the Serpent: Or – The Minding of Matter'. *Journal of Analytical Psychology*, 32(4): 359–381.

Santayana, G. (1910). *The Life of Reason or the Phases of Human Progress. Vol. 1: Reason in Common Sense*. New York, NY: Scribner.

Santayana, G. (1926). 'Normal Madness'. In *Dialogues in Limbo*. New York: Scribner.

Santayana, G. (1930). 'The Psyche'. In *The Realm of Matter: Book Second of Realms of Being*. New York: Scribner.

Smith, L. (1921). *Little Essays Drawn from Writings of George Santayana*. New York, NY: Scribner.

Winnicott, D. (1969). 'The Use of an Object'. *International Journal of Psychoanalysis*, 50: 711–716.

Chapter 17

Towards a psychoanalytic Spinoza

Reflections on his philosophy and the psychotherapeutic mind

Unpublished, 2006–2017[1]

Introduction

A passionate undertaking throughout my professional life has involved making my own psychodynamic emendations and amendments to Spinozan and neo-Spinozan concepts. The following represents a kind of 'work in progress' where I continue reconsidering, reworking and recycling these vital concepts. I am going to consider why and how I have found or made a particular active perspective, a relational attitude, out of Spinoza's concepts of the *conatus*, mind-body relations, passion and action and intuitive knowledge, that is, knowledge of the third kind. I shall discuss how I have adapted these concepts into psychodynamic language, including their representation in the psychopathology of difficult psychosomatic relations and how they help me psychosomatically re-order such confused and destructive internal and external relations. Destructive disorders of the self demonstrate a 'psychotic metaphysics' (Rhode, 1994) that can be understood from a Spinozan perspective. These Spinozan views are a vital part of my functional thinking and reverie in a particular inter-subjective environment. However, I do not expect my work to inform philosophy. Psychoanalytic theory and practice may benefit from some philosophy; as to how much or whether any philosophy can benefit from psychoanalysis, I cannot say.[2]

From a psychoanalytically interpretive perspective, Spinoza's philosophising was, *inter alia*, a profound way of making good sense and meaning out of the

1 This chapter derives from several versions of two unpublished but overlapping papers. 'Spinoza in Psychoanalysis: Reflections on his Philosophy and the Psychotherapeutic Mind' was originally presented on September 14, 2006, at the conference 'Wandering with Spinoza' at The Centre for Ideas at the Victorian College of the Arts, Melbourne. A later version was presented at a one-day conference, 'Psychoanalysis and Philosophy', at the Treacy Centre in Melbourne on February 27, 2010. The first draft of 'Towards a Psychoanalytic Spinoza' was dated 2009, the last amendments to a later version being made in March 2017 (Eds.).

2 I am not suggesting that Spinoza's task was proto-psychoanalytic, as proposed by Hampshire (1951), or that Spinoza's philosophical structural system pre-figured a Freudian topographic model (the invalidity of which has been shown by Deugd, 2004). Rather, I am discussing how I adapt and use certain Spinozan ideational processes in order to deepen and amplify my applied thinking.

DOI: 10.4324/9781003255826-18

apparent contingencies but actual necessities of external nature (*natura naturata et naturans*), of internal and interpersonal relations and also perhaps of the incomprehensible and emotional pain of his own losses and loneliness. However, I am not here intending to psychoanalyse Spinoza. That would be an act of intellectual arrogance and *déformation professional*, even an act of inquisitorial violence. Spinoza never asked to be analysed!

Before moving on to discuss how I make use of some of Spinoza's ideas, I acknowledge that, from a Spinozan perspective, everything I say is conditioned – as it must be for everybody – by my body-mind that is inherently natured, sexed and socio-culturally gendered as well as by my psychosomatic history and intimate relationships (Lloyd, 1994). More fundamentally, to carry the implications of Spinozan concepts into the personal and psychogenic position, as well as culturally and intellectually, all I think, feel and do has been conditioned by my own psychosomatic history and by my particular desires, pleasures, powers, failures in early and subsequent significant intimate relationships.

Psychoanalytic theories and practices are nowadays so scientifically, politically and socially criticised and doubted that they are almost dismissed as being beyond relevance. However, these shadows of psychoanalysis can at least be ameliorated and ethically answered through the radical perception of honest reflection and self-awareness.

I regard psychoanalysis as a mode of personal and interpersonal apperception, observation and reflection, a hermeneutic, interpretative system, a relational and potentially mutative art, not a science. It is an affective recreation and representation (through transference and countertransference), which affects both participants and may bring a change of psychic structure or 'relations of relations' which emerge and develop in the analysand. It is a particular framed 'thoughtful relationship' open to being worked upon so as to know and understand passive emotions and psychosomatic affects as they are experienced personally and interpersonally. This may lead to a deep emendation of psychic states, relations and behaviours. It is an activity aiming to increase agency by removing blocks, resistances and defences.

Psychoanalysis is about how we manage and order our core madness with normalising neuroses, philosophical systems, psychoanalytic theories, practices, frames and other formal rituals and arts. Thus, psychoanalysis, which is a very particular relationship, becomes a history in the making, re-structuring of forceful neurotic and psychotic processes. One of the co-ordinating processes that I use in this relational realm is a form of Spinozan 'reverie' as a means of thinking through, ordering and processing the other's infectious pre-verbal and pre-conceptual psychic confusion, changing unmanageable emotional chaos into functional order, which the psychoanalyst Wilfred Bion termed transforming 'beta fragments' into 'alpha functioning' (Bion, 1962, p. 36).

Throughout my professional life, alongside my clinical practice, I have continued to lecture on and write about the philosophical and intellectual lineage running from Spinoza to the immediate terrain of psychoanalysis and Jung. This line partly lies in the problematic but creative revision of Spinoza through German Idealism and Romanticism, which Beiser calls 'the romantic synthesis of Fichte and Spinoza, idealism and realism' (Beiser, 2003, p. 184). I have emphasised the following: 1) Lessing's, Mendelssohn's and Herder's 'refined pantheism' or 'dynamic panentheism' (that is, substance as the substantial organic force of all forces, *die Urkraft aller Kräfte*); 2) the Naturalistic ideals of Goethe; 3) the pantheism of Hölderlin, Novalis, Wordsworth, Coleridge, Shelley, Heine and other Romantics; 4) the problems of conscious and unconscious relations of subjective minds to other subjective minds (i.e. intersubjectivity) and to the world in Absolute Idealism (especially early Schelling); 5) the applied *Naturphilosophie* of 19th-century German psychologists; and 6) the philosophy of Santayana.

I have also incorporated more recent critical neo-Spinozan philosophy into my post-Freudian and post-Jungian thinking and practice. Here, I might mention the work of Hampshire (1994, 2002), Bennett (1984), Donagan (1988), Lloyd (1994, 1996), Deleuze (1988), Negri (1991, 2004), Montag and Stolze (1997), Montag (1999), Yovel (1999) and, in neuroscience, Damasio (2003).

In my teaching of this selective history of ideas, I try to emend this trajectory of somewhat self-centred Idealism by incorporating Schopenhauer's amoral, blind, impersonal Will, Nietzsche's moral relativism, Santayana's celebratory naturalism and scepticism and Sprigge's 'pantheistic idealism' (Sprigge, 2006) as necessary critical and adjunctive (sometimes disjunctive) concepts and visions.

Spinoza and Santayana

'The stone upon which Santayana built his cathedral was Spinoza', writes Kirby-Smith (1997, p. 25). The Spinozan stone is ultimately impersonal, lacking an emotionally striving architecture or any 'normally mad' purpose, and so is somewhat alienating because it is essentially just a representation of the eternal necessity of substance. Although a 'critical realist', Santayana tried to add the necessary human spirit, art and imagination to substance. However, Santayana's philosophical and poetic cathedral is still not friendly, fully relational or intimate, lacking common subjectivity and passion. It is even a bit inhumane and dwells too much in non-existent 'eternal essence'. In spite of his positive evaluation of and capacity for friendship, Santayana's idea of love remains universal rather than interpersonal.

On the other hand, this interpersonally rather detached, contemplative quality that Spinoza and Santayana share is yet surely a particular way of gaining valuable and rare perceptions and evaluations of the world. Above all, it offers the possibility of a 'good life' without false meaning: an acquiescence and a pleasure in the conscious realisation of our place in nature and a demonstration that creativity can arise out of this awareness.

Psychologically speaking, Spinoza and Santayana are not erotically relational, either inherently or temperamentally, and I think this is a problematic lack. Personally, I have had to add to Spinoza and Santayana my own necessities: the 'literary psychology' of Freud, Jung, psychoanalysis and its relational practice. This means that I am acutely attentive to persons and their subjectivities as infinitely differing and ever-changing. They continually dwell in that Spinozan realm which Deleuze calls a 'discontinuous volcanic line' that expresses 'all the angers of the heart' (Deleuze, 1988, p. 29).[3] This has to do with the psychosomatic reality of pain, frustrated desire, accident and loss, as well as lust, love, potent agency and joy.

Both these solitary philosophers were able to think their way through their 'abandonment-into-loneliness' and indeed to transcend it through intellectual and ideational reconstructive work. They made contemplation and the creation of an ontological world-view both a personal and, ideally, a common psychological and socio-cultural solution to passivity and misunderstanding. The problem remains that the Other is not allowed to be real as an object of desire and erotic curiosity and/or a disturbing, dangerous, contagious object.

I would say that in order to enjoy real intimacy, you had better take off your Spinozan spectacles and move out of your Santayana-inspired contemplative detachment when you go to bed with someone or when you find that you are in an urgent fight!

In my current psychoanalytic thinking, I have been making much of Santayana's idea of 'normal madness', which I have taken into my formulations about my clinical experience of intra-psychic and transferential relations. I have then brought these conceptualisations back again into my Spinozan *Anschauungsweise*.

Put over-simply, this Santayana, post-Spinozan idea is that it is madness to want or try to make the transient permanent, unchanging or eternal. And it is madness to try to make someone love you when they do not and perhaps cannot love you. Perhaps Spinoza implies something similar in his scholion to *Ethics* V, P. 20, although he is talking about passive desires and irrational attachments:

> [S]ickness of the mind and misfortunes take their origin especially from too much love toward a thing which is liable to many variations and which we can never fully possess. For no one is disturbed or anxious concerning anything unless he loves it, nor do wrongs, suspicions, and enmities arise except from love for a thing which no one can fully possess.
>
> (in Curley, 1994, p. 255)

In psychological terms, there is putting our madness to good use (Santayana, 1926) through necessary illusions, ideals, philosophical ideation or the recreation of beauty, or there are destructive forms of madness involving offensively acted out

3 Towards the end of Deleuze's second essay in *Spinoza: Practical Philosophy,* he notes how Spinoza's *Ethics* was written in two different times: 'The *Ethics* is a book written twice simultaneously: once in the continuous stream of definitions, propositions, demonstrations, and corollaries, which develop the great speculative themes with all the rigors of the mind; another time in the broken chain of scholia, a discontinuous volcanic line, a second version underneath the first, expressing all the angers of the heart and setting forth the practical theses of denunciation and liberation' (Deleuze, 1988, pp. 28–29).

defences against intolerable lack and impotent frustration. This can be seen in the 'impotent omnipotent' fantasy of the 'oedipal orphan'.

God as nature in Spinoza's *Ethics*

Don Garrett (2007), in a review of Steven Nadler's book on Spinoza's *Ethics*, shows how the *Ethics* offered a metaphysics that identifies God with nature while seeing everything in nature as progressing 'with absolute necessity . . . from equally necessary grounds or causes, in a way that leaves no room for contingency' (Garrett, 2007, p. 7):

> Thus, beginning with the attempted demonstration of the single-substance metaphysics that literally identifies God with Nature, Nadler considers in turn how Spinoza sought successively to establish the truth of universal necessitarianism and the absence of divine purpose [or providence]; the identity of mind and body; distinctive conceptions of knowledge and will [consciousness as part of natura naturans]; a comprehensive psychology of the emotions based on a fundamental drive to self-preservation [the *conatus*]; an ethics of reason, virtue and freedom; and an account of the way to blessedness and [immanent] eternality, if not personal immortality.
>
> (D. Garrett, 2007, p. 7)

To more fully amplify Garrett's summary: Spinoza's monistic metaphysics posits a single space-time entity whose local variations of forces, governed by pervasive natural laws, constitute physical 'objects' as states of the universe rather than as component parts of it. This means that the 'attributes' are how a substance is conceived since a single substance cannot consist of attributes or their modes. The one substance is perceived by humans in two ways (as mind and body), and also perceived infinitely by God.

By extension, from this monistic metaphysics, Spinoza proceeds to posit a relation between the mental and the physical, which entails the identity of the human mind with the human body. This is a treating of the mental and the physical as two fundamentally different dimensions of substantial being which all things, with all of their qualities, exemplify or express. The symbolic realism of this 'panpsychism' is compatible with the kind of 'incremental naturalism' (D. Garrett, 2008, pp. 18–19) that seeks to explain fundamental features of human thought, such as consciousness, representation and will, as sophisticated developments of features that pervade the natural world in a broad range of degrees, beginning with the very rudimentary, such as primitive organisms and 'the psychoid'.

Spinoza's conception of consciousness identifies the power of an idea to exert influence on an individual's self-persevering behaviour; the *conatus*. For Spinoza, freedom and responsibility, in the face of necessitarianism and the impossibility of actual free will, are based on the recognition of a causal determination through one's own determined nature that is attainable only in proportion to one's virtue.

Spinoza's God is not personal, purposive or transcendent, but is the omnipotent, omniscient, eternal and necessary law and cause of all things. The appropriate attitude to hold towards such a 'God-or-nature' is one of 'intellectual love' and 'acquiescence' of mind.

Spinoza's rational ethical aim is to transform harmful (passive) passions into an active shared pursuit of a rational and, thence, emergent intuitive knowledge about human beings and the rest of nature. Aaron Garrett (following Hampshire) sees this as an 'emendative therapy' (A. Garrett, 2003, p. 18) which turns a Spinozan 'passion into an action' by replacing 'an inadequate idea with an adequate idea' (A. Garrett, 2003, p. 88). Although we can say that Spinoza's three prime realities might be: no personal god, no immortality of the soul and no free will, Spinoza's aim in the *Ethics* is 'to lead readers . . . . to their own blessedness' (A. Garrett, 2003, p. 5). Hence, the 'ultimate goal of this emendation' is an ethics of 'how one ought to act in order to attain joy and blessedness' and to 'become what they are' (A. Garrett, 2003, p. 18).

I would summarise Spinoza's *Anschauungsweise* as follows: There is the eternal necessity of nature, and there are psychically necessary illusions; there is unconscious appetite and conscious desire; there is fear and disgust; there is attachment, love, loss and hate; there are strengths and weaknesses, pleasures and pains, joy and sadness, power and limitation; there are various degrees of ignorance and knowledge. But there is no personal God, no personal immortality (of consciousness or memory) and no actual free will; there can, however, be a subjectively or psychically real sense of freedom, most truly attained through rational and intuitive knowledge, a state that is very difficult to achieve, yet is possible. To put this in Spinozan Latin, '*Amor aeternae necessitatis naturae, summa laetitia et acquiescentia est*'. Wittgenstein also points to a form of eternity in the mutability of the present moment in Proposition 6.4311 of his *Tractatus Logico-Philosophicus*:

> If by eternity is understood not endless temporal duration but timelessness, then he lives eternally who lives in the present.
>
> (Wittgenstein, 1933, p. 185)

My Spinozan approach

In my adaptation of such Spinozan concepts psychoanalytically, it must be remembered that they are each part of a whole metaphysical system and, as such, are interdependent. In addition, what is known as Spinoza's geometric method is central to his therapeutic and ethical goals. Spinoza's form of argumentation is modelled on that of Euclid's *Geometry* as a series of definitions, postulates and axioms from which Spinoza's propositions are demonstrated to follow by logical deduction. The geometric form, content and the deductive argument of the *Ethics* (the full Latin title of which is *Ethica in ordine geometrico demonstrata*) belong together as a unified whole, as Aaron Garrett, Don Garrett and Steven Nadler all observe. For them, this formal order (*in more geometrico*) is uniquely suited to the content, medium and message, the three being inter-dependent. In other words, Spinoza's geometric form and method are intrinsic to the concatenation of content and argument that constitute the *Ethics*.

There is also an implicit issue here about top-down or bottom-up approaches. One can present theory as preceding subjective practical experience, thus creating both a lens through which to comprehend the raw data and also building a foundation and clear structure for the representation and interpretation of difficult ethical and/or psychological issues. Alternatively, one can acknowledge and present material through a form and method that systematically demonstrates that theory emerges out of and is motivated by the need to order problematic experiences.

For example, in the field of current Spinozan studies, Jenny Bunker (2006) has argued that, in spite of his top-down geometrical-deductive rationalist method and form, Spinoza's philosophy is empirically informed in a bottom-up 'embedded' way, which is significantly similar to Schopenhauer's embodied and experientially-based Idealism. Aaron Garrett (2003) has also described Spinoza's intrinsic 'emmet's inch' or bottom-up perspective as opposed to an 'eagle's mile' or top-down perspective in the *Ethics*. In what follows, I will be using both 'top down' and 'bottom up' approaches.

My approach is thus to move from setting out a theoretical structure to elaborating and then demonstrating the elements and their relations through practical psychodynamic experience. I do this for several reasons. One is that this approach reflects Spinoza's 'geometrical method' or deductive system without denying its experiential motivation and import. Another is because the psychological is hereby seen to demonstrate the practical usefulness of the established theoretical structure. In any case, I repeat: as a psychologist, I can only borrow philosophical ideas to help me; I certainly do not claim that psychology is needed by philosophers to help them with their philosophy.

I use Spinoza's philosophy and neo-Spinozan thinking to help me recycle madness and put it to good use: a Spinozan mind can be a psychoanalytic assistant. Spinoza's ethical naturalism and the *acquiescentia mentis* that can emerge through it also help me interpret and integrate unchanging pathological states in borderline persons, and paradoxically thereby sometimes enable the emergence of a new attitude of ironic understanding and acceptance, which is actually such a deep transformation that it seems like a structural change within the predetermined patterns of affect and behaviour.

Five Spinozan concepts

Five inter-related Spinozan concepts that are most useful to me in the analytic setting are as follows: 1) the *conatus*, 2) 'the mind as the idea of the body', 3) neo-Spinozan theories of 'emotions, passions and actions', 4) the issue of 'free necessity' and 5) 'intuitive knowledge'. I have extended and adapted these into a language of psychodynamic, inter-subjective and relational relevance, which I use as a lens to look through, onto and into psychic and psychosomatic dynamics.

As well as being both a concatenation of position, attitude or *Anschauungsweise*, Spinozan and neo-Spinozan thought is also, for me, a rigorous form of thinking itself: both Euclidian/deductive and constructive/creative. As such, it acts as an internal intellectual structure, a species of mental 'organ' that operates behind my functional or pragmatic intent.[4]

1 The conatus

For Spinoza, the *conatus* underlies all natural laws, including the laws of living organisms and, therefore, of our human drives, appetites, desires and defences. It is the inherent endeavour or striving to persist in being and 'the drive to self-maintenance, through degrees of complexity of interlocking parts, through balance of motion and rest in physical systems, through degrees of freedom and degrees of the power to act' (Hampshire, 2005, p. xxx). It is 'the drive for self-maintenance against disruptive forces coming from inside and outside the organism. All individuals are held together in their activities by this drive' (Hampshire, 2002).

The *conatus* is the striving to increase the power of action, 'a power to exercise powers, a power to acquire new powers' (Lloyd, 1996), 'a striving . . . for . . . an increase in power of action, which is what Spinoza understands joy to be' (Curley, 1988, p. 115).

The *conatus* is the essence of every finite thing (mode) to struggle to keep itself actualised and to endeavour 'to continue to exist in as perfect a form as possible' (Sprigge, 2006, p. 43); 'every actualised essence is always doing its best to keep itself actualised in as robust a form as possible' (p. 44). The *conatus* is an energetic process and is where mind and body come together, i.e. *conatus* is physical-matter-as-energy through which one 'substance' is represented as many 'modes', i.e. through which 'substance' individuates.

The *conatus* is related to the concept of the mind as idea of the body and, more generally, to corporeality and embodiment of bodies, body-bits and bodily relations, or in other words, the somatic. As Lloyd explains, 'Desire, joy and reason come together in the *conatus* of mind as idea of body' (Lloyd, 1996, p. 89). In other words, the *conatus* of mind is where I experience the expressed identity of mind and body, in my appetites and desires, my pleasures and pains, my joys and sadness. Furthermore, when the *conatus* is 'related to mind and body together, it is called appetite', which is seen by Spinoza as the very essence of a person (Lloyd, 1996, p. 74). A further differentiation is that we can consider 'desire' as conscious and 'appetite' as unconscious.[5]

4 This paper originally contained a lengthy section on the *jouissance* grid as a diagrammatic depiction. We refer the reader to Chapter Seven, p. 107 and Chapter Fifteen, p. 218 (Eds.).

5 Spinoza writes, 'Between appetite and desire there is no difference, except that desire is generally related to [people] insofar as they are conscious of their appetites. So *desire* can be defined as *appetite together with consciousness of the appetite* [*appetitus cum ejusdem conscientia*]' (Spinoza *Ethics,* Bk 3, prop. 9. in Marrama, 2017, p. 513; translation after Curley, 1994, p. 160).

In so far as the *conatus* is where emotions come together in the mind as idea of body, bodies and body relations, the *conatus* is particular to an individual, to one's personal relations and so to the development of subjective, intersubjective, social and cultural identities. The *conatus* as 'my *conatus*' is my own individual nature naturing (*natura naturans*) by striving to preserve and to power my idiosyncratic, and particularly embodied, emotional, rational, relational, social self among other selves: the *conatus* is 'psychosomatic individuation'.

The *conatus* is mind as idea of body, of other bodies and of body relations (and of bodymind emotions and memories). I add that the *conatus* is the 'psychoid' substance of mind-brain-body identity, the 'existential inertia' (Nadler, 2006a), which is an energetic self-preservation and is of both body and imagination, matter and idea, i.e. psychodynamically, the 'psychoid *conatus*'.

In some ways, the *conatus* seems related to certain metapsychological, psychophysical and psychodynamic constructs, such as: instinct, drive, the autonomic nervous system, the auto-immune system, the developmental process itself, the (Schopenhauerian) Will and the Nietzschean will-to-power, Freud's 'libido', Jung's 'psychic energy' and the regulating (healing) function of the Self, Bion's 'transformations in O'. However, it is unlike any of these in that it is a particular metaphysical concept of naturalistic immanence.

The *conatus* can be understood as 'a kind of existential inertia' (Nadler, 2006a, p. 195). As Nadler subsequently commented:

> By 'existential inertia' I mean something stronger than the Newtonian sense whereby a state of being of a thing (e.g., motion or rest) does not change unless acted on by a force. Rather, what I mean (on Spinoza's behalf) is that a thing will actively resist any externally-derived attempts to diminish its power of existing – much as any solid object will resist attempts to break it apart. Indeed, Spinoza seems to make an even stronger claim: that not only does a thing resist any attempts to break it apart, it will actively strive to pursue those things that aid its integrity and power. So 'inertia' might be taken to mean an active force to persevere in its state (of existing).
>
> (Nadler, 2006b)

The *conatus* is ruthless. Its actions are often convoluted and 'crafty', unconscious as much as conscious, and its impetus is ruthless. It is an imperative in the face of doubts, confusions and moral dilemmas; so it causes conflicts, including, in some extreme situations, suicide as a complex act of preservation of the ideal of the self.

The *conatus* also expresses itself through dreams, fantasies and images that are emotive, irrational, partial, even delusional, etc., although self-revealing. One can see these as forms of psychic self-preservation through unconscious work, and/or expressions of the psychic life of the psychoid *conatus*.

Speaking from a psychodynamic position, I would say that the *conatus* is the causal drive behind an ethically good life as well as behind neurotic and destructive defences, behaviours and relations. The *conatus,* as 'psychosomatic individuation', is an expression of desire, power and defence. I would incorporate the idea that people have subjective, fantasy-driven and conflicted ideas of their *conatus*: *conatus* as a subjective and varying psychic reality, a multiple and unconscious (as well as conscious) complex of psychic and psychosomatic fantasies and drives. However, according to a psychodynamic interpretation (which does not agree at all with Spinoza), it is sometimes possible that my idea of how to best preserve or restore a diminishing or lost 'good self' may be to kill my idea of my pained, shamed or sick 'bad self'. I would also say that 'my *conatus*' is my own individual nature naturing by striving to preserve and to power my idiosyncratic and particularly embodied, emotional, relational and social self amid other selves: the *conatus* is 'psychosomatic individuation'.

There is the developmental necessity of a cunning Hegelian resistance and opposition to self-preservation, a sense of pleasurable power gained through destruction, including destruction of the ideal (parental) good. This attack may be either a developmental necessity or a borderline defence.

Don Garrett (2002) argues that Spinoza's idea of the *conatus* can be validated by his premise of inherence, in which individual things (and their causal self-preservation) are understood as finite approximations of infinite substance. Nadler delineates how the *conatus* is related to motivation through the elements of will, appetite and desire:

> In the mind, an individual's conatus manifests itself as will – not an abstract faculty of willing . . . but the particular affirmations or negations that make up much of our thinking life. When the human being is considered as a composite entity constituted by a mind and a body, its conatus consists in appetite. When a person is conscious of the striving of his mind and body together, when he is aware of an appetite, it becomes desire. In both cases, the mind and the mind-body composite, the conatus is the motivational force that lies at the root of all a person's endeavours.
>
> (Nadler, 2006a, p. 199)

Therefore, it is also the motivational force which lies at the root of our defences:

> In the human body, conatus presumably manifests itself as the body's physical resistance to any attempt to change the ratio of motion and rest among its parts to the point of dissolution. In the mind, it is the conscious striving after those things that (as far as it can tell) promote its well-being and the well-being of the body on which its existence depends.
>
> (Nadler, 2006a, p. 200)

Conatus: a final summation

To summarise how I have been making use of the *conatus* in my work, it is firstly the impulse or endeavour for self-preservation of life and of an idea of my (good) self and my products and is, therefore, basically defensive. It is the endeavour or impulse to increase my powers for self-preservation and is the urge to express myself (creatively or, if necessary, destructively), which is an individuating of the *conatus*, and then to apply reason (thinking), responsibility (ethics) and healthy depressive scepticism (negative capability). Thence there may emerge 'intuitive knowledge' or 'selected facts' and provisional interpretation.

Secondly, however, the *conatus* for self-preservation can manifest as an impetus to destroy another (another *conatus*) and may itself be a victim of the destructive *conatus* of another. It can be paradoxical or counter-intuitive, for example, in acting upon the idea of preserving or restoring the good self by destroying the bad self through suicide, or can become pathologically paranoid or perverse because its defensiveness is affected by human unconscious and conscious emotional tensions and manoeuvres. This is the stuff of the forces, tensions and conflicts of the '*conatus* as *jouissance*'.

Thirdly, although I will not elaborate on this point, it is important to note that all these personal forces and qualities could also be said to apply to the *conatus* of different cultures. Here, I refer the reader to 'Herder's force: pluralism, expressivism, mind-body relations and empathy'.[6]

Fourthly, the *conatus* is a mere potentiality or latency until it is active and so becomes actual through different histories, languages, social orders, arts and religious and ethical systems.

Fifthly, the aspects I am particularly interested in are the forces, tensions and conflicts of the '*conatus* as *jouissance*' as they are manifest through primitive psychoid and psychosomatic affects in the transferential and countertransferential field.

To conclude: the *conatus* is an intrinsic psychoid and energetic striving for self-preservation and for the maintenance and increasing power of mental and physical activity and agency. This striving can be unconscious, conflicted, counter-intuitive and multiple; it is also interpersonal, relational and social; it incorporates the endeavour to make or find 'meaning' and thus also to make or find symbolisation; as well as pertinent to the human realm, the *conatus* is also 'panpsychic' or substantially absolute, and is, therefore, an aspect of our being 'part of nature'.

2 *The mind is the idea of the body*

Rosenthal paraphrases the implications of Propositions 11–13 of Part 2 of the Ethics thus: 'I exist in that I think as a body' (Rosenthal, 1989, p. 129). I add: 'I am an emotional and thinking mind in that I am a (human) body with a (human) brain among other bodies which affect me'. As we have seen,[7] Spinoza's concept of 'the mind as the idea of the body' helps me work through mind-body relations,

6 See Chapter Fifteen of this book where Herder's application of the *conatus* to culture is discussed (Eds.).

7 See Chapter Seven (Eds.).

psychosomatic identifications and problematic symbolic equations (Segal, 1950, 1957) arising out of faulty developments of the symbolising function. In such states, the mind *is* the body, and the mind as idea of the body is missing or has not yet been realised. The essential Spinozan position is that the mind and the body are to be understood univocally as two necessarily different apprehensions of that which we can also know rationally and by intuitive knowledge (of the third kind) to be a substantial unit.

Before reconsidering my adaptation of Spinoza's 'mind is the idea of the body', let us revisit other writers upon whom I have drawn in this regard.

Diane Steinberg defines and describes Spinoza's system of mind-body relations most clearly:

> As an idea . . . the mind bears an essential, but noncausal, relation to its object, the body. The essential linkage between the mind and body in Spinoza has three important aspects. In the first place the existence of the mind necessarily parallels that of the body . . . . The second aspect of the essential linkage between mind and body is that as an idea the mind is necessarily individuated by its object . . . . The third aspect of the essential linkage between mind and body in Spinoza is that mental processes and the abilities and limitations of the mind can be explained in terms of bodily processes and abilities and limitations.
>
> (Steinberg, 2000, pp. 35–36)

Charles Jarrett argues that Spinoza held an identity theory, not a dual aspect theory. To say mind and body 'are two different expressions of one thing' is a dual aspect theory. To say 'that the mind and the body are one thing that is expressed in two ways' is an identity theory. In the identity theory reading of Spinoza:

> 'Mind' and 'body' denote one thing, although conceived differently, rather than two things that are aspects or expressions of something else.
>
> (Jarrett, 2007, pp. 74–75)

Stuart Hampshire writes:

> The brain maps the body, and the mind maps the brain, and both would lose their representative function if they were broken down into their separate segments . . . But the property, say, which becomes salient is still kept within its context in the whole map, and the map still reflects the patterns of the brain.
>
> (Hampshire, 2005, p. li)

Translating this into the realm of psychosomatic analytic interaction, my particular (countertransferential) mind-body response to your psyche-soma maps your omnipotent but thwarted (transferential) mixture of desire-love and frustration-hate towards me (as it does to yourself and others) and maps the relations formed between us, which are also your internalised relations.

Previously, I formulated a psychodynamic, inter-subjective and relational application of Spinoza's metaphysical statement that the 'mind is the idea of the body' in stages of conceptual refinement.[8] Although, in the following, many of these stages are repeated, I also add some later thinking.

The emotional mind is the idea of the 'passions and actions' of the body and, thence, the subjective idea of the passions and actions of other bodies and other minds. The mind is the conscious and unconscious ideas of and concerns about what has happened, is happening and is going to happen to the body from the inside and from the outside; therefore, also what the body desires, is frustrated by and fears of itself and of others. All such 'ideas' of body/bodies are subjectively complex, fantastically distorted, semi-conscious or unconscious, but energetically affective, i.e. 'the idea of the body' implies that the mind includes unconscious phantasies of the body, bodies and body relations. The mind is an emotional ideation process of management (e.g. splitting, paranoid-schizoid – depressive thinking, etc.) of emotional psyche-soma relations to body, body-bits and other bodies. The mind thinks in order to manage the vicissitudes of emotional-physical needs, appetites, desires, frustrations and fears concerning other-minded (emotional and thinking) bodies and bits (breast, penis, etc.).

Mind-body-brain development and, therefore, the development of images and ideas, emerges out of the relations between personal/internal mind and other mind-body-brains, as well as with the contingencies of the material world as it affects the subject.

The mind is the psychic structural formation, the emergent image and idea (preconceptions, conceptions, phantasies, thoughts, words) of body, brain and environment, of biological, neurological and relational development. In other words, mind includes images, thoughts and words of the development of internal (intra-physical and intra-psychic) and external (inter-physical and inter-psychic) relations.

Putting the body first, one can say that we are embodied emotional minds, and our brains are our interactive and ideational minds. Here, I requote Santayana: 'Now the body is an instrument, the mind its function, the witness and reward of its operation' (Santayana, 1910, p. 206). The body is the matter of and for the mind; i.e. the 'body-and-brain' is the expressed material or corporeal aspect of the energetic *conatus*, the embodied desires, pleasures and pains of its mental aspect.

Subjectively, I am an emotional and thinking mind in that I am a body with an emotional and thinking brain among other similar bodyminds who affect me. All these psyche-somatic relations are as much unconscious as conscious. I come into being through other bodies and other body-minds and thus am inherently dependent upon them. As Mark Wartofsky writes,

> the dependency on other bodies, in a strange and dialectical sense, is the very condition of a body's activity, since its power to act is its power to affect other

8 See Chapter Seven (Eds.).

> bodies; as, in turn, the power to act of these other bodies is their power to act on this (my) body. The fundamental mode of the existence of human bodies, as individuals, is therefore a relational mode, or one of interaction.
>
> (1973, p. 338)

The clinical importance of these bodymind matters is that they affect my thinking about and working with the psychoid realm as a field of communication conveyed through the psychosomatic forces of infection and contagion in the transference and embodied countertransference. When the mind and the body are (or remain or become) conceptually and psychosomatically confused to the point of subjective identification, where there is concrete equation rather than symbolisation, the person is psychotically deluded.

Regarding the psychoid, as discussed elsewhere,[9] Jung implicitly uses a dual-aspect theory when he speaks of psyche and matter being two aspects of one thing, ultimately resting on 'irrepresentable transcendental factors' (Jung, 1970; *CW* 8, para. 418). Addison (2008) points out that although Jung drew on the earlier ideas of the psychoid as conceived by the vitalist Driesch and the psycho-physical parallelism of Bleuler (Addison, 2008, p. 3), the 'body and mind do not stand in a parallel relation but are two different aspects of one and the same thing, which falls under the scope of [Jung's] notion of the psychoid unconscious' (Addison, 2008, p. 5).

In terms of a Spinozan identity theory (dual-aspect monism), the psychoid would therefore be simultaneously both 'bodily matter and sense' and 'mental image and idea'. Body and mind are but different modes of 'bodymind' as a single substance.

3 *Passions, actions and relations: jouissance of the emotions and the conatus*

In Spinozan terms, the mind is the idea of the body, moved by desires, pleasures and pains (*cupiditas*, *laetitia* and *tristitia*). Spinoza's three primary affects are *tristitia* (pain), *laetitia* (joy) and *cupiditas* (desire). In relation to *laetitia*, there is also *gaudium* or gladness and *hilaritas* or cheerfulness. As Lloyd explains, *hilaritas* 'is a higher order joy . . . a pleasure of reflection that goes beyond the mind's joy in engaging in unimpeded activity in the here and now' (Lloyd, 1996, p. 90). I expand this into a wider complex of internal and interpersonal emotional relations (including ideas of bodies and body relations) that make for a *jouissance* of affects and the tensions between them. This *jouissance* I have understood as part of the *conatus*.

The innate 'psychoid *conatus*' further materialises and develops as it is met by and goes out to meet the world: parents and other people, appetites and desires, fears and shames, forces of the super-ego, external or environmental contingencies, etc., and so it develops and changes as it is nurtured, fed and affected, as it

9 For a final summation on the psychoid, see Chapter Eighteen (Eds.).

adapts and/or defends itself, as it flourishes, fights, flees or freezes. Thus, it moves into a dynamic multi-dimensional *jouissance* of increasingly complex desires, fears, pleasures, pains, powers and limits. Here, as explicated in earlier writings, my '*Jouissance* Grid' expresses through a two-dimensional diagram the dynamic psychic and psychoid affects, emotions or passions and their relations, which I use, like Bion's 'grid', to help me think through, clarify and order the psychosomatic beta disorder in the transference.[10]

To remind the reader, *conatus*-as-*jouissance* incorporates all affects and passions of the dual aspects of the psychoid 'bodymind'. *Conatus*-as-*jouissance* is non-binary. Emotions oscillate and are full of ambiguity and ambivalence: we can both love and hate the same person, simultaneously feel desire and disgust, love and hate. The dynamic relations depicted in the diagram are also simultaneously of the body and the mind, personal and interpersonal. There is a dynamic relationship between appetite/desire and disgust/fear, between pleasure and pain, joy and sadness, power and impotence, all of which are incorporated in the psychoid *conatus*.

A quotation from Spinoza's *Political Treatise*, written in 1675–1676, expresses something of the interpretive approach implicit in my '*jouissance* of passions' grid, as well as of the psychoanalytic attitude in general:

> I have laboured carefully, not to mock, lament, or execrate, but to understand human actions; and to this end I have looked upon passions, such as love, hatred, anger, envy, ambition, pity, and the other perturbations of the mind, not in the light of vices of human nature, but as properties, just as pertinent to it, as are heat, cold, storm, thunder and the like to the nature of the atmosphere, which phenomena, though inconvenient, are yet necessary, and have fixed causes, by means of which we endeavour to understand their nature, and the mind has just as much pleasure in viewing them aright, as in knowing such things as flatter the senses.
>
> (Spinoza, Gosset trans., 1993, p. 288)

Love as a passion

A principle espoused by Spinoza, Borges and others is that the highest form of love transcends our demands to have our love fully met and returned. Yet there also needs to be a place for ordinary human love, as between people, for poetic imagination and aesthetic sensibility, for ideas and experiences of beauty and ugliness and their essential relation to the ethical. This is a lack in the original Spinozan system, but which was perhaps recognised and addressed by Herder, Schlegel, Schelling, several German and English Romantic poets, Heine, Schopenhauer and in a very different way, by Santayana. As a good nominalist, I say, 'there's no such thing as love without lovers'.

10 See the *Jouissance* Grid and explanations in Chapters Seven and Fifteen (Eds.).

Spinoza suggests that nature, including human nature, is intrinsically neither beautiful nor ugly, neither good nor bad, except in so far as we subjectively judge it so. Nature (*natura naturata* and *natura naturans*) is as it is, in itself neutral. But we as humans do evaluate bodies: our own, those of others and of the world. We re-act to, act upon, re-form (or deform) and relate to such bodies and matters according to our conscious and unconscious ideas thereof. This adds an imaginative and aesthetic feeling-value to the system, which Spinoza may have considered to be inferior to rational thought, though surely not without its place in human nature, a real part of 'living well and rejoicing', which may also be part of 'natural human virtue'. Spinoza's radical virtue ethics may bridge this apparent split by being able to extend to an incorporation of aesthetics and poetics as active virtues.

The place of thwarted desire, fear, disgust, depression, anger and destructiveness, as well as the pain of loss, is as natural as is the place of our actively enhancing pleasures and powers. However, a rational, differentiated and creative use of our subjective feelings can be a virtue, a human 'good'. In this subjective-projective zone, there can either be empowering understanding, thought and action, which leads to enjoyment and to living well or better, or there can be unconscious, passive emotions, which lead to emotional pain for oneself and others.

The problematic resolution of the opposed relations between reason and imagination, between rational knowledge and sceptical irony, between realism/naturalism and creativity and/or between the stasis of the eternal necessity of nature and subjective developmental freedom were urgent and vital to the Spinozan-pantheistic controversy (the *Pantheismusstreit*) and to its development through subsequent Romantic and Idealist philosophers. This is our common psychosomatic ambiguity and our inherent 'romantic irony'. On one hand, there are the realities of love and imagination, which we relate to creatively while knowing that we are part of one nature, and on the other hand, there are our impossible longings, our separateness and having to acquiesce to the cruel laws of matter.

This is still a live psychoanalytic issue in that it translates into the psychological problem of the relations between ideas of a unity of common consciousness, empathy, identification and the separateness of other minds.

4 The problem of free necessity

For Spinoza, there is a tension between the freedom of choice which we may experience through our subjective sense of the *conatus* as autonomous and our being bound by the laws of nature. The sense of freedom of choice in a structurally, neurologically, biologically, physically and developmentally determined reality is the problematic matter of psychotherapeutic action. From the point-of-view of psychic reality, we have a necessary illusion of possible change (of understanding, choice and agency). 'Psychic reality' is also of the imagination and so is fictional. However, as Lloyd explains, Spinoza himself accepts that fictional imagination is part of the nature of the thinking mind and so is a natural and, therefore, necessary illusion (Lloyd, 2008). The contents of this natural psychic reality include inadequate ideas, opinions, fantasies, imaginings, projections, beliefs in a personal god, the immortality of the soul, freedom of choice, etc. Freedom of choice might be our psychic reality, and we may speak of free necessity, whilst physically (like all matter), we are actually part of determined *natura naturans*.

5 Knowledge of the third kind

Spinoza delineates three kinds of knowledge: the first from imagination (*imaginatio*); the second from reason (*ratio*); and third, intuitive knowledge (*scientia intuitiva*). The first, also called 'opinion', is derived from sensory experience that has been represented 'in a way that is mutilated, confused, and without order for the intellect' (Spinoza in Nadler, 2006a, p. 177). Knowledge of the second kind, Spinoza tells us in the *Ethics*, refers to how 'we perceive many things . . . from the fact that we have common notions and adequate ideas of the properties of things' (Spinoza in Nadler, 2006a, p. 178). The 'third kind of knowledge', as explained by Nadler (2001) is a 'purely intellectual intuition of the essence of things':

> This 'third kind of knowledge' – beyond both random experience and ratiocination – sees things not in their temporal dimension, not in their duration and in relation to other particular things, but under the aspect of eternity, that is, abstracted from all considerations of time and place and situated in their relationship to God and his attributes. They are apprehended, that is, in their conceptual and causal relationship to the universal essences (thought and extension) and the eternal laws of nature.
>
> (Nadler, 2001)

In the psychoanalytic context, I use 'selected facts', which emerge through the unconscious, pass through the primitive-psychosomatic, to become semi-conscious information. From there, they are processed through conscious fantasy, reverie, linking-thinking and interpretation as a form of Spinozan *scientia intuitiva,* which informs my analytic understanding and makes for a mutative language. Such intuitive knowledge, arising out of critical analytic thinking and reverie, may then be expressed through interpretations which effectively and affectively challenge a patient's apperception of basic lacks (or loss) of self, subjective and private non-existence. Thereby, they may 'catastrophically' change a person's psychic structure: the disturbing loss of the effectiveness of a defensive persona-mask and the slow but sure emergence of a '*conatus*-as-*jouissance* self'.

For Bion, the coherence of the selected fact was originally seen in its Humean sense of 'constant conjunction', that is, giving coherence that makes sense to the observer; eventually, though, the coherence was seen as already existing, waiting to be intuited. This is a sublation into thought through psychosomatic information, identification and memory or mind. It is knowledge emerging and arising out of subjective and interpersonal somatic and psychic experience, i.e. from psychoid beta-chaos, confusion and not-knowing, through animal faith and reasoning (thinking through feeling) to 'intuitive knowledge' and so to interpretation.

My psychoanalytic attitude as an ethical position

I will now summarise my psychoanalytic attitude in Spinozan terms. In the face of not really knowing what is going on, whether intra-psychically, psychosomatically and relationally, amidst the forces of these five areas just outlined (the *conatus*, body-mind relations, passions and actions, free necessity), yet still using thinking, feeling, imagination and reason, I may further a psychotherapeutic style of intuitive knowledge, of *conatus intelligendi* which is both aesthetic and ethical.[11]

This involves the development of the symbolising function and the imaginative making of personal meaning, yet without losing the eternal and absolute necessity of matter and the basic matter of contingent necessity. It involves irony, ambivalence and negative capability. Concerning Keats' concept of negative capability, which Bion applied psychoanalytically, (Keats, 1817 in Bion, 1970, p. 125), David Wood, in his book *The Step Back* (2005), also says:

> The step back marks a certain shape of philosophical practice, one that does not just resign itself to, but affirms the necessity of, ambiguity, incompleteness, repetition, negotiation, and contingency. I have revived Keats's expression negative capability to capture this array of concepts.
>
> (Wood, 2005, p. 4)

A Spinozan position incorporating these five interrelated deductive or interpretative ideas does a lot of work for me. My psychosomatically embodied and countertransferentially informed interpreting of difficult emotional disorders and their relations is helped by such a Spinozan mind. The use of Spinozan ideas, other philosophical systems and clinical theories is a lens. It need not be a defensive manoeuvre; it does not necessarily avoid the affectivity of the emotional psychic encounter. Paradoxically, such philosophical and clinical theory enables me to experience the intense storms of transferential and countertransferential psychosomatic passion more openly because it enables a muscular emotional receptivity, an informed reverie and a critically directed thinking, rather than a hard psychic brittleness.

As I have been arguing before, substance monism helps me negotiate borderline subject-object identifications, while dual-aspect theory helps sort out pathological mind-body confusions. The *conatus* is still at work, albeit perversely, in borderline manoeuvres for self-preservation.

11 See Chapter Seven where Clark links Yovel's hypothesis of the *conatus intelligendi* to the epistemophilic impulse and the selected fact (Eds.).

Dynamic Spinozan models of human passions and actions, as well as ideas of the proscribed limits to possible change, helps me acquiesce to and integrate that which is eternally unchanging and unchangeable to achieve a subjective and creative sense of freedom within a determined universe, even to enjoy the tension (the *jouissance*) between one's pleasurable powers and their hard limitations. At the same time, I hold an animal faith in the necessary illusion of free choice, in the psychic reality of a sense of agency and free will in the face of a determined actuality (unconscious mind, body, brain, family, history and other contingencies): 'free necessity'.

Spinoza's non-dualistic identity theory, that is, a form of dual-aspect monism, and his proto-Nietzschean moral relativism (contextualised in an ethical comprehension), enhances my alpha function and capacity for going-on-being in the face of psychosomatic beta-destructiveness, rage, disorder and toxic projective identifications in the borderline battlefield, as well as to sorting through regressions to the pre-symbolic, attacks on symbolising, confused and confusing symbolic equations and other problems with the symbolising function, but without myself defensively resorting to pseudo-symbolising.

Faults and failures to the symbolising function, such as concrete thinking and the inability to imagine, arise in particular when persons have not been able to mourn the separation from the physical object (mother), have not achieved a depressive understanding, cannot use fantasy as an 'as if' way to re-creative linking-thinking, and thus for them 'the psychic is made matter' rather than matter being 'imbued with psychic significance' (Britton, 1998, p. 138). Paradoxically or counter-intuitively, I find that an effective way to sort out failures to symbolise and the pathological materialising of the psychic, and so to create a mental environment through which a person may start to develop real symbolising, is for the analyst to 'think imaginatively' through a lens of a Spinozan mind-body identity theory.

The pre-symbolic is the primal identity of the Spinozan *Deus sive Natura*, God or Nature, of the psychoid and of the psychosomatic 'bodymind' substrate. Therefore, the basic pre-symbolic realm is not intrinsically pathological; rather, it is its non-development, mal-development or misuse that is pathological: the idea of the mind as the idea of internal and external objects, rather than the emotional and thinking mind being its objects, has not developed and so is confused and operates in states of pathological identification, in which the emotional and thinking mind is its objects. Drawing on Rhode's (1994) concept of psychotic metaphysics, I have described how borderline persons unconsciously demonstrate a radical metaphysics.[12]

A Spinozan *Anschauungsweise* or 'manner of apprehending things'[13] enhances my analytic understanding in such realms of borderline confusions of fantasy/reality, mind/body, self/non-self, destruction/creation. I use such Spinozan thinking both for

12 See Chapter Seven (Eds.).

13 For Heine, this 'manner of apprehending things' or *Anschauungsweise* was Spinoza's fundamental pantheism, which underlies and motivates his metaphysics, politics and ethics (Goetschel, 2004, p. 260).

the objects of this concern (the *conatus* as psychoid or psychosomatic libido, mind-brain-body relations, a psychology of relations of personal and interpersonal affects, his ethical naturalism, etc.) and for the pleasurable power of using such a reasoning and intellectual intuition. Thus, my *Anschauungsweise* is variously deductive, empirical and pragmatic. Or rather, simultaneously so, because (in a Spinozan sense) form, content and affect are identical.

My psychoanalytic use of Spinoza's concepts in practice (action)

I will now show how my Spinozan-inspired *Anschauungsweise* works in practice in my work with personality disorders, particularly focusing on the problems of thinking through confusing psychosomatic forces that are affective in these destructive transferential and countertransferential fields. The main problems with which I work are near-psychotic destructive borderline disorders, narcissistic defensiveness, severe damage to the self (loss of self), various forms of depression and anxiety, obsessional thoughts and actions and sometimes psychogenic autistic pockets. These also involve disturbances to the development of the symbolising function and, therefore, to disturbed internal and external relations and matters of identification. The *jouissance* dynamic and other Spinozan modes of thinking contribute considerably to my mental formulations, responses and interactions. For example, the *jouissance* of borderline persons is expressed through a defiant and driven form of the *conatus*, that is, in aggressive-defensive behaviours, moving through a concatenation of emotions, such as: (appetite and) desire > (lack and) frustration > (psychosomatic and) emotional pain > (impotent) anger > (projective identification and) active destructiveness-as-power.

Work with borderline personality disorders involves experiences from the psychoid realm, which, through states of identification and confusion, both personally and interpersonally, and even between mind and the world, demonstrate a primitive fused identity. Borderline states and relations unconsciously demonstrate that 'the mind is the idea of the body' in a confused, confusing and primitive way.

The analytic frame holds the ostensibly unwanted but inwardly called for healthy clarification and way out of psychosomatic confusion and disorder caused by the wrong oedipal victories. I can be hated and murdered because I am not enough, but I more than just survive: I am a self who perseveres and goes on being and so can reliably be there to be used by you in so far as I allow that to be so, but the price is the reality of my 'other-minded-ness' and the laws of love, war and separateness that I set.

Finally, I remember that it is 'me as their phantasy' that is envied, that my body and mind need not be made to identify with and suffer as the target of their psychosomatic missiles. I have a separate and healthier mind, and I know that I am a separate person. This analytic position of recognition of phantasy, of de-identification and of the reality of actual separateness is vital to the management of both destructive borderline forces and narcissistic adhesiveness.

The sometimes possible borderline achievement of mourning the limits of analysis (and all attachments and relations) can indeed become a movement to a truly muscular position beyond the grief for lacked and lost goods and beyond the recurrent destruction of all subsequent good objects. It may become a fiercely honest acceptance of the limits of their life to such an extent that it is accompanied by a recognition and knowledge of their angry loneliness and of the limits of their life's goods, which is also vitalising. However, the actively destructive forces still do go on to the very end and beyond: a perverse *conatus*.

In analysis with borderline 'beta matters', the analyst is often made to have or 'be' the mind, brain, body and the neurological energy for and of the other and thence to have to actively feel, think, observe, link, imagine, remember, mourn and interpret one's way through psychosomatic blocks, pains and passions. This is experienced bottom-up, from the autonomic system and, thence, processed through symbolisation and thought to a relational psychosomatic order, from beta chaos to alpha functioning.

Bion (1970) argued that the analytic attitude at the beginning of each meeting should be one of 'negative capability' (Keats, 1817, in Bion, 1970, p. 125), the analyst should be 'without memory, desire and understanding'. By this, he meant: without preconceived ideas based on subjective memories of previous history, without desire for ideal progress and change, and without believing you know an absolute truth, theoretically or even through experience (including that you both can understand as well as not quite know what is really going on). In this way our observations and interpretations can be challenging, radical and liberating.

As wounded healers, we heal through the survival, management and recycling of our own wounds as best we can, putting our madness to good uses!

Final musings on my Spinozan *Anschauungsweise*

The substance of psychosomatic activity is psychoid, beta-elemental and psychotic. The learnt languages and thinking of the inter-related mind-brain-body activities may organise this substance into valuable creations as well as normal neuroses and/or pathological. 'Beta bits' are transformed into 'alpha functioning' by thinking, feeling (and imagining) out of and through our internal and interpersonal psychosomatic or emotional frustrations.

Intuitive and rational thinking about (reflecting on and understanding of) ideas of ideas, affects and passions in the analytic relationship is an alpha functioning of beta pre-order and disorder. It is a useful ordering of the substantial primitive-beta reality which precedes and goes on actively being even after any ordering.

As we have seen, for Spinoza, mind and body are two different perceptions of one activity. In the *massa confusa* of borderline and other personality disorders, this Spinozan principle is acted out through projective identification, communication and information by psychic evacuation, infection, invasion, destruction and/or seduction and, in narcissistic cases, which are, *inter alia*, a defence against borderline fear, defeat and anger, we are instead subject to adhesive identification and extractive introjection.

In analysis with 'borderline beta matters', the analyst is sometimes made to have or become the mind, brain, body and the neurological energy for and of the other and thence to process, feel, think, link, interpret, observe, explore, imagine and recreate our way through the psychosomatic blocks, passions and pains.

Conclusion

My Spinozan *Anschauungsweise* helps order 'mad' internal and interpersonal relations and mind/body identity confusions in psychotherapeutic work with borderline disorders. Thus, too, my analytic thinking and action are helped both by a conjunction of a Spinozan process of deductive reasoning as well as by certain Spinozan matters of objective perception and attention. I use Spinozan ideas as 'transitional objects', incorporating realms of both ideational thinking and emotive imagination, separate and infected, focusing on details and open to intuition, internally related to imagination and idea, externally related to matter, other bodies and minds, let alone being simultaneously both knowing and unknowing.

I would suggest that a naturalistic Spinozan approach to our thinking, feeling, imagining and acting in this peopled world (and in analytic relations) may sometimes help us mourn and make out of our normal madness, loneliness and melancholia something emotionally better and a psychosomatic life that is more realistic and joyful. An increase of self-awareness and irony is sometimes possible through a strong and real enough (analytic) relationship. Such a relation emerges from and reinforces a sense of personal reality and a more realistic idea of the other-peopled-world, which in turn also enables an acceptance or integration of the reality of other minds, the limits of personal control and an acquiescence to natural contingencies. This is surely a psychological realisation of a neo-Spinozan naturalism and an ethical attitude towards necessity.

Personal and interpersonal psychosomatic relations can sometimes be experienced, as Hampshire said, 'in present curiosity and enjoyment, in the company of this body and now' (Hampshire, 1994, p. 10). However, I would add that they are sometimes also experienced through the identifications and communications of intolerable psychosomatic lacks and handicaps in the dangerous but lively company of very difficult 'bodymind' confusions now.

It is out of a bedrock of atheistic naturalism and scepticism that there emerges our world of passionate attachments and emotional pains, love and hate, companionship and loneliness, a sense of beauty and of ugliness, of virtue, reason and ethics, of wilful destruction and imagination, the making of meaning, memory and mourning and all other such psychic realities or fantasies. So, too, our human condition (all of us being determined parts of a determined universe) incorporates the necessary and pleasurable illusion of free will and creativity. I think that this hard natural foundation is structurally essential to a healthy development of the latter subjective qualities.

To mix the languages of Spinoza, Santayana and Bion, I would say that a psychically healthy and ethical life depends upon us dismantling the defensive use of idealism and fantasies of absolute knowledge and of progressive teleology. Rather, we may try to apprehend ourselves as part of nature and understand our judgements with anti-egotistic relativism, pluralism and an ironic scepticism. Through a good enough therapeutic relationship, we may be able to psychically 'recycle' the disorders that arise out of our experience of fateful contingency, relating actively to our internalised family, to our own and other people's emotional minds and bodies, remembering and mourning our loves, hates and hurts, realising that the management of lacks and failures can be as mad (though necessary and understandable) as their maddening objects or conditions, integrating a healthy acquiescence to the limits of psychosomatic permanence: that is, to our mortality and to other supra-personal realities. In this way, we may think through apparently unthinkable frustrations, limitations and pains, and our difficult endeavours may increase our active enjoyment of this embodied life in the face of a wonderfully meaningless universe.

References

Addison, A. (2008). 'Reframing the Unconscious: A View of Jung's Psychoid Unconscious Then and Now.' *Paper Given at Journal of Analytical Psychology Conference*, 10 April, 2008, Orta, Italy. Unpublished.

Beiser, F. (2003). *The Romantic Imperative: The Concept of Early German Romanticism*. Cambridge, MA and London: Harvard University Press.

Bennett, J. (1984). *A Study of Spinoza's Ethics*. Cambridge: Cambridge University Press.

Bion, W. (1962). *Learning from Experience*. Northvale, NJ: Jason Aronson.

Bion, W. (1970). *Attention and Interpretation*. London: Tavistock.

Britton, R. (1998). *Belief and Imagination: Explorations in Psychoanalysis*. London: Routledge.

Bunker, J. (2006). 'Spinoza as Empiricist'. Lecture based on PhD, Presented at the 'Wandering with Spinoza' Conference at the VCA Centre in Melbourne, Australia; 13–15 September 2006.

Curley, E. (1988). *Behind the Geometrical Method: A Reading of Spinoza's Ethics*. Princeton, NJ: Princeton University Press.

Curley, E., ed. and trans. (1994). *A Spinoza Reader: The Ethics and Other Works*. Princeton, NH: Princeton University Press.

Damasio, A. (2003). *Looking for Spinoza; Joy, Sorrow and the Feeling Brain*. Orlando: Harcourt.

Deleuze, G. (1988). *Spinoza. Practical Philosophy*. Translated by R. Hurley. San Francisco: City Lights.

Deugd, C. de (2004). 'Spinoza and Freud: An Old Myth Revisited'. In *Ethica IV: Spinoza on Reason and the 'Free Man'*. Y. Yovel & G. Segal, eds. New York: Little Room Press.

Donagan, A. (1988). *Spinoza*. Chicago: Chicago University Press.

Garrett, A. (2003). *Meaning in Spinoza's Method*. Cambridge: Cambridge University Press.

Garrett, D. (2002). 'Spinoza's Conatus Argument'. In *Spinoza: Metaphysical Themes*. Olli I. Koistinen & John I. Biro, eds. Oxford: Oxford University Press.

Garrett, D. (2007). 'All Necessarily So'. Review of S. Nadler, *Spinoza's 'Ethics.' Times Literary Supplement*, 19 October 2007, 5455: 7–8.

Garrett, D. (2008). 'Representation and Consciousness in Spinoza's Naturalistic Theory of the Imagination'. In *Interpreting Spinoza: Critical Essays*. C. Huenemann, ed. Cambridge and New York: Cambridge University Press.
Goetschel, W. (2004). *Spinoza's Modernity*. Madison, WI: University of Wisconsin Press.
Hampshire, S. (1987). *Spinoza*. Harmondsworth: Penguin (Original work published, 1951).
Hampshire, S. (1994). 'Truth and Correspondence in Spinoza'. In *Spinoza By 2000: The Jerusalem Conferences. Volume II: Spinoza on Knowledge and the Human Mind*. Y. Yovel, ed. Leiden: Brill.
Hampshire, S. (2002, October 24). 'The Spinoza Solution'. *The New York Review of Books*, 49(16): 55.
Hampshire, S. (2005). *Spinoza and Spinozism*. Oxford: Clarendon Press.
Jarrett, C. (2007). *Spinoza: A Guide for the Perplexed*. London: Continuum.
Jung, C. (1970). 'On the Nature of the Psyche'. In *The Structure and Dynamics of the Psyche*. Vol. 8 of *The Collected Works of C.G. Jung*. R. Hull, trans. 2nd edn. London: Routledge & Kegan Paul.
Kirby-Smith, H. (1997). *A Philosophical Novelist: George Santayana and the Last Puritan*. Carbondale: Southern Illinois University Press.
Lloyd, G. (1994). *Part of Nature*. Ithaca, NY: Cornell University Press.
Lloyd, G. (1996). *Routledge Philosophy Guidebook to Spinoza and the Ethics*. London: Routledge.
Lloyd, G. (2008). *Providence Lost*. Cambridge, MA: Harvard University Press.
Marrama, O. (2017). 'Consciousness, Ideas of Ideas and Animation in Spinoza's Ethics'. *British Journal for the History of Philosophy*, 25(3): 506–525.
Montag, W. (1999). *Bodies, Masses, Powers: Spinoza and His Contemporaries*. London: Verso.
Montag, W. & Stolze, T., eds. (1997). *The New Spinoza*. Minneapolis: University of Minnesota Press.
Nadler, S. (2001). 'Baruch Spinoza'. In *Stanford Encyclopaedia of Philosophy*. https://plato.stanford.edu/entries/spinoza/ (accessed 24 October 2008).
Nadler, S. (2006a). *Spinoza's Ethics: An Introduction*. Cambridge: Cambridge University Press.
Nadler, S. (2006b) Unpublished correspondence to Clark, 4th April, 2006.
Negri, A. (1991). *The Savage Anomaly: The Power of Spinoza's Metaphysics and Politics*. Trans. M. Hardt. Minneapolis: Minnesota University Press.
Negri, A. (2004). *Subversive Spinoza:(Un)Contemporary Variations*. Edited by T. Murphy; Translated by T. Murphy, M. Hardt, T. Stolze and C. Wolfe. Manchester: Manchester University Press.
Rhode, E. (1994). *Psychotic Metaphysics*. London: Karnac Books.
Rosenthal, H. (1989). *The Consolations of Philosophy: Hobbes' Secret, Spinoza's Way*. Philadelphia: Temple University Press.
Santayana, G. (1910). *The Life of Reason or The Phases of Human Progress. Reason in Common Sense*. London: Archibald Constable & Co.
Santayana, G. (1926). 'Normal Madness'. In *Dialogues in Limbo*. New York: Scribner.
Segal, H. (1950). 'Some Aspects of the Analysis of a Schizophrenic'. *International Journal of Psycho-Analysis*, 31: 268–278.
Segal, H. (1957). 'Notes on Symbol Formation'. *International Journal of Psycho-Analysis*, 38: 391–397.
Spinoza, B. (1993). 'A Political Treatise'. In *A Theologico-Political Treatise and A Political Treatise*. R. Elwes, ed., A. Gosset, trans. London: Dover edition.
Sprigge, T. (2006). *The God of Metaphysics*. Oxford: Oxford University Press.
Steinberg, D. (2000). *On Spinoza*. Belmont, CA: Wadsworth.
Wartofsky, M. (1973). 'Action and Passion: Spinoza's Construction of a Scientific Psychology'. In *Spinoza: A Collection of Critical Essays*. M. Grene, ed. Garden City, NY: Anchor Books.

Wittgenstein, L. (1933). *Tractatus Logico-Philosophicus*. With English translation by C. K. Ogden and F. P. Ramsay. London: Routledge & Kegan Paul.

Wood, D. (2005). *The Step Back: Ethics and Politics after Deconstruction*. Albany, NY: State University of New York Press.

Yovel, Y., ed. (1999). 'Transcending Mere Survival'. In *Spinoza by 2000: The Jerusalem Conferences. Volume III: Desire and Affect: Spinoza as Psychologist*. Y. Yovel, ed. New York: Little Room Press.

Chapter 18

Why (and how) psychoid relations matter

Unpublished, May, 2018[1]

Introduction

As psychoanalysts, we work with both neurotic and more psychotic unconscious phantasies and defensive relational manoeuvres which patients have developed in order to survive and live with a deeply disturbing and disordering early environment. We work 'mind-to-mind' – that is, with words and other communications about internal and interpersonal relations, desire and disgust, attachment and loss or lack, passion and shame. These are re-constellated in the regressions, dependencies and familiarities of the transference/countertransference and thereby, the provisional making and recurrent re-making of symbolic meaning. Clinically this involves a necessary prioritising of the subjectively affective (and effective) mind and its unconscious phantasies and relations. 'Mind and mind-to-mind' (imaginative, emotional and thoughtful minds) are the starting premises of our metapsychology. This is a technical requisite for our taking psyche as a projective, emotive, ideational, phantasy-making and phantasy-moved mind; for a developmentally normal, healthy and necessary differentiation of mind and body; and for our symbolic understanding.

The rest of this paper follows on from a 'yes but'. There is an ontological (rather than metapsychological) alternative to our conceptual and practical dualism of mind and body: namely by apprehending psyche as psychoid. This is a distinctively Jungian concept, which I have been building on and qualifying.[2] Jung was perhaps philosophically more of a Kantian/post-Kantian Idealist than I am. I have

1 An earlier version of this paper was given as an ANZSJA training seminar on September 1, 2017, in Auckland. Clark also worked on this paper in preparation for a conference in Ascona in July 2018; the last editorial changes were made on May 18, 2018 (Eds.).

2 Addison (2009) points out that it appears that Jung had already mentioned the term 'psychoid' in his first meeting with Freud in 1907, going so far as to suggest the unconscious be given the name 'psychoid'. Addison also traces the etymology of 'psychoid' as deriving from 'psyche' as meaning spirit, soul, breath, breath of life and the Greek suffix *-oeide* 'related to *eidos*, meaning shape or form or what is seen'. Thus the term 'may express an attempt to convey something about the manifest shape or form of the spirit, soul or mind, animated by the breath of life'. At the same time, related terms such as Latin *psychicus* have 'material and bodily' associations (Addison, 2009, p. 126) (Eds.).

DOI: 10.4324/9781003255826-19

an 'animal faith' in the primacy of matter and body, although such a given nature, such an inherent bio-structure, is subsequently nurtured, so bringing about a 'developed structure'. I also suggest that the psychoid manifests a vital interpersonal affectivity. Analytically, we are always working with mind as the subjective emotional meanings that we both derive from and give to bodily relations. My task is to conceptually heal the split between the mind and the body, without thereby confusing fantasy and reality or ideational and sensory-somatic realms, etc. However, a developmental confusion of fantasy and reality (and a confusion of zones) is symptomatic of the affective disorders of borderline patients.

The psychoid, like an ever-present pet dog, has forever been my faithful companion, close, intimate, irritating and demanding. As I describe more fully in the following chapter,[3] personal body-issues drew me to live in India in my late teens, where I first studied the body-denying Jains, then the body-valuing Parsee Zoroastrians. But later, at university, my schizoid fascinations with the body suddenly became urgent when my 'pet dog' savaged me with serious physical illness. This problematic 'matter with body' eventually pulled me into analysis. This difficult, omni-present dog refers to the psychoid soma and the meanings of its matters and developmental relations and includes the 'mind as the idea of the body', or 'soma' (body processes and body relations). It is the subject and object of unconscious and conscious developmental meaning/meaning-making. The majority of my publications, seminars and presentations over the years did not only emerge out of difficult clinical relations working with (and being worked over by) destructive borderline patients and their infectious, primitive, psychoid projective identifications. They also relate to my own on-going psyche-soma preoccupations.

Clinical theory must not be top-down but rather arise out of problematic therapeutic experience as well as personal experience. In *Faces in a Cloud* (1993), Atwood and Stolorow argue that much clinical theory is predicated on an over-arching metapsychology, but this metapsychology is often clinically irrelevant. I mostly agree, although I also think that ontology does have a useful place in our theory. However, although the matter of the meanings given to the psychoid and difficult somatic relations has preoccupied my clinical thinking, I now do also wonder: so what? My assertion of the 'primacy of matter and body-matter' sometimes seems to be banal. What clinical difference does such a basic materialist predicate make? Why bother to discuss the psychological apprehension of body as *soma*, as a unit of emotional meaning, as *Leib* rather than *Körper* or *physis* (here drawing on the early 19th-century Swiss philosopher Ignaz Troxler)? What is clinically useful about a recognition that the psyche and all psychic relations are actually and always psychoid? Maybe this conversation with you will be a conduit through which to find out whether any personal, theoretical and clinical relevance arises out of consideration of 'the psychoid'.

Going back over what I have thought, written and spoken about for well over 40 years, I realise how repetitive I am, how mono-toned (monotonous?). In the

3 See Chapter Nineteen (Eds.).

terms of Isaiah Berlin (1953), I am a hedgehog, not a fox: 'a fox knows many things, but a hedgehog knows one important thing'. Except, as I say, I'm not quite sure that my one thing is even important. Perhaps I only know one rather obvious thing.

Throughout my writings, I have been reusing case examples from previous papers because I do not wish to make public any recent case stories that should remain private and true to our discreet analytic relations. Nor do I wish to create fictionalised cases out of a collage of different clinical exchanges from different patients since doing so treats persons and events as typical and vaporises difference and uniqueness. I have recycled the deidentified/fictionalised cases of Pat,[4] Rose,[5] Jim[6] and Christine[7] since these first three cases have to do with transferential/countertransferential relations, acted out at a primitive, pre-symbolic and regressed psychoid level, and Christine depicts well the phenomenology of narcissistic relations. Although such clinical cases are of extreme psychosomatic and relational disorder, the psychoid and somatic are affective in all our therapeutic work relations. Indeed, it is substantially active for all of us, always.

To cite but one here, working with Pat involved both my not knowing what was going on but eventually coming to understand our 'consubstantial psychoid relations' and Pat beginning to symbolise and co-ordinate her terribly disordered somatic self. Pat was pathologically and chaotically unsure of her identity or, rather, identities. She lied and re-told matters about herself many times, was wildly unpredictable and was full of radical contradictions and alterations. She had psychogenic issues of repulsion arising out of a zonal confusion of fantasies and imaginings about her insides, vagina and stomach and their juices and contents. She was abjectly ashamed of her 'revolting bodily processes'. Such disgust also applied to others, especially women's bodies, which she 'really hated', and to men's sperm, which she found initially 'delicious' but then 'utterly foul': the desired and the disgusting are two responses to the same part-object. She was ashamed and furious that she was revealing these 'mad issues' to me.

How and why the psychoid matters

As I suggested previously, I retain some ambivalence about the role of any kind of pre-given theory in the clinical encounter. Given that caveat, I will now discuss some of my theoretical foundations: the *how* in my title. I proceed by first thinking philosophically before moving into the psychological (which is more imaginally, poetically and emotionally to do with relational experience). This is the *why* in my title. But, as already said, my construction and use of theory have arisen out of having to think about difficult clinical and affective psychosomatic,

4 See Chapter Five (Eds.).
5 See Chapter Seven (Eds.).
6 See Chapters Seven, Nine, Ten and Thirteen (Eds.).
7 See Chapters Nine, Thirteen and Sixteen (Eds.).

mind-body relations, which are personal and interpersonal, and which are more immediate and literally vitalising than metapsychological theory. It is a *sine qua non* that theory is internal and private and never spoken in an analytic relationship. It is part of my hidden analytic sub-structure. Furthermore, my writings are a continuation of my 'thinking through', aided by my internal helpful companions: Spinoza and Santayana above all, but also many other philosophers, analysts and many analysands.

My conceptual use of philosophy and the history of ideas, of ontological systems, is not, as such, clinically informative. It merely helps me think clearly and observe critically. Top-down theory can be a clarifying lens and give the practitioner a sure procedural footing. Some of us enjoy it for its intellectual worth and stimulation. It also disturbs my comfortable ideas and my 'knowing'. So, although theory is often used as a defensive disengagement, as an anti-relational, dissociative, schizoid defence against borderline murderousness (and against my countertransference hate of narcissistic falseness), it can help me think through difficult clinical problems.

I have written extensively about my use of Spinoza, my indebtedness to neo-Spinozan scholars and also George Santayana. Here, I draw on Santayana's organic psyche and on recent scholarship on Santayana. Of particular significance for me have been the writings of Michael Brodrick in 'Santayana's Amphibious Concepts' (2013), John Lachs' *On Santayana* (2006) and Jessica Wahman's 'Why Psyche Matters' (2006), which has influenced my own title for this chapter.

Santayana's organic psyche

I begin, however, with Santayana himself. Santayana elaborates upon a materialistic lineage where *psyche* and *physis* are both organic. This lineage is Epicurean (Santayana especially admired Lucretius), lives on through Spinoza's philosophy and thence becomes the naturalistic narrative of his own ontology. The psyche is 'that habit in matter which forms the human body and the human mind' (Santayana, 1922, p. 221). It encompasses our biology, neurobiology, functions and processes of self-preservation. As Martin Coleman explains,

> psyche is the self that one immediately cares about and is more essentially the body than the body itself. While psyche is not material, it is the organisation of matter in living creatures or the 'habit in matter' reproduced in organisms after their kind. The life of psyche is observable and a topic for biological study, and its behaviour and the events that influence it belong to the realm of matter.
>
> (Coleman, 2009, p. 199)

In Santayana's own words:

> The psyche is a natural fact, the fact that many organisms are alive, can nourish and reproduce themselves, and on occasion can feel and think . . . The machinery of growth, instinct, and action, like the machinery of speech, is all physical:

> but this sort of physical operation is called psychical because it falls within the trope of a life, and belongs to the self-defence and self-expression of a living organism . . . She is a mode of substance, a trope or habit established in matter.
>
> (Santayana, 1972, pp. 331–332)

In the *Realm of Spirit*, Santayana writes that 'the self-maintaining and reproducing pattern or structure of an organism, conceived as a power, is called a psyche' (Santayana, 1972, p. 569). He also wrote, in a letter to A. A. Roback in 1952, that 'The psyche is the life of the body with all its functions more or less combined to evoke consciousness and action' (in Kriss, 1952).

Psyche as an amphibious concept

The authors to whom I now turn all help in various ways to clarify what Santayana meant by this concept of psyche as a natural fact, power or mode of substance. I begin with Michael Brodrick, who likens Santayana's understanding of how 'some events encompass two different natures, the physical and the phenomenal' to that of 'amphibious creatures' who cover 'both water and land'. Furthermore, 'the most amphibious concept developed by Santayana' is that of the organic and epiphenomenal psyche (Brodrick, 2013, p. 246). Thus, Santayana's psyche is amphibious.

Examined from without, psyche is 'the self-maintaining and reproducing pattern or structure of an organism, conceived as a power'. The inner nature of psyche, on the other hand, is that of a 'moral unity' that consists of impulses, feelings, perceptions, memories and, in some cases, concepts (Brodrick, 2013, p. 247). In psychological terms, this 'amphibious' conception of the organic psyche is an understanding of body and its processes as primary but inherently incorporating other emergent epiphenomena such as consciousness, subjectivity, ideation, feeling and attachment. As Brodrick further observes:

> A theory of mind-body relations based on the concept of psyche as amphibious avoids the traditional mind-body problem, rendering epiphenomenalism and the other classic theories of mind-body relations obsolete. Even better, it acknowledges our experience of physical and mental facts as fully compatible while also acknowledging our experience of them as different and distinguishable.
>
> (Brodrick, 2013, p. 248)

To thus describe the psyche as 'amphibious' is a representation of Santayana's critical Spinozism, a dual-aspect theory where body and mind (and thereby body-mind relations) are apprehended as being different properties, or 'attributes' (and 'modes') of a unit of 'total natural events' (Brodrick, 2013, p. 248). The 'amphibious psyche' is a psyche conceived as having dual identities (identity dualism), a representation of Spinoza's two attributes of 'the single substance' (substance monism), and these two attributes each have infinite and finite 'modes'.

Psyche, spirit and mind-body relations

I now move on to John Lachs, who points out that Santayana's view of mind-body relations is markedly different from Descartes. Body is viewed as 'primary, substantial, continuous reality' whereas mind is the 'evanescent product of physical changes'. Santayana further distinguishes psyche from spirit; psyche (or soul) referring to 'the human organism' and spirit to 'consciousness' (Lachs, 2006, p. 46). He continues:

> This soul is not an immaterial principle or being but the very essence of natural, biological life. Santayana describes it as the physical structure, drives, and habits that constitute the organism as an extended activity-pattern in space and time.
>
> . . . Though physical in nature, the psyche's function is primarily moral, distinguishing good from bad and fighting for what it sees as right. It struggles to survive and flourish, sometimes successfully and sometimes against overwhelming odds. When the organism is extinguished it is the psyche that dies; having an organ no longer, spirit (or consciousness) simply follows suit.
>
> (Lachs, 2006, p. 47)

Thus, for Santayana, spirit and psyche are distinct concepts. As Coleman explains:

> Spirit is different from psyche and lies outside the realm of matter, yet it depends on psyche. Spirit – 'the actual light of consciousness' – is called forth by the sensitivity of psyche and is a culmination of psychic activity . . . Spirit is impotent in the material realm even as it observes the changing shapes of the material flux. Spirit is an expression of that flux and cannot deny its material basis.
>
> (Coleman, 2009, p. 198)

Lachs also points out that for Santayana

> material reality is . . . 'out of scale' with our senses: On the human level, we categorise the real in terms native to us and paint it in hues that, without us, it does not display. This is why Santayana calls consciousness a 'normal madness,' a distortion of the facts that is natural, everyday, and unavoidable for creatures in our situation.
>
> All of our conscious life suffers from this imaginative miscolouration.[8]
>
> (Lachs, 2006, p. 50)

Why psyche matters

If the material, natural and organic psyche is discerned as being where *natura naturata et naturans* (natural matters) are kept alive and are given narrative

8 On the disjunction in scale between the human senses and material reality, Lachs refers to Santayana, 1972, p. 274 (Eds.).

(literary) meaning, then the issue is where and how does this 'psyche' fit in the monistic unit of Santayana's four 'Realms *(attributes)* of Being'? In 'Why Psyche Matters', Wahman shows how critical the concept of psyche as material is to Santayana's ontology: 'Far from a tangential add-on to his four realms of being (essence, matter, spirit, and truth), the material psyche is fundamental to his understanding of what human existence entails' (Wahman, 2006, p. 133). Santayana poses two realms of being: spirit and matter. Spirit refers to conscious awareness. Psyche is part of matter as the principle of animation. Psyche is the 'organising principle of a living material being', a 'mode of matter' (Wahman, 2006, p. 134). Psyche is the animating force of a material body (Wahman, 2006). This has direct implications for psychotherapy, its art of interpretation and emphasis on metaphorical and symbolic thinking:

> The epistemological consequence of Santayana's recognition of psyche as a material principle obscured from conscious awareness is that psychological knowledge becomes a project of interpretation, a translation of the objects of awareness into explanatory metaphors. These metaphors may be the systematic models of physiology or the more openly mythological conceptions of psychotherapy.
>
> (Wahman, 2006, p. 143)

Santayana's solution to mind/body dualism is to place 'both elements on the side of matter' (pp. 143–144). Psyche, as matter, forms both 'the human body and the human mind' (Santayana, in Wahman, 2006, p. 143). However, instead of a mind/body duality, there is a dualism between spirit (consciousness) and psyche:

> But the dualism between spirit and psyche remains intact . . . In distinguishing between spirit and psyche as different realms of being, he is able to acknowledge how wholly transcendent to our conscious mind much of what we call our 'self' actually is.
>
> (Wahman, 2006, p. 144)

In *Narrative Naturalism,* Wahman explains how 'in Santayana's naturalist ontology spirit has no causal power: it illuminates and witnesses things that are of interest to psyche, but in itself possesses no agency' (Wahman, 2015, p. 109). Consciousness (spirit) has no generative effectivity: it is an observer and witness, always subjective and partial, sometimes mad, but also imaginative and symbolic and, as such, often useful to psyche. Indeed, it is out of the organic matter of psyche that consciousness emerges. It is only the 'organic psyche' (i.e. the psychoid *conatus*) that has active power, is effectual and originary. However, through its relations to matters of the 'psychoid *conatus*', the urges, panics and delusions of consciousness can drive us somewhat mad!

Santayana's psyche and spirit

As we have seen, a key element of Santayana's anti-transcendental epistemology is the distinction between psyche and spirit. Psyche is the animating principle of matter, whereas spirit denotes conscious awareness, the 'actual light of consciousness falling upon anything' (Santayana, 1972, p. 331). As Wahman puts it, 'Psyche, then, is the thinking, perceiving, intending, and willing organism; spirit, by contrast, is nothing more than the awareness of these energies as the organism goes about its daily life' (Wahman, 2015, p. 102). Wahman, citing Santayana's *Scepticism and Animal Faith* (Santayana, 1923, p. 147), observes how for Santayana, psyche is part of one's 'material being' and that

> instead of equating my self with my actual awareness, 'I must thicken and substantialise the self I believe in, recognising in it a nature that accepts or rejects events, a nature having a movement of its own, far deeper, more continuous and more biased than a discoursing mind: the self . . . is a living psyche'.
>
> (Wahman, 2001, p. 2)

For Santayana, 'psyche is the animating force of a material body that by some ultimately inconceivable miracle, produces spirit as an epiphenomenon of itself. Consciousness is wholly other to the matter which produces it, yet depends on it for its very existence' (Wahman, 2001, p. 2, citing Santayana, 1972, p. 335). Wahman also notes that:

> According to Santayana, matter is the substrative foundation . . . that grounds conscious reality. He describes it as being in continual flux and claims that, occasionally, this flux of material forces forms vortices, that is, organises itself into certain self-maintaining habitual patterns. In such cases, matter becomes life. This organization, this principle that organises material force into life – any kind of life – is a psyche. At the level of the human organism, the psyche is 'that habit in matter which forms the human body and the human mind'.
>
> (Wahman, 2001, p. 3, citing Santayana, 1922, p. 221)

My psychoanalytic use of dual-aspect substance monism, property dualism and Santayana's materialism

Using a combination of Spinozan monism, Santayana's organic psyche and the psychoid *conatus*, I would say that there is one Substance which we identify through two Attributes (out of infinite unknown attributes) i.e. the aspects of Extension and Thought. Thence, out of these two, we further identify (or 'modify') many modes. Sometimes, the two attributes are 'used' as if they are different for an applied or practical reason, such as the property dualism utilised in psychoanalytic theory and practice. However, the *conatus* and Santayana's organic psyche, or what I call the 'psychoid *conatus*', sublates this dualism back into a substantial monism.

As a psychotherapist, it may be useful to think and interpret as a 'property dualist'. Yet I can also understand and know the world, including the human world, as a dual-aspect substance monist. From a subjective perspective and an analytic position, I (necessarily) think and act (interpret) as a 'property dualist', working through and on the mind and its ideas. However, I am simultaneously a substance monist and a dual-aspect theorist, for whom the mind is the idea of the body: our fantasies, feelings, thoughts, our particular brains, bodies and all material things are modal attributes, expressions or aspects of a single substance. I also incorporate Santayana's assertion of the primacy of matter, of matter as substance and of consciousness (mind) as an epiphenomenon, as I do his elaboration of Spinoza into 'the body is an instrument, the mind its function, the witness and reward of its operation' (Santayana, 1910, p. 206). The clinical relevance of understanding of psyche as 'organic' (or as Aristotle put it, the 'entelechy of a natural organic body', Aristotle, *De Anima*, Bk. 2), as a 'psychoid matter' depends upon the various narratives and the literary psychology that we construct about it, how we symbolise it and thereby the way we use it interpretively.

Damasio on the *conatus* and neurobiology

Another writer whose work has helped me formulate my theoretical ideas in recent years is the neurobiologist Antonio Damasio. Damasio has a long-standing interest in Spinoza's work and cites both Hampshire and Nadler in the acknowledgments to his *Looking for Spinoza: Joy, Sorrow and the Feeling Brain* (2003, p. 337).

Damasio interprets Spinoza's *conatus* as related to striving, endeavour and tendency. Spinoza discusses how everything 'strives to persevere in its own being' and this striving is its essence. Damasio suggests that Spinoza's *conatus* 'implies that the living organism is constructed so as to maintain the coherence of its structures and functions against numerous life-threatening odds' and that:

> The conatus subsumes both the impetus for self-preservation in the face of danger and opportunities and the myriad actions of self-preservation that hold the parts of a body together. In spite of the transformations the body must undergo as it develops, renews its constituent parts, and ages, the conatus continues to form the same individual and respect the same structural design.
>
> What is Spinoza's conatus in current biological terms? It is the aggregate of dispositions laid down in brain circuitry that, once engaged by internal or environmental conditions, seeks both survival and well-being.
>
> (Damasio, 2003, p. 36)

Damasio links feelings, the 'mind as idea of body' and the *conatus* as follows:

> Feelings are perceptions, and I propose that the most necessary support for their perception occurs in the brain's body maps. These maps refer to parts of the

> body and states of the body. Some variation of pleasure or pain is a consistent content of the perception we call feeling.
>
> (Damasio, 2003, p. 85)

Damasio's hypothesis is

> that a feeling is the perception of a certain state of the body along with the perception of a certain mode of thinking and of thoughts with certain themes. Feelings emerge when the sheer accumulation of mapped details reaches a certain stage.
>
> (Damasio, 2003, p. 86)

In regard to the relationship between the *conatus* and what he calls 'somatosensing maps', Damasio writes:

> The origin of feelings is the body in a certain number of its parts. But now we can go deeper and discover a finer origin underneath that level of description: the many cells that make those body parts and exist both as individual organisms with their own conatus and as cooperative members of the regimented society we call the human body, held together by the organism's own conatus.
>
> The contents of feelings are the configurations of body state represented in somatosensing maps . . . Finally, we can add that the living cells that constitute the somatosensing brain regions, as well as the neural pathways that transmit signals from body to brain, are not likely to be indifferent pieces of hardware. They probably make a critical contribution to the quality of the perceptions we call feelings.
>
> (Damasio, 2003, pp. 132–133)

In regard to Spinoza's writings on the body, Damasio quotes a translation of Spinoza's six postulates from Part II of the *Ethics* as follows:

1 The human body is composed of a number of individual parts, of diverse nature, each one of which is in itself extremely complex.
2 Of the individual parts composing the human body some are fluid, some soft, some hard.
3 The individual parts composing the human body, and consequently the human body itself, are affected in a variety of ways by external bodies.
4 The human body stands in need for its preservation of a number of other bodies, by which it is continually, so to speak, regenerated.
5 When the fluid part of the human body is determined by an external body to impinge often on another soft part, it changes the surface of the latter, and, as it were, leaves the impression thereupon of the external body which impels it.

6 The human body can move external bodies, and arrange them in a variety of ways.

(Spinoza, cited in Damasio, 2003, pp. 210–211).

As we have seen, Damasio does a persuasive job of showing how Spinoza's postulates could be compatible with contemporary neurobiology.

A cautionary word about neuroscience

Whilst acknowledging the explanatory value of neuroscience, I argue that, in the context of psychotherapy, neuroscience is best understood as being both a) the object of systematic observation, measurement and experiment (the formulation, testing and modification of hypotheses) and b) as an imaginatively and therefore a psychologically usable narrative. To hold this double apprehension enables both positions to qualify each other and so mitigate absolute reductionism on the one hand and ethereal fantasy on the other. As a reminder, my own psychological position entails utilising 'property dualism' within a form of 'substance monism'.

Psychological change

This is an appropriate place to reconsider the tricky matter of inherent, neurological and/or structural limits to the degree of possible behavioural and emotional change. To what extent are there determined personality characteristics (which is more than typology)? Some persons seem to have been born with an intense form of sensitivity and so a latent propensity to develop a psychogenic personality disorder. Their sensitivity, emotionality and nervousness are often seen by parents and others as 'over-sensitivity'. The distressed and 'difficult' child is often not understood or accepted and if, for various reasons, they are not as easy to love, they may feel unlovable. And so the psychogenic builds on 'the given' and 'the given' is over-determining matter and the primacy of body. Such given emotional and behavioural conditions are evident diagnostically as well as countertransferentially when working with angry borderline behaviour and other personality disorders.

As we know, neurologically, a person is much determined by the amygdala, the hippocampus and the prefrontal areas. The latter does not belong to the traditional limbic circuit, but its intense bidirectional connections with the thalamus, amygdala and other subcortical structures account for the important role it plays in the genesis and expression of affective states. Is this the brain area we are really working with psychotherapeutically, especially in the field of personality disorders? This matter of neurological determination is surely pertinent to our consideration of the psychoid in our interpretive and relational practices. Some basic knowledge of the relevant neurobiology helps me with my heteropathic understanding and management of strong affective reactions, such as of complementary countertransferential maternal feelings of hate in Winnicott's sense (Winnicott, 1949).

There are other determining body-matters and their ever-changing conditions, such as the effects of different hormones and varying hormone levels and other such metabolic conditions. To say more about these is beyond the scope of my competence, so I here merely indicate their obvious relevance.

As we drop further into psychosomatic experience, a reminder that my use of the more or less synonymous terms 'psychosomatic', 'psyche-soma unit', 'bodymind' (Grotstein, 1997) and 'psychoid *conatus*' are idiosyncratic and not axiomatic. Strictly speaking *soma* (as distinct from *physis*) already means body and body relations as subject and object of meaning, rather than anatomy and physiology. Following Winnicott, one can locate the self in one's body, the body being the root of development, out of which evolves the psychosomatic partnership. Self is a body-self, 'psyche here means the *imaginative elaboration of somatic parts, feelings and functions*, that is, of physical aliveness' (Winnicott, 1954, p. 202).

For Jung, the psychoid was a concept applicable to virtually any archetype, expressing the essentially unknown but experienceable connection between psyche and matter, a sort of Schopenhauer or Von Hartmann unconscious 'Will' which is partly unknown and unknowable, partly experienceable because a personally embodied 'thing in itself'. However, I suggest that the psychoid is simultaneously both 'bodily matter and sense' and 'mental image and idea'. At the psychoid level, body, image and idea are a unit, experienced or expressed with and through dual aspects, the different 'attributes' of a single substance ('substance monism') or, in the human animal, of a 'bodymind'. I also understand 'the psychoid realm' as being simultaneously both an object for scientific investigation and phenomenologically as a symbolic 'as if', a unit of meaning, i.e. as both organic function and as intuited idea or symbol of instantiated phenomena. This means that the 'psychoid realm' (or 'psychoid processes' or 'psychoid substance' or my 'psychoid *conatus*') can itself be conceived, apprehended and comprehended from a dual-aspect perception. My idea of the psychoid *conatus* (where *conatus* means the inherent striving for self-preservation, self-regulation and an increase in self-power) is derived from Santayana's use of 'organic psyche' as a reiteration of Spinoza's *conatus* (Kirby-Smith, 1997). Sometimes, I oscillate between a dual-aspect theory (Spinoza) and a critical belief in the primacy of matter and body, that mentation is emergent and so a secondary epiphenomenon (Santayana). Hence my neologism, 'the psychoid *conatus*'.

However, I am now more inclined to say that this doubly conceived or doubly identified 'substance' is ultimately (or basically) the supra-personal reality and force of matter or body and that this is the adamant fatefulness of our biology, our living, mortal bodies and that of others in our world. And thence from body-matter first come the various typical (rather than 'archetypal') emotive, poetic meanings we give to matter, body, other bodies and embodied-ness. Out of these bodily matters emerge the typical and common energetic aspects of our world, life, experience and relationships, and from which we make our narratives, fantasies, imaginings and images, our myths, poetry and music. It is the primacy of matter and our own bio-matter that gives the necessary impetus to the emergence and unconscious formation of the so-called 'archetypes per se' and thence to the 'archetypes', or, as I prefer, 'image schemas'. Body matter, body process and neurobiology are the foundations of our structural (and relational) development, bottom-up.

More psychologically, I interpret Santayana's 'psyche' as 'a material system' which incorporates the emergence, development and on-going flux of self-regulating and self-preserving (psychoid) processes, i.e. the 'psychoid *conatus*'. The psychoid *conatus* can, therefore, be understood as the psyche-soma's auto-immune system, including its autonomic nervous system. It can be further understood as an epiphenomenon of our general organic (bio-physical, physiological and particularly our neurological) functioning, which is self-maintaining, self-preserving and self-enhancing, psychically desirous (hungry, competitive, aggressive) and/or fearful and defensive, as well as adaptive.

Finally, I also emphasise that will-power and even reason are basically as much driven by the psychoid *conatus* as are fear and panic (fight, flight and freeze). So are appetite and desire (to possess and/or devour) in so far as reason has to do with self-preservation by using a wider comprehension than just an ego-centric focus. So, as well as apprehending the body as a thing of bio-matter and functional physiological processes, the *conatus* is also the raw force that generates the emergence of our thinking. We can and do also apprehend body as a unit of meaning, or the meanings we give to body and bodily relations, to mind-body relations, to the 'bodymind', to psychosomatic relations, to body as a subjective object and as a subjective 'event': i.e. body as soma. We all somatise, and (as Segal says) that which we somatise, we may yet be able to symbolise.

Our clinical issue, then, is: how to help the patient become open to the possible emergence of affective linking and memory and so to symbolisation in the face of adamant or repetitive somatisation. By somatisation, I mean somatisation as a defence against both the patient's pre- and anti-symbolic limitations and against the furious somatic force of primitive borderline acting out. Then our task is the therapeutic survival of, management and, thence, relatively healthy movement of these stuck and mutually painful psychoid processes and relations.

My six basic hypotheses are as follows:

1 The psychoid is our common 'amphibious' nature.
2 The psychoid is the primary and ultimate unit which is substantially omnipresent under all subsequent developments and differentiations.
3 It is also the super-ego's responses and reactions to physical and unconscious impulses and forces that drive us mad, not the natural unconscious forces themselves, unless, of course, such forces are actually psychotic and delusional.
4 All affect, all emotion is physical (as well as mental); psychic matters are psychoid matters; i.e. you cannot reduce the body (and its emotional meanings and memories) to anything else, certainly not to a generative 'mind'.
5 All psychoid processes are affectively interpersonal (as well as personal).
6 Understanding psyche as 'organic' or as a 'psychoid matter' has clinical relevance depending on how we symbolise and use this understanding interpretively.

Within this psychoid and pre-verbal relational field, both the analyst and the analytic relationship itself functions as an active container, a 'receptacle-processor', a 'bodymind' and a 'thinking breast' into which pre-symbolic beta matter and internalised confusion are evacuated. It is also a conduit for urgent communication, often sickening or seductive, sore or sexual (it stirs the teeth, muscles, genitals) and so demands internal recycling into a more integrated co-ordination and a separation out of identification into differentiation. Hopefully, through this recycling and differentiation, the lacks, losses and limitations that were once experienced as intolerable can be mourned and linkages made so there may emerge a more realistic symbolic functionality.

I am trying to link the psychotic transference to the psychoid to the psychosensory, psychosomatic or embodied countertransference, especially in borderline and regressed relations to the primitive psychic in-formation and projective identification as urgent communication, to intuitive knowledge or 'selected facts' and the analyst/analysis 'actively containing' and processing the 'separation needs and demands' of psychosomatic beta-confusion and symbolic equivalence. An analyst is not just 'a container', but an 'active container'. This may be another way of naming the analyst as 'a thinking breast', though as a poetic metaphor, it carries a slightly different sense. We can see (and sense) the primitive and fierce actions of *conatus* most clearly in the savagely raw and primitive manoeuvres of borderline acting out/acts, including acts of perverse destructiveness and self-destructiveness which paradoxically aim to assert an ideal of self and to express and communicate most acutely and urgently that self's lacks, wounds and desperate needs. It is even through such acts and events that the 'psychoid *conatus*' can yet be understood as the engine of emergent self-consciousness.

Psychoid processes are essentially embodied and embodying and are primitively emotional and feeling, and yet thence may become the raw engine of thought-making and meaning-making. This is where 'mind' is most obviously 'the idea of the body'. All this is but an ontological concept, i.e. a provisional and hypothetical languaging of our human condition or way of being. The next level (less general and more subjective) is about how this becomes individuated. I would say individuated in or through *jouissance* or 'passions'.

By 'passions' I mean:

- Desires and sufferings;
- Satisfactions and frustrations;
- Desires, lusts, loves;
- Fears (fight, flight, freeze), disgusts (which are often directed towards the same objects as lusts), hates (stop, attack, kill).

'Lust and disgust', as two impulse-reactions to the same object, are manifestations of the more physical-bodily level of 'love and hate'. As primitive responses to primitive part-objects, they are easily and often split in a schizoid, pre-ambivalent way. This is not always a matter of developmental stuckness or regression;

pre-ambivalence is not always pathologically paranoid-schizoid. It is also naturally and necessarily 'as it is' and can and should be accepted 'as is' because raw body matter is always the natural basis of the cooked and remains and is never lost through the cooking. All these passions are normal affects of the psychoid and psychosomatic *conatus* and their sometimes maddening affects as they tangle and struggle, get tensely stretched, torn and pushed around by the conflicting forces of the super-ego (and conscience), e.g. guilt and deep existential shame.

Retreat, psychogenic autistic dissociation, angry depression and borderline behaviour are defensive responses to a lack of primary love, parental hate (murderous envy), disgust, fear, bewilderment, 'perverted love' (incestuous lust) or disconnected indifference. Angry depression, malignant narcissism and, above all, borderline hate make for the most psychosomatically poisonous relational realms. Here, I refer the reader to reconsider Jim and his cathedral dream.[9]

Why is the psychoid so evident in borderline behaviour and relations?

As we have seen, those suffering severe borderline disorders live in a primitive, regressed, pre- and anti-symbolic state where symbolisation, reflection and reason are precluded by somatisation, where mind and body, fantasy and reality, self and other are often not yet differentiated, where frustration cannot be tolerated and so where appetite and desire are compulsively and impulsively acted out. Beta states are most fiercely, forcibly, actively and affectively released and communicated through primitive, psychoid, psychosomatic and infectious projective identifications, through the expression of murderous hate and/or desperate seduction.

Angry and destructive borderline persons are well able to discern and attack the therapist's particular vulnerabilities and complexes. This may be so, but is it not just as possible that the therapist's weak points are most touched, evoked and reactively hurt by a projective expression of a more general murderous envy and hate of an entire person?

From the therapist's side, this implies that, under such conditions of primitive projection and infection, one is not able to maintain and utilise one's own symbolising function. The therapist's own psychoid vulnerability disables the capacity to reflect symbolically. The wounded healer is ever re-wounded (a masochistic and melancholic repetition) by projective identifications and psychosomatic infections through the 'Achilles' heel', zones of inherent and developmental weakness. Thus, a state of 'hysterical identification' may be engendered. This calls for a recycling of the therapist's weak points, putting them to better use and so even making them points of strength.

Fiercely hungry borderline predators are well able to discern and target my particular psychosomatic vulnerabilities, complexes and weaknesses. However,

9 See Chapter Seven (Eds.).

embodied countertransferential information is received through such wounds and so is paradoxically also my 'strongly' reactive zone from which I am made to work. These vulnerable and 'weak' parts are where, analytically, we resort to our most acutely alert, 'most clever' psychosomatic defences. Certainly, it is where my psychoid *conatus* is at its most self-preservatory, my mind is at its most imaginative, crafty and intelligent, and so where I can operate in a dangerous field of infectious personality disorders most affectively. As a wounded healer, I can say that my permeability is both a personal curse and a therapeutic blessing.

As borderline persons simultaneously both evacuate their internal 'bads' and communicate desperately, they thereby kill the good parent/analyst and projectively 'make' the bad/failed parent/analyst. A common example of such destructiveness is a regression to a very close, even seductively needy baby. That baby then becomes a lethal, murderous baby-bomb. Borderlines may ostensibly love their desires and, therefore, their bodies, but they are also unconsciously angry and frustrated, afraid and disgusted with their bodies, bodily functions, internal processes, appetites and limitations and similarly with the desires of other people's bodies: their ambivalent desires for other people's desires. Often their enactments, aimed at fantastically re-controlling their bodies, are through addictive behaviours which are actually out of control.

The critical analytic issue for us is how to manage and move on from our analytic states of 'hysterical identification', from our mixed-up near-psychosomatic beta-states, which infect us at a pathological (if not near psychotic) and primitive psychoid level. What affective and constructive therapeutic actions can there be in this field of borderline destructiveness and in conditions of primitive psychoid attack, infection and contagion? How do we survive in these realms? Are we unconsciously masochistic, as if unconsciously asking, 'Love me for my ability to make your cruelty and my suffering at your hands, apparently pleasurable and enjoyable, and certainly good for you?' Apart from the possibility of not starting in the first place, or perhaps deciding not to take on borderline patients at all (that is, if you can recognise them to be so before you both have started and so cannot stop), then the best management and technical self-preservation involve increasing the frequency of weekly sessions and using the couch. The latter may be used as a substitute body for relational attack and abuse, but this is better than assaults onto and into the analyst's psychosomatic self, which needs the best analytic manoeuvres that it can make for healthy self-protection and other attacks on the frame. But the couch ought not be used by the analyst as a defensive, relationally evasive and affectively distancing decoy. Rather, it allows space for the analyst to be able to think and for the patient to feel free and undirected. But with cases of relentless borderline destructiveness, 'feeling free' does not hold for long, and so these patients often make the couch their object of abuse. With Pat, Rose and Jim, the couch became the analyst's body and environment, as well as mother's, father's and the whole-wide-world's frustrating, over-containing conditioner, and so hated and furiously rejected: a body to hurt and smash, if it could be.

What I have just said is about practical, technical therapeutic action. Subjectively, it is more an issue of what I do with my internal positioning. How might one facilitate a degree of (structural) change, and how does one survive in a not-too-defensive or false way? I think that an immediate countertransferential issue, on the other but complementary side to my responses to borderline hate and attack of all goods, is my response to their desperate erotic hunger, their devouring desire. In this realm, I ask myself: do I desire the other's desire, am I indifferent to their desire or am I repulsed by their desire? Or do I oscillate between such affective internal responses? This is as much countertransferentially informative as my reaction to their murderous attacks. As I also said in my accounts of my work with Pat, Rose and Jim, although interpretations cannot be well-received in a field of fierce and furious psychotic transferential attack, interpretations still need to be given, if only to make manifest the analyst's relative psychosomatic health. This separateness, presence of mind, capacity to think and so forth will itself be enviously attacked, though, as Fordham (1974) says in 'Defences of the Self', beneath the attack, the analyst's good and able self may be taken in and assimilated by the patient at a deeper (distant, split-off, unconscious) level. Or not.

There is still the issue of how to think, let alone interpret, when one's analytic capacity is petrified and frozen by the seeming life-threatening intensity of the attacks and the poisoned arrows of borderline projective identifications. Perhaps we could see this as a form of paralysed embodied countertransference. If I am not psychosomatically defeated, my analytic position becomes as follows: I am here to be transferentially fantasised, imagined, sensed and experienced as an attentive listener, a thinker, a linker, an 'as-if-er' (symboliser) and ultimately an Other. It is as if communicating to the patient that I am going to let you transferentially (and sometimes actually) apprehend and get to know my separate, different mind, my strong psychic foundations and structure, my relatively robust 'bodymind' based on a healthy psychoid *conatus*. These internal and interpersonal qualities may be taken in by you and made psychosomatically and symbolically real in such a way as to become your own goods.

Again, I must consider my own defences against murderous hate and, beyond these defences, our useful therapeutic management of psychosomatic attack, infection and identification. The analyst's defences against projective and murderous invasions and infections include: retaliation, evasion, falling asleep, autistic/schizoid dissociation or defensive detachment, including defensive forms of reverie. Here, I reiterate Plaut's warning that analytic *rêverie* can sometimes involve sentimental idealisation that attempts to escape the reality of the unchanging destructiveness of the other (Plaut, 1994, p. 254).

A non-defensive position and 'therapeutic action' (Lear, 2003) that may move us out of our analytic states of 'hysterical identification' towards a healthy separateness is, I believe, acquiescent acceptance by the analyst of the limits to knowing. Over-knowingness and over-interpretation can be a defensive act of violence. Analytically, we can never know; we can only interpret, and the other remains ultimately unknowable. A state of acute observation, active receptivity, intuitive reflection, heteropathic empathy and critical thinking may lead to linking and interpretation. Rather than using precocious interpretations which foreclose on themselves, not knowing leaves me open to the current reality of psychoid pains and pleasures, with imagination, critical thinking and provisional, transient meaning-making.

There is an appropriate form of non-defensive analytic detachment when it involves a sense of normal healthy separateness and an analytic position of observation, gathering of information and a 'space' to think critically and constructively. The contemplative analyst as 'thinking observer' is ultimately thinking about 'both us and the other' and is not in a solipsistic, autistic bubble. Such detachment is part of a necessary separation and mourning; part of normal, healthy difference. This is a matter of the analyst being real and, at times, more martial than erotic.

With those suffering borderline disorders, I try to offer a particular, demanding and psychosomatically difficult analytic relationship through which, out of the beta disorder, there may emerge a partial process of symbolisation and a greater degree of responsibility: a recycling and putting the violent, sickening, self-defeating defences of their damaged and desperate psychoid *conatus* to a more constructive and creative use: a reason-incorporating psychoid *conatus*.

A long and deep analytic relationship becomes a personal and interpersonal history of war, as well as of *agapē*, a shared relation that is ultimately worthy of 'remembrance' including a remembrance of inevitable disappointments and necessary disillusionments, limits, failures and impermanence. It is a relationship to be mourned, the free necessity of limits accepted and, *inter alia*, to be celebrated and lived beyond. The rituals of the analytic frame may have ended, but at another level, internally and in living memory, they go on being, for both of us are changed. But this might still be a little idealistic because, with borderline persons, their tendency to compulsively act out savage, erotic and destructive psychoid forces may only be partially ameliorated by a greater capacity to reflect, reason and symbolise. Perhaps this is all we can hope for, and perhaps then, a 'good-enough' ending.

References

Addison, A. (2009). 'Jung, Vitalism and "the Psychoid": An Historical Reconstruction'. *Journal of Analytical Psychology*, 54: 123–142.

Atwood, G. & Stolorow, R. (1993). *Faces in a Cloud: Intersubjectivity in Personality Theory*. Oxford: Jason Aronson.

Berlin, I. (1953). *The Hedgehog and the Fox: An Essay on Tolstoy's View of History*. London: Weidenfeld & Nicolson.

Brodrick, M. (2013). 'Santayana's Amphibious Concepts'. *Transactions of the Charles S. Peirce Society*, 49(2): 238–249.

Coleman, M., ed. (2009). *The Essential Santayana: Selected Writings*. Bloomington: Indiana University Press.

Damasio, A. (2003). *Looking for Spinoza: Joy, Sorrow and the Feeling Brain*. New York: Harcourt.

Fordham, M. (1974). 'Defences of the Self'. *Journal of Analytical Psychology*, 19(2): 192–199.

Grotstein, J. (1997). '"Mens Sane in Corpore Sano": The Mind and Body as an "Odd Couple" and an Oddly Coupled Unity'. *Psychoanalytic Inquiry*, 17(2): 204–222.

Kirby-Smith, H. (1997). *A Philosophical Novelist: George Santayana and the Last Puritan*. Carbondale: Southern Illinois University Press.

Kriss, R. (1952). 'As Student and Teacher, Santayana left Mark on College' [Obituary for George Santayana]. Harvard Crimson. www.thecrimson.com/article/1952/9/30/as-student-and-teacher-santayana-left/ (accessed 17 February 2023).

Lachs, J. (2006). *On Santayana*. Belmont, CA: Wadsworth.

Lear, J. (2003). *Therapeutic Action: An Earnest Plea for Irony*. London: Karnac Books.

Plaut, F. (1994). '"Critical Notice" on Bion's *Cogitations*'. *Journal of Analytical Psychology*, 39(2): 253–262.

Santayana, G. (1910). *The Life of Reason or the Phases of Human Progress. I. Reason in Common Sense*. New York, NY: Scribner.

Santayana, G. (1922). *Soliloquies in England and Later Soliloquies*. New York, NY: Scribner.

Santayana, G. (1923). *Scepticism and Animal Faith: Introduction to a System of Philosophy*. New York, NY: Scribner.

Santayana, G. (1972). *Realms of Being*. One-Volume Edition with a New Introduction by the Author. New York, NY: Cooper Square.

Wahman, J. (2001). 'The Meaning of Self-Knowledge in Santayana's Philosophy'. *Overheard in Seville – Bulletin of the Santayana Society*, 19: 1–7.

Wahman, J. (2006). 'Why Psyche Matters: Psychological Implications of Santayana's Ontology'. *Transactions of the Charles Sanders Peirce Society*, 42(1): 132–146.

Wahman, J. (2015). *Narrative Naturalism: An Alternative Framework for Philosophy of Mind*. Lanham: Lexington Books.

Winnicott, D. (1949). 'Hate in the Counter-Transference'. *International Journal of Psycho-Analysis*, 30: 69–74.

Winnicott, D. (1954). 'Mind and Its Relation to the Psyche-Soma'. *The British Journal of Medical Psychology*, 27(4): 201–209.

Chapter 19

The matter of an oddly embodied mind

My spiritual travels with a faithful but savage 'pet dog'

Unpublished, February, 2019[1]

Unless an autobiography represents its subject in creative ways (entertaining, poetically affective, intellectually challenging) it risks being a self-defeating defensive manoeuvre revealing the writer as exhibitionistic and narcissistic, or merely as plain boring. I am a rather private person, or so I have been told, and psychoanalysts are trained to avoid 'self-disclosure'. Therefore, what follows is forged against both my nature and my nurture. All autobiography also says something consciously and unconsciously about the nature and import of memory and identity. And, of course, any autobiography, like all memory and recounted history, is highly selective.

My story must, therefore, have a contextual theme and a spine. What follows is a 'psychosomatic' (and perhaps 'psychoanalytically thinkable') autobiography. This is a narrative of how and why, in my late teens, my affective body issues drew me to live in India for a year: firstly, ostensibly to study the body-denying Jains, and then secondly, as a reactive antidote, to engage with my long-standing fascination with the Parsee Zoroastrians, who, in contradistinction, valued body and matter.

Both during and immediately after going on to study anthropology at the University of Cambridge, schizoid fascinations with the body suddenly became real and urgent. I was hit by serious physical illness, which was an underlying and highly problematic 'matter with body' that eventually pulled me into analysis. A neurofibroma and a major operation on my spine drew me to Nietzsche, Jung and psychoanalysis.

Later, feeling the need to move my critical thinking away from over-idealisation of Jung (especially wanting to qualify his post-Kantian Idealism and Romanticism), I discovered Spinoza. I was also inspired by Stuart Hampshire's writings on Spinoza and other neo-Spinozan writers. In turn, this critical Spinozism led me on to Santayana. I relished both Spinoza and Santayana as cheerful realists. Both were also God-intoxicated atheists, affirming naturalism. Or rather, if Spinoza as a substance monist was 'God-intoxicated', then the materialist-naturalist Santayana was

1 Unpublished paper first presented at a residential on life writing at the Centro Incontri Umani, a centre for cross-cultural understanding, exchange and research in Ascona, Switzerland, in July 2018.

DOI: 10.4324/9781003255826-20

certainly an atheist 'in love with the symbolic life of religion', especially Catholicism, although, as he said, without any dogma. A remark variously attributed to Bertrand Russell, Robert Lowell and Santayana himself was: 'For Santayana, there is no God and Mary is his mother'.

Santayana also wrote: 'My atheism, like that of Spinoza, is a true piety to the universe and denies only gods fashioned by men in their own image, to be servants of their human interests' (Santayana, 1922, p. 246). In regard to mind-body issues (as I often quote), Santayana emended Spinoza's proposition that 'the mind is the idea of the body' into the more epiphenomenal (also more 'spiritual') idea that 'the body is an instrument, the mind its function, the witness and reward of its operation' (Santayana, 1910, p. 206).

Together, Spinoza, Santayana and Jung eventually led me to postulate a dual-aspect (idea and body) 'psychoid *conatus*', a phrase that intentionally incorporates the concepts of all three thinkers. This pragmatic dual-aspect attitude allows for the necessary property dualism of psychoanalytic theory and practice but still also realises the substantial unity of the 'bodymind'.

My idea of my body (that is, my bodily processes and body relations) has been the subject and object of my unconscious and conscious developmental meaning-making. The matter of my body and its affective relations has been like an ever-present pet dog, a faithful companion: both intimate, enjoyable and playful, as well as irritating, demanding and difficult, apt to snap and bite. My adolescent self (and my self beyond adolescence) lived in, or rather was lived by, a world of imagination and ideas, by epistemophilic curiosity, by day-dreams and desires, by fears of the all-seeing eye of the superego. In other words, I was what Jungians would call a *puer aeternus*. Below these fairly 'normal' neuroses, I was being driven by the somatic psyche's basic function of self-preservation and survival, by innate psychophysical forces of development and attachment, by animal instincts and impulses, appetites and defences. However, this is all fairly common and typical. So, let me now move from the general and theoretical into a more particular and personal story.

At school, I developed a passionate fascination with comparative religion. No doubt this was a reaction against my Anglican upbringing and an unconscious oedipal rebellion against my church-going father, especially when I developed an adolescent interest in a variety of world religions ranging from Islam to Jainism. Something else was also operative: a rebellion against my own body and its impulses, based largely on fear of these zones and processes. I was drawn to images of Norway, the searing beauty of its mountains and fjords, its stave churches and its language, and then to images and ideas about India, especially the asceticism of the Jains. This latter interest was, to an extent, symptomatic of an unconscious wish to escape difficult ideas, impulses and processes of my bodymind.

My fascination with India was aesthetic, spiritual and intellectual. India was, for me, an idealised country and culture: its scenery, architecture and rich variety of religions. Edward Mary Joseph Molyneux's illustrations of Francis Younghusband's *Kashmir* particularly caught my romantic imagination (Younghusband, 1909), and my reading in comparative religion was an intellectually exciting realm of challenging, anti-conventional ideas. These splits, idealisations and dreams were basically melancholic in nature.

When I was interviewed for entry to Kings College, Cambridge to read Social Anthropology, I was encouraged to actualise my somewhat ambitious proposal to go to India for a year to study and write up a report on the Jains. It was thereby deemed that I did not need to take the usual entrance exam.

However, as I began to suggest previously, these fascinations were largely fantastic and schizoid. Ethereal spirit looked down on matter. To understand spirit as a natural, sometimes exciting, sometimes frightening intellectual and imaginal epiphenomenon, a product of the matter of body, biology and neurobiology, would have been anathema, and any such realisation was repressed and split off by my magically disembodied mind.

And so I went to India for over a year, an innocent abroad, guided by youthful enthusiasm and folly. My trip out to India began in a somewhat unreliable cargo ship, the 'Coromandel', with a truly novelistic collection of passengers and crew. After several initiatory alarums and excursions, I docked in Karachi before flying on to Delhi.

Here was the shock of the real India – the smells, the colours, the sounds and the seething movement! I was initially employed teaching English at the Doon School in Dehradun for two to three months. Accompanying pupils on trips to Mussoorie, bicycling to Hardwar and Rishikesh, the life and air and scent of these hill towns and the spectacle of the Himalayas were a gloriously real realisation of my images of Kashmir. And they still haunt me to this day.

I then travelled around India with the next colonial teacher imported to teach at the Doon School, a very tall, fair-haired young Scotsman who, one might say, was remarkably different from me. Whilst I valiantly tried to 'blend in with the Indians', this tall Scot wore a sort of panama trilby hat. Nevertheless, to say the least, we saw a lot together: many places and people, including tea plantations and tea planters. After we parted, he to take up his stay at the Doon School, I was at last alone. I consider this next phase to be my 'Kim-esque' journey along the Grand Trunk Road.

Here follows a much abbreviated selection of my exploits. An incredibly happy time visiting Simla and a trip to Dalhousie on the edge of Kashmir added to the realisation of my mountain dreams and, indeed, still inform my actual dreams.

After a month-long stay with a most hospitable (or rather a most tolerant) Sikh family in Ghaziabad (where I was caught up in a local election process), I eventually arrived at the Dilwara temples of Mount Abu. But this, my great goal, turned out to be a terrible shock. Many of the more important *Śvētāmbara* Jain monks did not speak English, some no longer spoke at all and some were in a process of *Sallekhanā*, or fasting to death. This was difficult to witness. In fact, I realised that I was totally unprepared. I did not know what to ask, even if they had spoken (at all, let alone English), and other than the Jain architecture, I did not know what to look at or look for. My own food was minimal. There was also a sacred python in a cave that I had to walk past every evening. I rather feared he, too, might well be very hungry. Suffice it to say, I was out of my depth physically, culturally, intellectually and emotionally.

I wrote nothing. I had failed in my task as a budding anthropologist, and so I fled, but carried by a young person's fickleness, I quickly moved on, initially to Udvala and then back to Delhi.

Two immediate developments followed. In order to support myself, I led a life of petty crime. I also became fascinated by the Zoroastrianism of the worldly Parsees, no doubt as a matter-loving and body-loving antidote to the life-denying and body-denying Jains. This interest eventually bore fruit as part of my training exams in Zürich several years later, where my main source was Zaehner's 1956 *Teachings of the Magi*. However, my naive life of petty crime went badly wrong. I found myself money-less and very lonely. The Parsees of Malabar Hill looked after me with extraordinary generosity at Christmas time but let me know that any attempt to get inside their practices and sacred places was proscribed.

I travelled on to Lucknow and on to the South, witnessing the great monolithic Gommateswara statue of Bahubali in Shravanabelagola in Karnataka, endless beautiful tea plantations, a 'Staying On'[2] woman in 'Ooty', Cochin and its tiny Jewish community.

On a memorial tomb in Madras Cathedral, I found and decided upon the name of any future daughter I might have: Amelia. The tombstone read *Tomb of Amelia Boileau, née Adam, died 2nd Nov. 1833*. Both my son and my daughter have travelled to India, perhaps to an extent following in their father's footsteps and perhaps arising out of my stories (and my daughter sought out and found the original tombstone that had inspired her name).

Thereafter, my progress became increasingly tough. Whilst sleeping rough and homeless in a bus shelter in Calcutta, a bus stop I shared with a prostitute and a leper, I collapsed in agony. The saintly leper took me to Mother Theresa, from whence I was rescued by an English businessman, with whom I stayed as a bedridden patient for a month. I convalesced in a beach house in Puri in Orissa. This was the beginning of what was revealed four years later to be the first symptoms of a neurofibroma in my spine.

Eventually, after over a year away, I sailed home via South Africa. The very painful and debilitating symptoms of the neurofibroma returned and nearly crippled me over the entirety of my last year at Cambridge. At the same time, I became aware of another idiosyncratic physical reality. I realised that I had severe scoliosis, unnoticed until then; a structural fault which, as well as shaping me to be an immanent representation of Richard the Third, has caused me perennial aches, pains and back problems.

At university, my main intellectual passion was Walter Kaufmann's writings on Nietzsche, which reinforced my war on paternal Christianity. I wrote (a disastrous)

2 'Staying on' is a reference to colonials who 'stayed on' in India after Indian independence, as depicted in Paul Scott's 1977 novel *Staying On* (Eds.).

final thesis on Nietzsche and Max Beckmann. I also fell properly and madly in love for the first time. However, my split-off body issue proved to be the stronger force of destiny. After finishing Cambridge (and whilst working at Christie's), my increasingly agonising illness caused by my neurofibroma reached a crisis and, delirious with pain, I finally broke down physically and was taken by ambulance to hospital in London.

The years of crippling physical symptoms, a major spinal/central nerve operation to remove the neurofibroma and my slow recuperation were psychosomatically both deforming and formative. Throughout my time in hospital, both before and after the operation, I read and re-read Thomas Mann's *Joseph and His Brothers* (1933). This vivid re-telling of the biblical story of Joseph symbolically represented my own descent into the pit of near-death and my eventual rebirth. The illness – and the Joseph story – led me to Jung, into psychoanalysis and into my own analytic vocation.

Personally encouraged by Ingaret Gifford and Laurens Van der Post, I went to Zürich where I underwent an analytic training (in both Zürich and then also in London) and then started my practice as an analyst.

However, through learning from experience and critical clinical thinking, I increasingly came to question many seeming fundamentals of Jungian psychology. This disillusionment was more to do with some elements of classical 'Jungian psychology' (content, symbols and knowing) rather than with Jung's own psychology (such as awareness of necessary limits, symbolising and unknowing).

I studied and later taught the philosophical ancestry of Jung's psychology, particularly from Kant through Absolute Idealism, Schelling and 19th-century German psychiatry. I had moved from Nietzsche into a mixed fascination and fight with Absolute Idealism. It was hence, through an increasing critical scepticism and naturalism, that I came to find a very different philosophical home in the world of Spinoza and Santayana, as well as many neo-Spinozan thinkers and scholars of Santayana, such as Jessica Wahman's use of Santayana in her 2015 book *Narrative Naturalism*. I also began to read against Jung, in other psychoanalytic clinical literature and in philosophy.

Through over 40 years of analytic practice that has particularly involved the treatment of severe borderline personality disorders, I have been developing my clinical and theoretical ideas on the psychoid *conatus*. This is where philosophy and psychology come together, and this is also where practice and personal matters come together.

Initially, I used Jung's psychology, or rather my idealisation of its impersonal, 'archetypal' aspect, as a further defence against my own psychosomatic realities. Through my unconscious blindness and schizoid distortions, my subject, my ongoing task, remained the rescuing of the denied and lost body. Yet amid the neurotic denials and splits, there was a curative or re-balancing pull. Part of the Zürich training entailed the study and examination of a personally chosen theme from comparative religion. I chose Zoroastrianism. As well as a study of its theological, mythological and other details, I was particularly concerned to emphasise that

Zoroastrian dualism was not a dualism of mind and matter or mind and body, unlike Manicheism, let alone certain denominations and interpretations of Christianity (I would add, not all, and not inherently). For Zoroastrians, as well as the earth and matter, both the body and its life were inherently 'good' (although 'evil' could infect either).

Expressing a different aspect of this theme, I wrote my training thesis on the Wild Man and the Green Man (Clark, 1977) as symbolic representations of the healthy 'earthing' and embodying of the ethereal, schizoid *puer*: a covert description and account of myself and of my own analytic experience. I increasingly became both theoretically and clinically critical of the archetype and idealising glorification of the 'wise' Jung: my reactive and rebellious father complex was (and still is) affective and active.

Through my time of training, belatedly but vitally, I found that it was above all the desires, fears and passions (using the word 'passion' in both of its meanings) of relationships that made my body, and my body with bodies, become more real and alive. I was reminded that my mind is not only my idea of my body but also my idea of my body with other people's 'bodyminds', and that I am affected by and am affecting other people's 'bodyminds', let alone by my various ideas of what other people are thinking of my body!

It is worth mentioning here three published examples of this theoretical, clinical and personal interest. In 1996, I published a clinical paper entitled 'The animating body: psychoid substance as a mutual experience of psychosomatic disorder'.[3] In 2006, I published 'A Spinozan lens onto the confusions of borderline relations'[4] and in Copenhagen in 2013, I gave a paper entitled 'Why and how psychoid relations matter', which was later published in 2015 as 'Psychoid relations in the transferential/countertransferential field of personality disorders'.[5]

Continued critical studies of the dual-aspect substance monism of Spinoza and the naturalistic ontology of Santayana give this organic and clinical development an intellectual and aesthetic architecture.

However, it was and is not only intellectual. Another bodily fascination drew me to seek out a certain zone of voyeurism. I went to Africa, attracted there by the desire to watch hippos. They fascinated me as forces of non-reflexive embodiedness and of loud bodily processes, both individually and collectively. I saw tourists (including myself) as curious and excited voyeurs of ultra-sensuality, affectively evoking our/my body-identifying, body-responding mind: indeed, the mind as idea of the body and of bodies in action and interaction. Thus, my difficult but omni-present 'animal', my 'pet dog' (and perhaps my 'wild hippos'), that is, the psychoid *soma* and the meanings of its matters and developmental preoccupation throughout my adult life.

3 See Chapter Six (Eds.).
4 See Chapter Seven (Eds.).
5 See Chapter Sixteen (Eds.).

As said in earlier papers, substance monism but with a dual aspect (idea and body) understanding of the psychoid *conatus* allows for the property dualism of psychoanalytic theory and practice. In borderline clinical relations, the psychoid *conatus* is the conduit through which infectious communications, seductions and destructions occur. It is also where a more real, truer and authentic self may be realised.

This psychoid *conatus* is the matter and the 'essence' of my history, my realm of on-going reflection, value and action. Its realisation has been deepened and substantiated through long-term work with the interpersonal affects of the psychoid (psychosomatic affects) in analytic relations with the forceful and infectious projections of destructive borderline persons. In regressed and primitive states, the psychoid and the autonomic nervous system are the conduit for psychosomatic communication.

I now see my therapeutic work in the borderline field as originally being an unconscious attempt to 'cure', in the sense of 'putting to better use', my own narcissism. More generally, the clinical relevance of this understanding of psyche as 'organic' as a psychoid matter depends upon the various narratives and the literary psychology that we construct about it, how we symbolise it and thereby the way we use it interpretively.

And, finally, I do not want to glorify the reality of the psyche as being only a force for teleological healing: the forces of self-preservation of the psychoid psyche are themselves complex and paradoxical, and they entangle with other conative forces and ideas. The psyche and its parts can be destructive and self-destructive as well as constructive.

At this point in my history, my psychoid *conatus* is a matter of natural *aging*, of body (and possibly mind) slowing and decaying. It is late autumnal, becoming winter. My body cannot keep up with the ideas, impulses and desires of the mind. After all, the mind is an ever-changing idea of an ever-changing body. For me, it is now the *conatus* of 'keeping on going'.

The psychoid *conatus* is part of *natura naturans* . . . nature naturing in Spinoza's sense.[6] Like my scoliosis and other fateful truths, it is always a crooked timber and can never be straightened by a fallacious belief in the organic existence of the ideal. Believing such an ideal to be objectively real is the normal madness of taking the pathetic fallacy literally rather than as poetic metaphor.

A rider: I have told my story as though it had a thread, and its thread led somewhere definite; as though it had a purpose or meaning, a teleology. But I have merely formed this narrative, made meaning, purpose or neat order out of a selective telling of but a section of my life. It is a wrought and distorted story, with much omitted and much forgotten. It is surely partial. Memories of past persons, relationships, events or scenes are never about a reliably constant object. They are

6 *Natura naturans* or 'nature naturing' is a Latin term coined in the Middle Ages and taken up by Spinoza to mean the self-causing activity of nature. See *Ethics* Part 1, Prop. 29, Scholium (Eds.).

feeling-toned images that, due to a variety of unconscious forces, appear, disappear and re-appear, ever changed and changing. Memory and, therefore, identity are not firm. There can be no absolute and final reductionism. Santayana said that autobiography is an aspect of 'literary psychology', perhaps poetically valid, but never an absolute truth. Slightly misquoting himself, he ended his novel *The Last Puritan* thus:

> After life is over and the world has gone up in smoke, what realities might the spirit in us still call its own without illusion save the form of those very illusions which have made up our story?
>
> (Santayana, 1936, p. 602)

And so I end this short 'memoir' with the fuller and earlier quote, make of it what you will:

> But, if his sense for the eternal had been absolutely direct and pure, he would have seen the eternal in the figments of sense . . . And though the world would laugh at him, the angels would not; for after life is done, and the world is gone up in smoke, what realities may the spirit of a man boast to have embraced without illusion, save the very forms of those illusions by which he has been deceived?
>
> (Santayana, 1936, p. 89)

References

Clark, G. (1977). *The Transformation of 'Spiritual Image' and 'Instinctual Shadow' into 'Instinctual Spirit': Pan, Wild Man, Green Man, and Animals as Symbols of the Instinctual Shadow of the Introverted, Spiritually-Fascinated 'Puer' and of Its Transformation.* Diploma Thesis, C. G. Jung Institute, Zürich.

Curley, E., ed. and trans. (1994). *A Spinoza Reader: The Ethics and Other Works*. Princeton, NJ: Princeton University Press.

Santayana, G. (1910). *The Life of Reason or the Phases of Human Progress. I. Reason in Common Sense.* New York, NY: Scribner.

Santayana, G. (1922). 'On My Friendly Critics'. In *Soliloquies in England and Later Soliloquies*. New York: Scribner.

Santayana, G. (1936). *The Last Puritan: A Memoir in the Form of a Novel.* New York: Scribner.

Scott, P. (1977). *Staying On*. Chicago: University of Chicago Press.

Wahman, J. (2015). *Narrative Naturalism: An Alternative Framework for Philosophy of Mind.* Lanham, MD: Lexington Books.

Younghusband, F. (1911). *Kashmir: Described by Sir Francis Younghusband*. Painted by E. Molyneux. London: Adam & Charles Black (Original work published, 1909).

Zaehner, R. (1956). *Teachings of the Magi: A Compendium of Zoroastrian Beliefs*. London: Allen and Unwin.

Last jottings[1]

JUDITH PICKERING AND GEOFFREY SAMUEL

On Sunday, February 24, 2019, Giles was admitted to hospital feeling very ill. A week of tests revealed late-stage, metastatic liver cancer. In hospital, with only a few weeks to live, Giles jotted down some vital aphorisms in a tiny diary, which reveals much of what was essential to him.

A Zoroastrian saying he wrote out in capitals was HUMATA HŪXTA HUVARŠTA, three Avestan words encapsulating the ethical goals of Zoroastrianism as 'well thought, well said, well done' or 'good thought, good word, good action'.

There were many quotes about joy, such as 'all joy wants eternity' (Nietzsche). And 'There cannot be too much joy – it is always good' (Spinoza IVP42). Another Spinozan saying in Latin was: *Amor aeternitatis naturae, summa laetitia et ultima acquiescentia est*. Again, a rough translation is 'the love of the eternity of nature is the highest of joys and the final acceptance'. Of this last, he spoke of *acquiescentia in se ipso*, as in, 'acceptance of what one is'.

Spinoza's word for joy, *laetitia*, is related to *acquiescentia*. Giles spoke much in his dying days of *acquiescentia*. This, for him, was not a passive emotion as is sometimes implied by the English word acquiescence, but more a sense of deep contentment, self-knowledge and acceptance. Some scholars of Spinoza (LeBuffe, 2010, pp. 22–23, 198) translate *acquiescentia* as self-contentment or even self-esteem. For Spinoza, *acquiescentia* is related to blessedness, a form of *acquiescentia* of mind that arises out of the intuitive knowledge of God, and it is the highest form of joy or *laetitia* (LeBuffe, 2010, p. 200). A passage Giles wrote out by hand in his diary by LeBuffe explains:

> As Spinoza presents it, the knowledge of God is knowledge, primarily, of oneself and, secondarily, of other things. Without this knowledge, a mind may not consciously desire to persevere in being. That is why Spinoza claims that the knowledge of God is the most useful thing to the mind . . .

1 We gratefully acknowledge the generosity of Giles' family for providing us with these precious and vital elements of Giles' life and last days.

DOI: 10.4324/9781003255826-21

> He claims that the knowledge of God is the highest good, however, not because it is instrumental to perseverance, but because it is also the best among those goods that we seek for their own sakes. It is *acquiescentia in se ipso*, the highest form of *laetitia*.
>
> (LeBuffe, 2005, p. 243)

This is also related to knowledge of the third kind or intuitive knowledge and also to self-awareness. Knowledge of God is the highest good, self-contentment (*acquiescentia*) is also good and *acquiescentia* is the highest form of *laetitia* (LeBuffe, 2010, p. 198). The highest *laetitia* arises out of the highest *acquiescentia*, which, in turn, arises out of knowledge of God, that is, of the third kind. The day before he died, Giles was heard to murmur in the night 'acquiescence high'.

There was a scribble in his diary about the connections between the *conatus intelligendi* as the quest for infinity; essence, desire, *conatus*; enhancing our powers (self-enhancement); the *conatus intelligendi*; the desire for eternity as a quest for infinity and how all these are related to meaning and self-integration.

There was a quote from Antoine de Saint-Exupery:

> A rock pile ceases to be a rock pile the moment a single man contemplates it, bearing within him the image of a cathedral.
>
> (Antoine de Saint-Exupery, p. 327, 1942)

Regarding his long-lived concern to transcend mind-body dualism through dual-aspect substance monism, he had written out the passage he had so often quoted in his writings: 'The body is an instrument, the mind its function, the witness and reward of its operation' (Santayana, 1910, p. 206).

Another jotting from Spinoza's *Ethics* was *Omnia praeclara tam difficilia quam rara sunt*, which can be translated as 'all things excellent are as difficult as they are rare'.

Pointing to being a 'God-intoxicated atheist' he also wrote out the following passage from Santayana:

> My atheism, like that of Spinoza, is true piety towards the universe and denies only Gods fashioned by man in their own image, to be servants of their human interests.
>
> (Santayana, 1922, p. 246)

Giles was always acutely aware of human limitations and also wrote down George Santayana's dictum of religion as representing 'the love of life in the consciousness of impotence'.

He also wrote out a few poems about death and immortality: one was 'Some are Afraid of Death' by the poet Richard Church, in which the poet describes how one's last breath might be like a sigh of contentment, as when kissed by a lover. Another was a quote from William Wordsworth's 'Intimations of Immortality':

Our birth is but a sleep and a forgetting;
The Soul that rises with us, our life's Star,
Hath had elsewhere its setting,
And cometh from afar;
Not in entire forgetfulness,
And not in utter nakedness,
But trailing clouds of glory do we come
From God, who is our home:
Heaven lies about us in our infancy!
(Wordsworth, 1837, p. 388)

In his last week, he made known his requests for 'a joyful celebration of my life', which also can be seen to reveal the essence of his life. He asked for a table to be set up with photos of his beloved family and, amongst the photos, a few key symbolic objects: a *Nequid Pereat* paperweight, a primitive Polish picture of Spinoza, a little brass frog and a tiny antique Buddhist statue of Mahākāla which his mother had given him in a Christmas stocking when he was a little boy.

Nequid Pereat (let nothing perish) is a clock outside Wells Cathedral, a place of pilgrimage for Giles, who never failed to visit during trips to England. The original expression derives from St John's Gospel. The clock from Wells from 1310 has two knights who strike the bells with their pikes as an instruction not to waste precious time but also that nothing ever is lost but resides within the Alpha and Omega of God's Eternity. Giles said of *Nequid Pereat* 'the ironic ideal and the last words'. He said this about his own death as if to reassure us all that 'nothing perishes' in the eternity of God.

The little brass frog was, for him, a good luck charm which he held whenever good luck was needed: mostly for close ones rather than himself. The statue of black Mahākāla, a Dharmapāla, or protector of the Dharma, was a sacred icon for him, again held in his hand when facing life's challenges.

He wanted to include the poem 'The Wonder of the World' which Giles attributed to 'BB' (Denys Watkins-Pitchford), but in fact is by Janet Loxely Lewis (Lewis, 1981). Some lines are said to be taken from a gravestone:[2]

The wonder of the world,
The beauty and the power,

2 The origins of these lines are obscure. Lewis notes that they came from an old Swedish gravestone and had been quoted by the American naturalist Olaus J. Murie of Moose, Wyoming. They were recorded independently by the English poet Denys Watkins-Pitchford ('BB'), who prefaced all his books with these lines. A short biography on the BB Society's website describes them as 'taken from an old Cumbrian gravestone', www.bbsociety.co.uk/bb-biography accessed March 1, 2024.

The shapes of things,
Their colours, lights and shades,
These I saw.
Look ye also while life lasts.

He wanted two excerpts read out. The first was from *The Life of Reason: Reason in Religion* by George Santayana:

> The feelings which in mysticism rise to the surface and speak in their own name are simply the ancient, overgrown feelings of vitality, dependence, inclusion; they are the background of consciousness, coming forward and blotting out the scene. What mysticism destroys is, in a sense, its only legitimate expression. The Life of Reason, in so far as it is life, contains the mystic's primordial assurances, and his rudimentary joys; but in so far as it is rational it has discovered what those assurances rest on, in what direction they may be trusted to support action and thought; and it has given those joys distinction and connection, turning a dumb momentary ecstasy into a many-coloured and natural happiness.
>
> (Santayana, 2014, p. 166)

He also wanted to have included the closing passage from Isaac Bashevis Singer's short story 'The Spinoza of Market Street' in which the central character, Dr. Fischelson, an eccentric Polish Jew and Spinoza scholar living in Warsaw during the First World War, contemplates the eternity of nature and achieves his own version of Spinoza's *acquiescentia* (Singer, 1962, pp. 23–24).

Requests for hymns included 'Abide with me' by Henry Francis Lyte. One wonders whether when in hospital, as he felt that 'other helpers fail and comforts flee,' he sought 'help of the helpless' in 'Abide with me'. While aware of how 'change and decay' were all around him, Spinoza's God was perhaps one of the unchanging principles that might abide with him.

At the brink of death, he cried out 'acquiescence high', perhaps an inkling of:

Where is death's sting? Where, grave, thy victory?
I triumph still, if Thou abide with me.

Hold Thou Thy cross before my closing eyes;
Shine through the gloom and point me to the skies.
Heaven's morning breaks, and earth's vain shadows flee;
In life, in death, O Lord, abide with me.

(Lyte, 1861)

Another request was for the hymn 'Dear Lord and Father of Mankind'. The poem is by the American Quaker poet John Greenleaf Whittier and is an excerpt from a longer poem, 'The Brewing of the Soma', written in 1872. Giles had a rare first edition of Whittier's book *The Pennsylvania Pilgrim*. He loved the lines, 'Speak through

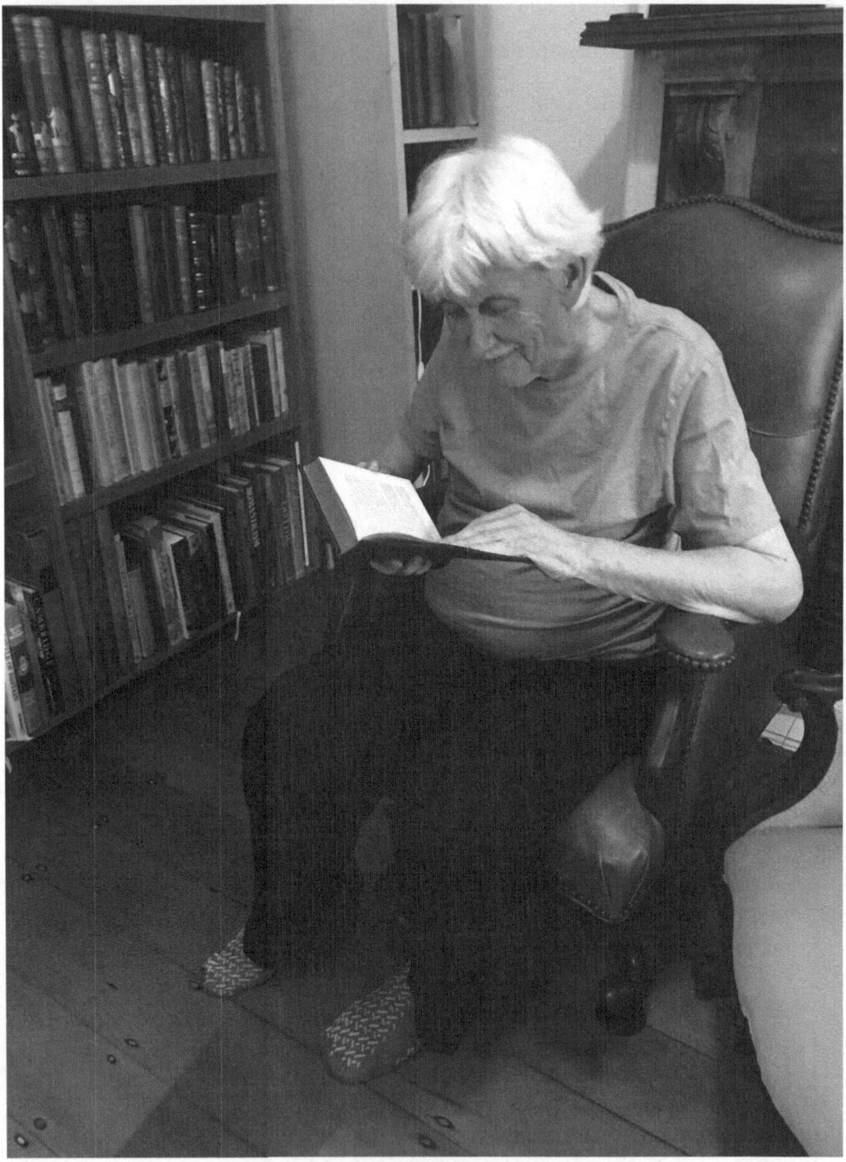

Figure 20.1 Giles Clark at home in his library of rare books a week before he died

the earthquake, wind and fire, O still, small voice of calm'. Above all, he loved the line: 'the silence of eternity, interpreted by love'.

The last words of our 'God-intoxicated atheist' spoken before taking his last breath were:

'I want God!'

References

Curley, E., ed. and trans. (1994). *A Spinoza Reader: The Ethics and Other Works*. Princeton, NJ: Princeton University Press.

de Saint-Exupery, A. (1942). 'Flight to Arras III'. Lewis Galantière, trans. *The Atlantic Monthly*, March, 1942 Issue, pp. 313–333.

LeBuffe, M. (2005). 'Spinoza's *Summum Bonum*'. *Pacific Philosophical Quarterly*, 86(2): 243–266.

LeBuffe, M. (2010). *From Bondage to Freedom: Spinoza on Human Excellence.* Oxford and New York, NY: Oxford University Press.

Lewis, J. (1981). *Poems Old and New, 1918–1978*. Athens, OH: Ohio University Press/Swallow Press.

Lyte, H. (1861). 'Abide with Me'. In *Hymns Ancient and Modern*. W. Monk, ed. London: Novello and Co.

Santayana, G. (1910). *The Life of Reason or the Phases of Human Progress. I. Reason in Common Sense*. New York, NY: Scribner.

Santayana, G. (1922). 'On My Friendly Critics'. In *Soliloquies in England and Later Soliloquies*. New York: Scribner.

Santayana, G. (2014). *The Life of Reason or the Phases of Human Progress. III. Reason in Religion*. Cambridge, MA: MIT Press.

Singer, I. (1962). *The Spinoza of Market Street*. London: Secker & Warburg.

Whittier, J. (1872). 'The Brewing of the Soma'. In *The Pennsylvania Pilgrim and Other Poems*. Boston: James R. Osgood.

Wordsworth, W. (1837). *The Complete Poetical Works of William Wordsworth*. H. Reed, ed. Philadelphia: James Munroe and Co.

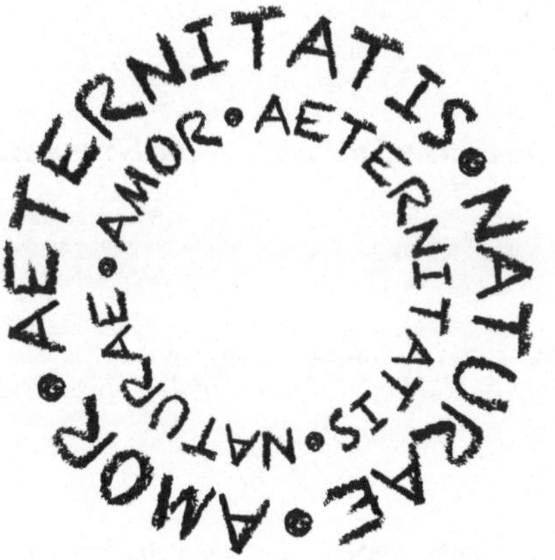

A Bibliography of works by Giles Clark

JUDITH PICKERING AND GEOFFREY SAMUEL

This list has been compiled from documents of which we are aware. It is not complete. Giles also wrote a thesis on Nietzsche and Max Beckmann at Cambridge University, but we have no further details.

1977

The Transformation of 'Spiritual Image' and 'Instinctual Shadow' into 'Instinctual Spirit: Pan, Wild Man, Green Man, and Animals as Symbols of the Instinctual Shadow of the Introverted, Spiritually-Fascinated 'Puer' and of its Transformation. Diploma Thesis, C. G. Jung Institute, Zürich.

1978

'A Process of Transformation: Spiritual *Puer*, Instinctual Shadow and Instinctual Spirit'. *Harvest Journal*, 24: 24–39.

1981

'Review of G. Adler, *Dynamics of the Self*'. *Journal of Analytical Psychology*, 26(4): 365–367.

1983

'A Black Hole in Psyche'. *Harvest Journal*, 29: 67–80.

'Review of P. Berry. *Echo's Subtle Body*'. *Journal of Analytical Psychology*, 28(4): 392–395.

1984

'Review of A. Samuels, *Dethroning the Self*'. *Journal of Analytical Psychology*, 29(3): 298–299.

'Review of E. C. Whitmont, *Return of the Goddess*'. *Harvest Journal*, 30: 134–136.

1987–88

'Animation through the Analytical Relationship: The Embodiment of Self in the Transference and Counter-transference'. *Harvest Journal*, 33: 104–114.

1988

'Review of L. Zoja and P. Hinshaw (eds.), *The Differing Uses of Symbolic and Clinical Approaches in Practice and Theory*'. *Journal of Analytical Psychology*, 33(1): 85–89.

1991

'Review of R. H. Hopcke, *Jung, Jungians, and Homosexuality*'. *Journal of Analytical Psychology*, 36(2): 249–252.

1995

'How Much Jungian Theory Is There in My Practice?'. *Journal of Analytical* Psychology, 40(3): 343–352.

1996

'The Animating Body: Psychoid Substance as a Mutual Experience of Psychosomatic Disorder'. *Journal of Analytical Psychology*, 41(3): 353–368.

'Jung's Philosophical Ancestors'. Temenos Seminars, Canberra, 20 April 1996. Unpublished.

1999

'Mind-Body Intimacies and Pains'. Unpublished.

2006

'A Critical History of Ideas as Relevant to Analytical Psychology'. ANZSJA Training Seminar. Canberra. Unpublished.

'Mind-Body Matters with Clinical Case Examples'. ANZSJA Training Seminar, Canberra. Unpublished.

'The Psychotic Core, Defences and the Development of the Symbolising Function: Narcissistic Relations and the Failure of the Symbolising Function as Un-Recyclable Pathology'. ANZSJA Training Seminar, Melbourne. Unpublished.

'Recycling Madness'. Unpublished.

'A Spinozan Lens Onto the Confusions of Borderline Relations'. *Journal of Analytical Psychology*, 51(1): 67–86.

'Spinoza in Psychoanalysis: Reflections on His Philosophy and the Psychotherapeutic Mind'. Conference paper: *Wandering with Spinoza*, Melbourne, September 2006. Unpublished.

2007

'Dreams and Dreaming'. Unpublished.

'Personal Shocks and Analytic Shocks'. ANZSJA Training Seminar. Unpublished.

'Projective Identification'. ANZSJA Training Seminar, Canberra. Unpublished.

'The Psychotic Core, Defences and the Development of the Symbolising Function'. ANZSJA Training Seminar, Melbourne. Unpublished.

'The Training Process'. ANZSJA AGM. Unpublished.

'Using a Jungian Inheritance of Lack and Loss: Psychosomatic Infection, Mourning and Irony in the Analysis of Borderline Relations'. Lecture for the 150th anniversary of Freud – November 2006. *Psychoanalysis Downunder*. 7A. www.psychoanalysisdownunder.com.au/issue-7a

2008

'The Active Use of the Analyst's Bodymind as it is Informed by Psychic Disturbances'. In *The Uses of Subjective Experience*. A. Dowd, C. San Roque and L. Petchkovsky, eds. E-book: ANZSJA. https://anzsja.org.au/wp/wp-content/uploads/2016/04/ANZSJA-UsesOf-SubjectiveExperience.pdf

'Disturbances to Symbolising Processes'. ANZSJA Training Seminar, Sydney. Unpublished.

2009

'ANZSJA as Will and Idea'. Unpublished.

'Difficult Passions: Desires and Destructions at Our Core'. Canberra Jung Society, Canberra. Unpublished.

'On Architecture'. Darghan Street Dialogues, Sydney. Unpublished.

'Romantic Catastrophes and Other Vital Realities'. ANZAP Saturday Morning Seminar Series: 'A Symposium on Love', Sydney. Unpublished.

'Self-Preservation and Repetition: The Defences of Dangerous Desire and Shamed Appetite'. ANZSJA Training Seminar, Melbourne. Unpublished.

2010

'The Abuse of an Object'. ANZSJA Training Seminar, Melbourne. Unpublished.

'Borderline Envy, Hate, Rage, Destruction, Cruelty and Murderousness in the Transference and Counter-Transference'. ANZSJA Training Seminar, Melbourne. Unpublished.

'Decay and Death'. Darghan Street Dialogues, Sydney. Unpublished.

'The Embodied Counter-Transference and Recycling the Mad Matter of Symbolic Equivalence: a Re-evaluation of Samuels' Idea of the "Embodied Counter-Transference"'. In *Sacral Revolutions: Reflecting on the Work of Andrew Samuels: Cutting Edges in Psychoanalysis and Jungian Analysis*. G. Heuer, ed. London: Routledge, pp. 88–96.

'On Borderline Pathology'. ANZSJA Training Seminar. Unpublished.

'On Evil, Sadism, Power and Perversion'. Darghan Street Dialogues, Sydney. Unpublished.

'On Psychosis'. ANZSJA Training Seminar. Unpublished.

'Phenomenology of the Analytic Response or Position to Borderline Forces'. Unpublished.

'Spinoza and Psychoanalysis'. Conference paper, 'Philosophy and Psychoanalysis', Melbourne. Unpublished.

'Unconscious Structures and Defences'. Professional Development Seminar, Christchurch. Unpublished.

'Unconscious Structures and Defences, and How an Analytic/Psychotherapeutic Relationship May Challenge and Change Some of Them'. ANZSJA Professional Development Seminar, Christchurch, New Zealand. Unpublished.

2012

'Herder's Force: Pluralism, Expressivism, Mind-Body Relations and Empathy'. In *Montreal 2010. Facing Multiplicity: Psyche, Nature, Culture Proceedings of the XVIIIth Congress*

of the International Association for Analytical Psychology. P. Bennett, ed. Daimon Verlag, pp. 1222–1233.
'Narcissists and Borderlines'. Unpublished.

2013

'From Pain to Pleasure and Back Again: *Jouissance* and a Best Possible Life'. Unpublished.
'On Narcissism'. ANZSJA Training Seminar. Unpublished.
'Why Train'. Unpublished.

2014

'On Symbolising and Not-Symbolising'. ANZSJA Training Seminar, 5 July 2014. Melbourne. Unpublished.
'Somatising, Symbolising and Not Symbolising'. ANZSJA Training Seminar. Unpublished.
'Splitting and Somatising: A Case of Disordered Symbolising and Precluded Empathy'. ANZSJA Training Seminar, Melbourne. Unpublished.

2015

'Analytic Relations with a Focus on The Psychoid'. ANZSJA Training Seminar, Auckland. Unpublished.
'A Personal Reflection on Jungian Analysis Now'. ANZSJA Training Seminar, Auckland. Unpublished.
'Phenomenology of Borderline Communications'. Unpublished.
'Psychoid Relations in the Transferential/Counter-Transferential Field of Personality Disorders'. In *Copenhagen 2013: 100 Years On: Origins, Innovations and Controversies. Proceedings of the 19th Congress of the International Association for Analytical Psychology*. E. Kiehl, ed. Einsiedeln: Daimon Verlag, pp. 850–859.
'Random Thoughts on my Psychoanalytic Values and History'. Unpublished.

2016

'On Borderline Urgencies and the Case of Hellie'. Unpublished.
'On Working with Loss and Defeat'. Unpublished.
'Thoughts on Jungian Analysis (and Psychoanalysis) Now'. Unpublished.

2017

'11 Points regarding Narcissism'. Unpublished.
'On Normal Madness'. Unpublished.
'Towards a Psychoanalytic Spinoza'. Unpublished.

2018

'The Matter of an Oddly Embodied Mind: My Spiritual Travels with a Faithful but Savage "Pet Dog"'. Ascona Life-Writing Residential, July 2018, Ascona, Switzerland. Unpublished.
'Why and How Psychoid Relations Matter'. Unpublished.

Index

Fictionised Clinical Cases